Strategies
for Teaching Nursing

Strategies
for Teaching Nursing

THIRD EDITION

Rheba de Tornyay, R.N., Ed.D., F.A.A.N.
Professor, Community Health Care Systems
Dean Emeritus, School of Nursing
University of Washington
Seattle, Washington

Martha A. Thompson, R.N., M.S.N., M.A.Ed.
Professor
Department of Nursing
San Jose State University
San Jose, California

A Wiley Medical Publication
JOHN WILEY & SONS
New York · Chichester · Brisbane · Toronto · Singapore

Library of Congress Cataloging in Publication Data:

de Tornyay, Rheba.
    Strategies for teaching nursing.

    (A Wiley medical publication)
    Bibliography: p.
    Includes index.
    1. Nursing—Study and teaching. I. Thompson,
Martha A.   II. Title.   III. Series.   [DNLM: 1. Education,
Nursing. 2. Teaching—(methods. WY 18 D482s]
RT71.D38   1987   610.73'0711   86-19060
ISBN 0-471-01197-5 (pbk)

Printed in the United States of America

10 9 8 7 6 5 4 3 2 1

Preface

In this third edition of *Strategies for Teaching Nursing* the purpose of the book remains as before—to help teachers of nursing learn more about their options for helping students meet educational objectives. We have added new material, incorporating current references. Portions have been deleted, clarified, or rearranged to provide a closer relationship between the theoretical material and the actual teaching of nursing students. Emphasis remains on the importance of the teacher selecting a variety of teaching strategies based on characteristics of both students and teachers and is directed to teachers who are trying to expand their repertoire of teaching strategies, those who are learning to teach, and those who teach nurses and nursing students in a variety of situations.

Living with scarce resources has become a way of life for college teachers, and funding deficits are a reality that will remain with us in the years to come. In many institutions class size is increasing rather than decreasing, as most faculty and students would prefer. We have added two chapters, "Teaching with Guided Design" and "Teaching in the Clinical Setting," that we hope will help teachers to work more effectively with groups of students.

The book is divided into three parts. The first part discusses the components of teaching in which the teacher is a reinforcer of desired behaviors in students, uses examples and models to explain concepts, seeks simulated work situations, and helps students to develop the psychomotor skills needed to practice nursing. The second part discusses the skillful combining of teaching components into four specific teaching strategies: the lecture, the seminar, guided design (an exciting new development), and clinical teaching. The third part of the book discusses several strategies used to individualize instruction, such as learning modules, learning contracts, and computer-assisted instruction.

The underlying assumption for this book is that teaching skills can be learned. Because teachers of nursing may enter a teaching career with neither the prerequisite trial of competence nor experience with the tools for teaching, they may tend to teach as they themselves were taught. We hope that our book will help them as well as experienced teachers to see new ways to help their students achieve objectives. We do not accept the old adage that "teachers are born, not made." Nor do we believe that effective teaching can be based solely on a "bag of tricks." Teaching skills are performance behaviors and must have rational reasons for being selected. We have, for that reason, included the learning principles relevant to each of the teaching techniques we describe in the hope that we will have helped to bridge the gap between theory and practice.

RHEBA DE TORNYAY
MARTHA A. THOMPSON

Acknowledgments

We wish to acknowledge the helpful reviews and suggestions for this third edition made by the following colleagues: Michele Fox, Anne Loustau, Suzanne Malloy, Betty Mayer, and Sharon Wahl. We thank Gail Hauk and Helen V. Sadowski for their excellent assistance with research for this revision. The contribution of Sharon Eaton and Grace Davis for the chapter on psychomotor skills is appreciated. We want our friends and families to know how grateful we are for their patience and support during the time we were working on this revised edition.

Without our students this book would never have been written. They have been the testing grounds for the strategies we discuss. They continue to provide the challenges and joys we experience as nursing instructors.

RHEBA DE TORNYAY
MARTHA A. THOMPSON

Contents

PART 1

THE COMPONENTS OF INSTRUCTION

1

Employing Reinforcement

Reinforcement is a major condition for most learning. It is among the most powerful procedures used in teaching. Reinforcement techniques can be varied to provide different effects depending on the types of learning we want students to acquire. Because of its importance we have chosen to consider this component before the others.

As a learning theory, reinforcement has its roots in Thorndike's *Law of Effect*. From his studies dealing with cats, rats, and humans, Thorndike formulated general laws from his laboratory data. The *Law of Effect* (Thorndike, 1911) states:

> Of several responses made to the same situation, those which are accompanied or closely followed by satisfaction will, other things being equal, be more firmly connected with the situation so that when it recurs, they will be more likely to recur; those which are accompanied or closely followed by discomfort will, other things being equal, have their connections with that situation weakened, so that when it recurs, they will be less likely to recur.

Stimulus-response (S-R) learning theory explains behavior in terms of the association between stimulus and response. Learning is represented in terms of the systematic changes in S-R associations. The term reinforcement is used to refer to the events that strengthen responses.

DEFINITION OF REINFORCER

A *reinforcer* is anything that strengthens behavior and increases the probability of its recurrence. There are, of course, both positive and negative

3

reinforcers. In the teaching-learning process both positive and negative reinforcers are incentives for students. Put in its most simple terms, a positive reinforcer is a positive reward. A negative reinforcer is a negative reward—a stimulus that gives relief from something unpleasant. Examples of positive reinforcement include praise, smiles, money, prizes, being recognized, doing a task well, and other pleasurable responses from others. Examples of negative reinforcement include relief from pain or discomfort. A student will learn to make a response that will enable her or him to escape an uncomfortable situation.

Although external incentives may be important, especially in the early stages of learning, most students are quite able to monitor their own actions. The most productive incentives are those that are internally controlled. Learners try to solve problems and make decisions from among alternative points of view or courses of action. Whenever they are faced with a problem or the need to make a decision, they automatically try to resolve the issue. Such challenges help focus thought and motivate toward the finding of solutions to problems. The "carrots" provided by external incentives are less important in motivating the learner.

Fuhrmann and Grasha (1983, p. 69) point out that although reinforcement is deemphasized by cognitive theorists, it is not completely ignored. Rather than viewing reinforcement as a variable that automatically influences our actions, these theorists are interested in how beliefs and thoughts modify the influence of reinforcement. For example, students who are intrinsically interested in learning or performing certain tasks may lost interest if they are offered rewards for doing what they want to do anyway. It may appear to them that rewards are controlling their behavior. How a particular reinforcer affects students depends on what they believe it represents. Beliefs and values modify the effects of reinforcers.

Modern behaviorists strike a balance between the role of external stimuli and the ability to use thoughts to control actions. They discuss the role of externally administered rewards and punishments in influencing behavior, but they also focus on how individuals self-monitor, self-regulate, self-reward, and self-punish actions.

The traditional view of reinforcers has been modified in recent years. Behaviorists are more willing to consider a wider range of stimuli as reinforcers. Thus, researchers now believe that the chance to socialize with peers, and other things that are described later in this chapter, will motivate individuals to take certain actions.

Teaching applications stress the use of positive reinforcers or rewards. Aversive stimuli, such as frustration, anger, and anxiety, have too many negative effects to make them useful to teachers. Furthermore, there are ethical issues regarding the use of unpleasant stimuli to influence a student's behavior.

EFFECTS OF POSITIVE REINFORCEMENT

In employing reinforcement, the teacher, of course, must know what behaviors are to be reinforced. It is the correct answer? Is it thinking through a difficult problem, even when the answer is only partially acceptable? Is it participating in a classroom discussion? Is it performing a task smoothly? Is it being willing to tackle a difficult task? Is it being willing to try again after making a mistake? Is it being willing to share one's own ideas? Is it being willing to share one's own feelings?

The older educational research literature abounds with examples of the effects of positive reinforcement. In a study (Verplanck, 1955) designed to test the influence of reinforcement on students' verbalization of opinions, each time a student began a statement with such phrases as "I think . . ." or "I believe . . ." or "It seems to me that . . . ," the experimenters used such reinforcers as "You're right" or "I agree with you" or rephrased the student's statement. They nodded, smiled, and utilized other nonverbal positive reinforcers to indicate their approval. When reinforced in this way, the students tended to volunteer their opinions more readily. When the reinforcers were withdrawn by the experimenters by ignoring the remarks of the students, or by such statements as "I certainly disagree with that," the number of opinion statements made by the students sharply decreased.

Anderson, White, and Wash (1966) were interested in determining whether praised students would perform better than reproved students. Further, they wished to test the hypothesis that school achievement was a critical variable in the effects of praise and reproof. They tested the following two hypotheses:

H_1 Praised students will perform better than reproved students.

H_2 Reproved low achievers and praised high achievers will perform better than praised low achievers and reproved high achievers.

The subjects for their study were university students in a course in educational psychology. An objective test of the subject matter was utilized as the criterion test. In addition, an objective test in mathematics was used to determine if behaviors would be transferred to a different

subject area. Results indicated that there was greater achievement incre-
ment in performance in both subject areas when praise was used rather
than reproof with both the low achieving student and the high achieving
student. Their findings lend support to the notion that praise may assist
in the transfer of learning from one area to another.

The previous two studies were selected to illustrate one of Hilgard's
(1956, p. 486) principles of learning: learning under the control of reward is usually preferable to learning under the control of punishment;
and learning motivated by success is preferable to learning motivated by
failure.

Let us now turn to some of the ways in which positive reinforcement
is employed. The more obvious verbal ways are by saying "good" or
"fine" or "yes" when a student responds. The more obvious nonverbal
ways are by nodding, smiling, moving toward the student, and generally
looking pleased. Additional reinforcing behaviors include calling the
student by name, writing the student's comments on the chalkboard, or
repeating comments and referring back to what a student has contrib-
uted. Statements such as "That indicates careful thinking on your part,"
Your comments showed good grasp of principles," "It is apparent that
you have included information gained from your other courses," and "I
like the initiative you showed in your nursing care today" not only act as
positive reinforcers for students, but also indicate the kind of behavior
the teaching is rewarding. Teachers sometimes comment that the student has displayed creativity or originality in a term paper and yet fail
to be specific about the reasons for reaching that conclusion. When a
student solves a problem in an inventive way, a comment telling how the
actions show originality helps to guide this behavior for the future and
fosters repetition.

A very powerful reinforcing behavior is a request from the teacher
for a student to share successful experience with others. For example,
telling a student "I am impressed with the nursing care you gave today
in working with a patient demonstrating multiple nursing care problems
and hope that you will share your care plan with others" gives the student recognition and prestige with classmates. It is, of course, essential
to recognize the achievements of each student in the group rather than
always turning to the better student, as tempting as it may be.

A very major problem for every instructor is determining what, in
fact, constitutes positive reinforcement for an individual student. Reinforcement can be highly personal. The old phrase "different strokes for
different folks" applies here. A reinforcer for one student may affect

another student quite differently. We know that individual differences in people mean that rewards to the individual are closely tied to their own value system. Whereas praise, recognition, and encouragement are universally valued, the quantity of reinforcement is an unknown factor for effectiveness with each individual student. Mild praise can be strongly reinforcing to a student whose failures may have been outnumbering successes, while high praise may be relatively ineffective for the student who consistently achieves honors. Another factor to consider is that the effects of many events are transitory. A reinforcer for a given student at one time may not be the one for another time. Glaser (1969) makes the point that when attempts are made by teachers to allow students more participation in decision making, it may be initially reinforcing for students to receive more power to act on their own. But later many may feel that they do not want to make decisions and the effect loses its power.

CLASSIFICATION OF REINFORCERS

Tosti and Addison (1979) have attempted to classify educational reinforcement in a systematic way in order to help teachers identify what may serve as a reinforcer for some students, at least some of the time. Although their list appears to be most applicable for classroom teachers in grades 1–12, the general categories could well be applied to college classes in nursing. Their taxonomy includes the following:

I. *Recognition*
   Praise
   Certification of accomplishments
   Formal acknowledgements (awards, testimonials, letters of recommendation)
   Informal acknowledgements (private conversations, "pat" on back)
   Publicity (note in school newspaper, public press)
II. *Tangible rewards*
   Grades
   Food (free lunch)
   Prizes

III. *Learning activities*
Opportunity for desirable enrichment assignment ("honors" class)
More interesting, or more difficult, clinical assignments

IV. *School responsibilities*
Opportunity for increased self-management
Opportunity for more participation in or more frequent decision making
Acceptance of suggestions for improving curriculum
Greater opportunity to select own goals for learning experiences
Greater opportunity to control own schedule and set own priorities

V. *Status indicators*
Appointment as a peer tutor
Having own space (study carrel, desk)

VI. *Incentive feedback*
Increased knowledge of examination scores
Knowledge of individual contributions (helping others)

VII. *Personal activities*
Opportunity to engage in special projects
Extra time off

It is important to point out that reinforcers will motivate students only if they are contingent upon learning performance. The reinforcer must be the result of, or must be directly linked to, student accomplishments. Tosti and Addison (1979) aptly point out that the indiscriminate use of reinforcers may result in happy students but may not result in *productive* students. Again, it is exceedingly important that the instructor constantly keep the instructional objectives in mind in determining what to reinforce.

It is relatively easy for teachers to practice giving positive reinforcement when students are correct. But what should be done about a wrong response? Obviously, teachers do not wish to reinforce an incorrect answer. The way in which students are told that they are wrong is important here. Ignoring the response really doesn't tell what the error is; rather, it leaves students wondering whether they are right, partially right, or what. When teachers say, "No, that's really not it," they let students know they are not on the right track. It is possible to reward students for trying, as well as let them know that they are not right. In other words, it is possible to be accepting of the person while rejecting the idea or response presented.

EFFECTS OF NEGATIVE REINFORCEMENT

Essentially, a negative reinforcement is punishment. Punishment is the removal of a positive reinforcer and the addition or substitution of an aversive stimulus. When an individual student is ignored or ridiculed in any way, the teacher's behavior serves as negative reinforcement. We have all observed classrooms where the students are reluctant to volunteer ideas or responses. This occurs when individual students have experienced embarrassment or rejection or have failed to be heard. Not only will the embarrassed student be reluctant to participate again, but other students will tend to withdraw in the fear that the same treatment will be forthcoming to them.

Mager (1968) makes an eloquent case for what he terms positives and aversives in developing attitudes toward learning. Following his list of what he terms "universal aversives," every nurse can probably trace reactions to specific clinical areas or nursing care problems to the way she or he was introduced to material or taught in the courses that related to these areas. Painful learning occurs when cramped into small working quarters or having to hold instruments until one's wrists hurt. Confusion happens when excessive noise is present or when directions cannot be heard. Fear and anxiety occur when, by word or deed, students are told that it is doubtful if their actions will lead to success or that the grades will reflect the fact that almost no student is superior. Frustration is common when too much information is given too rapidly or too soon to be absorbed by the learner. Students are made to feel insignificant when the teacher ignores a student's question. Teaching one thing and testing another leads to dejection among students. The list goes on and on and is, indeed, a sad commentary on the educational process.

How to achieve a beneficial balance in the use of punishment and reward for adult learners is not clear-cut. There is some evidence that if an individual receives some aversive stimulation along with positive reinforcement, the punishment procedure may actually strengthen the positive response. This is most clearly demonstrated by the methods employed by some stop smoking clinics, in which a mild electric shock treatment is administered preceding any positive comments to deter the clients from smoking. Be that as it may, it is highly unlikely that any nursing instructor should involve such drastic techniques to foster learning!

POSSIBLE REASONS FOR FAILURE TO USE POSITIVE REINFORCEMENT

Given the fact that there is overwhelming evidence supporting the generalization that reinforced responses tend to be repeated in given situations, whereas nonreinforced responses tend to be discontinued, it is interesting to speculate on the reasons why nursing instructors too often fail to reinforce desired behaviors. Possibly it may be linked to the prevalent notion that praise will spoil a child, and this notion carries forward to the adult learner. It must be fresh in the memory of any nurse that when the instructor did *not* say something it meant everything was all right. As nursing instructors, we are quicker to point out what improvement a student needs rather than reinforce the worthy behavior. Somehow, we expect the student to experience intrinsic motivation, and we are overconvinced at times that the student really does not need to be told when doing well. One might wonder how many nursing students have changed majors because of inadequate support in terms of positive reinforcement during the early nursing experiences. Nursing is difficult enough to master, and the novice nurse cannot help but feel inadequate (one might say the same for the experienced nurse!) much of the time.

KNOWLEDGE OF RESULTS AS REINFORCER

A very major reinforcing event for a student is knowledge of results. In practicing motor skills, knowledge of results assists in improving the skill. Nursing students frequently find out if they have performed a nursing procedure correctly by the results achieved. For example, if the student neglects to replace fluid with air while withdrawing fluid from a sealed vial by means of a syringe, the student soon learns by the difficulty in withdrawing the fluid that the pressure within the vial has been reduced. This example illustrates one of Hilgard's (1956, p. 487) learning principles. He points out that information about the nature of good performance, knowledge of one's own mistakes, and knowledge of successful results aid learning. Practice is valuable to the student only when there is knowledge of results.

This idea of knowledge of results has implications when we provide students with information about the correct answers following a written examination. Many years ago, the effect of grading examinations was studied in high school science courses (Curtis & Woods, 1929). Tests consisting of 100 objective-type items were administered to a large number of high school students. The teachers followed four different procedures in returning the tests, as follows:

1. Teacher read the correct answer while each student corrected his own paper. Discussion followed.
2. Teacher marked wrong responses, but wrote nothing else on the paper. Papers were returned and discussed item by item.
3. Teacher wrote in all corrections, and papers were returned and treated as in Number 2 above.
4. Teacher wrote in all corrections, but when papers were returned only specific questions asked by students were discussed.

The test was repeated the next day and 6 weeks later to determine short-term and longer-term retention. A consistent pattern of merit for the four methods was demonstrated. Number 1 was most effective; Numbers 2 and 3 were equal; and Number 4 was poorest.

Whereas this last example illustrates the effect of immediate feedback for a content-oriented approach, it is possible that immediate feedback may be contraindicated for some teaching strategies.

In the learning and problem-solving divisions described by Bruner (1966), the problem-solving cycle is called trial-and-error, means-end testing, trial-and-check, hypothesis testing, and many others. The problem-solving cycle involves the formulation of a test of trial, the operation of the testing procedure, and the comparison of the results of the test with some criterion. Bruner points out that knowledge of results is useful, depending on when the learner receives the corrective information. For example, if knowledge of results occurs too early in the problem-solving sequence, it may be ineffective, either because the learner cannot understand the implications of the feedback information, or because it actually interferes with learning for oneself.

Timing for knowledge of results feedback may be important. Sullivan, Schutz, and Baker (1971) found that immediate knowledge of results of a multiple choice item was more effective than a delayed-feedback procedure when given to ROTC cadets in a university program. Their study gives credence to the effects of letting students score their own classroom tests in order for the knowledge of results to be provided immediately.

Knowledge of the importance of supplying feedback has provided the impetus for the technological innovations in instruction that will be discussed in Part 3. There is no question that programmed instruction and computer-assisted instruction aid learning, not only by allowing the student to progress at an individual rate, but because of their ability to provide immediate feedback through the knowledge of results of actions.

GRADES AS REINFORCERS

Whereas grades are considered one of our most important motivational devices, there appears to be an incredible lack of research on the effect of grading on student learning. We all know that grades are important to students. We know for certain that most students are motivated to get sufficiently high grades to remain in college. The nursing student who aspires to graduate school is motivated to get grades high enough to unlock the door to further education. Grades can bring about the kind of learning the instructor desires. If teachers base their grades on memorization of details, then students will memorize the text to receive the positive reinforcement of a good grade. If students are rewarded for integrating and applying principles, then they will try to acquire such ability. Grades can be utilized as an incentive for learning, as they can provide positive reinforcement for students. Using grades chiefly as a threat may produce avoidance through negative reinforcement.

In addition to grades as rewards, classroom structures that administer rewards to students on a systematic, ongoing basis should be sought. Perhaps the most widely used method is the establishment of contracts with students. Contracts involve the students' performance of certain activities to earn points that are later "cashed in" for a grade. Students know in advance exactly what is expected for a particular grade. The rewards are divided into smaller units, with each unit providing reinforcement to the student for completing it. Contracting with students will be discussed more fully in Chapter 14.

PROVIDING CONDITIONS TO FOSTER POSITIVE REINFORCEMENT

One way of providing positive reinforcement is by seeking experiences for students so that they will succeed. The old adage of "nothing succeeds like success" is really helpful. By providing instruction in incre- ments we can allow for success most of the time. We do not simply place students in situations we know they cannot handle. We build up to the more difficult nursing situations, if that is at all possible. We recognize that students were not ready to tackle a given nursing situation if they find themselves in one, and we help them with their problem-solving techniques so that they learn how to cope with the problem on their own. We give the student some control over the selection and sequencing of the instruction. Probably most important of all is when we can express genuine delight in the student's success. The idea to be conveyed by the teacher is "I know you can do it," rather than "prove to me that you can achieve."

Brodie (1969) points out that there may be a difference of perception between student and teacher. Students may interpret lack of response from the instructor as negative reinforcement. They may express in- ability to please the teacher no matter what is attempted. The teacher, on the other hand, may actually have thought that the student was doing a good job, and failure to comment may have meant there was no criti- cism. Therefore, it is important to remember that the lack of a positive response is, in fact, negative reinforcement.

The instructor who provides experiences with a prediction of success for the student helps the student store a backlog of success that can compensate for later failures and thus provide a tolerance for failure. The very nature of nursing practice is such that we hardly have to go out of our way to seek experiences that will cause feelings of inadequacy for the nursing student. These occur regularly enough in the day-to-day nursing experiences. By helping students to accentuate the positive, we help them cope with their failures in a constructive way.

GROUP REWARD STRUCTURE

We have focused on individual rewards in this chapter. However, in nursing, as in other professions, effective performance frequently re- quires the cooperative performance of a group of professionals. The effects of cooperative, competitive, and individual reward structures on performance have been systematically studied during the past 50 years with, unfortunately, not uniform results. Slavin and Tanner (1979) de- fine a reward structure as a set of rules under which rewards are dis- tributed to individuals contingent upon their performance. A *cooperative* reward structure is one in which individuals depend on one another's performance to be rewarded, as in a collaborative project. A *competitive* reward structure is one in which one person's success requires another's failure, such as in competitive sports. An *individual* reward structure is one in which the connection between a person's behavior and the earned rewards does not depend on any other person's performance.

Because it is important to help nursing students toward the goal of cooperation, nursing faculties should seriously consider rewarding students for cooperative behaviors. Slavin and Tanner (1979) found in their study, which was designed to investigate the conditions under which a cooperative reward structure increased productivity and learning more than did an individual structure, that students in the cooperative reward structure groups performed at a higher level in terms of initial learning and retention than did the students in the individual reward groups. The study focused on reading comprehension as one of the traditional learning tasks in high school and, hence, may not be directly transferable to the learning tasks of nursing. Nevertheless, it behooves every nursing instructor to develop some learning activities in which the entire group is rewarded for the activity, if cooperative behavior as a learning objective is to be rewarded.

There is still another factor that merits emphasis. Research supports the conclusion that cooperative reward structures are more positively associated with "social connectedness" than are the other structures (Slavin, 1977). This is a term that social scientists use to describe the degree to which an individual feels attracted to others and feels and acts a part of a valued group. These social dimensions include interpersonal attraction, friendliness, positive group evaluation, helpfulness, and other positive feelings towards colleagues. Certainly these attributes are important to foster in the neophyte nurse. However, that these behaviors are not always developed is clearly observable when one views the overt and covert behaviors and attitudes of some nurses at work and the attitudes of coworkers toward one another. Increases in mutual attraction as a consequence of a cooperative reward structure have been obtained by a number of investigators in studies that have employed different group sizes, tasks, ages, and durations, yet the finding of greater interpersonal attraction occurring with a cooperative rather than a competitive structure has persisted (Slavin, 1977). Abundant evidence exists reinforcing the importance of a cooperative setting, characterized by a positive, mutually supportive group climate.

SUMMARY

Reinforcement is a needed condition for learning and a powerful procedure used in teaching. The effects of positive reinforcement have been amply documented in the educational literature. In order to foster positive attitudes and behaviors in students, instructors should become sensitive to the ways in which they provide feedback to their students. Praising the desired behavior helps to ensure that it will be repeated.

The importance of positive reinforcement is summarized eloquently by Sister Maura Eichner, the recipient of the Theodore M. Hesburgh Award, the highest teaching award given by the Association of Catholic Colleges and Universities (Ingalls, 1986). She said this:

> In teaching, to give praise is to give what a student needs: confidence, courage, whatever. I think that is the heart of the matter. When writing comments on students' papers, or voicing comments in the classroom, it is important to find the one point that was the best in what the student had to say. You have to be honest, but I try to balance whatever is going to be negative with something positive.

2

Explaining Through Examples and Models

Explaining is an essential part of teaching. To explain is to make something that is not known or understood by students understandable. Some teachers explain aptly. They seem to get to the heart of the matter with just the right terminology, examples, and organization of ideas. Others, unfortunately, get themselves and others all mixed up. They use terms beyond the level of comprehension of their students; they draw inept or inaccurate analogies; or they employ concepts and principles that cannot be understood by students without their understanding the very thing being explained. Teachers can either go beyond students' comprehension, or they can bore their students by giving ideas beneath the level of student expectations.

Outstanding college teachers are able to explain ideas and the connections between them in ways that make eminently good sense to the uninitiated. Most students who receive consistently clear presentations will be able to define, illustrate, and compare and contrast concepts correctly.

An educational system is basically a communication system. It involves a flow of information from the *transmitter* (teacher) to the *receiver* (student) by going through *channels* (language). The transmitter and receiver must agree on the definitions used in the communication process in order to communicate. Therefore, no matter how scholarly the teacher's explanations may be, they are to no advantage to the student if they do not communicate meaning, clarify an issue, or help to relate to previous experiences.

USE OF EXAMPLES

The most common way that teachers explain is by the use of examples. Examples are necessary to clarify, verify, or substantiate concepts. An example helps the student to understand the nature or character of the issue being examined. It may be a smaller part of the issue. An example is, in fact, a sample of the whole. Suppose we want to explain to students that all body actions are dependent on the integrity of the moveable body parts. One example, or part of this generalization, would be that hip and knee joints must be altered from flexion to extension in order for a person to stand erect. The effective use of examples includes the following suggestions.

Begin with Simple Examples and Progress to More Complex Ones

By simple we mean what is simple to the student, not to the teacher. There are times when an extreme example may better illustrate a point rather than a more subtle one. To help students to understand and recognize behavior, it may be easier to recognize symptoms in a patient hospitalized specifically because of depression when the symptoms of sleeplessness, anorexia, muteness, and immobility are pronounced rather than expecting the student to recognize the more subtle symptoms of a postpartum depression. Another example might include using, as illustration of principles, simple nursing measures to relieve sleeplessness rather than the more sophisticated measures required for the patient with complex nursing problems.

Select Examples Relevant to Students' Experience and Knowledge

This follows the oft-repeated principle of learning—that of proceeding from the known to the unknown. The use of simple, everyday examples can illustrate scientific principles in easy, understandable terms and assist in comprehension, retention, and transfer of such principles. Suppose we wanted to understand the generalization that protein matter coagulates faster when wet heat is used rather than dry heat. By using an example well known to all students, such as it takes less time to boil an egg than bake one, we are selecting from an experience common to all students. In discussing the family as a sociological unit, if we draw on students' knowledge of families they have known, we are again utilizing their own experiences as examples.

Relate Examples to the Principles or Ideas Being Taught

Informing students that, in most cases, a patient's breathing will be eased if the patient is placed in a sitting position may foster rote learning. If, on the other hand, the principle that breathing is eased when the chest cavity is enlarged by allowing gravity to pull on abdominal organs, as *for example* when a patient is placed in a sitting position, will place the focus on the principle rather than on the example. All teachers have had the experience of having students remember *only* the example while forgetting the principle it illustrated.

Check to See if the Objectives of the Lesson Have Been Achieved by Asking Students to Give Examples That Illustrate the Main Point

This feedback mechanism allows the teacher to ascertain if students understand the main points or principles of a given concept under discussion. Asking students to share experiences that exemplify the concept under consideration not only helps other students to broaden their understanding, but reinforces learning and promotes transfer.

USE OF EXAMPLES TO GENERALIZE

When students learn to generalize, they are essentially organizing their experiences so that they are meaningful and useful to them. Such organization is important in terms of both retention and transfer. Generalizations can be developed in two ways. The first is by deduction, when a generalization or rule is given to a student and the student deduces examples from the generalization. One such example would be if students were told that an individual whose circulatory system is able to compensate for a decrease in oxygen supply by increasing blood flow is better able to tolerate hypoxia than a patient whose circulatory response is defective or lacking. Following this generalization, students would be asked to *deduce* examples that illustrate this principle.

In the inductive process, the student begins with a set of observations and, based on observations, develops or induces a generalization or principle to predict or explain the pattern of relationships observed. For example, if the teacher wished students to induce the generalization about toleration of hypoxia, students might care for patients who exemplify the principle, such as a patient who has had a sympathectomy, a patient with generalized atherosclerosis, and so forth.

Both deductive and inductive processes promote learning. Deductive learning assists the student in the testing of theory and its application to the solution of problems. Inductive learning helps the student to generalize concepts and theories from experience.

Comparing and contrasting examples are effective teaching strategies following content sampling. When students are asked to seek similarities and differences among examples to find principles and generalizations it assists them in the future use of the concepts under discussion. This way of learning to generalize also helps students in organizing material for themselves.

MODELS

The patient care study can be used as a means of comparing the nursing care needs of a specific patient to the specified possible needs as described in a textbook. Viewed in this way, the care study is an example of a larger body of alternative patterns for nursing care. Selection of content for the nursing curriculum can be derived from the nursing care problems selected as representative of the knowledge required for meeting the nursing care needs of many individuals and families. In this latter example, the problems can be derived inductively in order to determine the general content for the nursing course. The specific nursing care problems represented by the problem models are utilized as problem-solving vehicles to assist students in the decision-making process.

A model helps the student to integrate data. One specific type of model is the replica. A replica is a scaled construction that reproduces features of the original. It may be scaled down or be a mock-up of the original. The latter is utilized when something small, for example, a cell, is made more tangible and understandable when blown up. A large replica of the human cell helps the viewer to see relationships of the individual parts, which a microscopic picture or flat plate could never accomplish. Models of this type are frequently used in teaching to assist students in viewing parts of the body not readily seen in perspective without this aid. For example, a mock-up of the human ear is used to illustrate the flow of fluid when the outer canal is irrigated. The replica serves as a pictorial or physical representation of parts or the total under inquiry. The replica serves mainly to describe a static condition, a thing, or a dynamic system at a particular instant of time. The scaled down or scaled upward model can be worked with more easily than the object or system it represents.

Another type of model is termed *analog* model. An analog employs the properties of a familiar system in order to represent the properties of the system under inquiry. It utilizes analogy for explaining something by comparing it with something else. The analog model is frequently used in research. The comparison of the human brain to a computer model has been made in order to guide the systematic inquiry of human problem solving. The behavioral sciences have modeled their inquiry by comparison with biological science models. To further clarify, suppose that biological theory of cell growth were used as a model for social growth. Relatively precise meaning has been given to anabolic and catabolic processes in cell growth theory. By giving correspondingly precise meaning to the building and deteriorating processes of human institutions, a one-to-one correspondence is approximated, and we would have the necessary conditions for using cell growth theory as a model for institutional theory. The analog model, unlike the replica, can be utilized effectively to describe, explain, and represent dynamic systems. It is more general than the replica, and as such it can be representative of many different processes.

The third type of model is the symbolic model, which is most frequently utilized in teaching. Symbolic models are intangible except as sounds from a speaker or word on a paper. Words are symbolic models as the word brings the image of what it conveys to the receiver. Mathematical symbols and formulas likewise constitute symbolic models.

USE OF SELF AS ROLE MODEL

In addition to the use of models to explain and clarify teaching, the use of self as a role model in the teaching of nursing cannot be underestimated. Learning from role models is called identification.

Identification has long been prominent in theories of socialization because it explains how individuals learn new behavior and social roles. A number of principles have been proposed for the choice of a model for identification. Persons may be chosen as models because they frequently reward the learner or because the learner experiences vicarious rewards from their model. The nursing instructor who is praised by a patient or is observed to have assisted in providing comfort to a patient may be selected as a role model by the nursing student who vicariously receives pleasure from the instructor's nursing skill. Persons may be chosen as models because they are envied as recipients of rewards from others. Finally, persons may be chosen as models because the learner perceives traits in the model similar to his or her own.

Mager (1968) points out that modeling behavior is exceedingly important in the achievement of attitude objectives. The often stated phrase "Actions speak louder than words" is relevant here. Particularly in the clinical area, nursing instructors have the opportunity to behave in ways in which they wish their students to behave. Instructors are truly the living audiovisual examples of what they are trying to convey to their students.

ILLUSTRATIONS

The old cliché "A picture is worth a thousand words" is well known to all. The need for illustration is inherent in the teaching process. Illustrations not only supply missing objects or aspects of a given topic, but they eliminate the need for a continuous effort to recall what has been said before. How would you describe correct body mechanics for lifting an object from the floor by using words alone? Imagine having to give your students a mental picture of the lower intestinal tract without using diagrams or illustrations.

The age of television has emphasized this as a visual age. Most people find it difficult to understand purely verbal concepts. In general, people feel more secure when things are visible and they can see for themselves. Visual memories are longer than auditory memories.

The use of photographs, videotapes, diagrams, slides, and transparencies all enrich the teaching-learning process. There is much material from which to choose; so much material, in fact, that it can cause the nursing instructor to become confused and perplexed in selecting appropriate materials to illustrate the principles being taught.

SUMMARY

Effective teaching requires effective communication. The use of examples, models, and illustrations assists students in proceeding from what they know and have experienced to something new. Examples help students to apply principles and generalizations to specific instances.

3

Using Simulation and Games

Simulation and games for teaching have been used for many years. War games date back centuries and are still used for training military personnel. Most readers are no doubt familiar with the use of flight simulators for training military and commercial pilots, space simulators for training astronauts, and automobile simulators for driver education.

The idea of using simulation and games in formal education is also not a new one. Games were mentioned in educational writings as early as 1775 (Knight, 1949). James (1908) encouraged teachers to make learning more activity oriented. More recently, other educators have argued that vicarious experience and acting on what has been learned are important parts of the total learning situation. Common sense support for the value of experiential learning techniques is found in the writings of Mark Twain who said, "A fellow who takes a bull by the tail once gets as much as sixty or seventy times the information as one who doesn't."

Such views required that education shift its focus from the mere transmission of content to one of bringing theory and real-life experiences closer together. Further, with extensive proliferation of knowledge it became important to help learners develop skills of inquiry and problem solving that would increase their effectiveness in coping with future situations. Increasingly, then, experiential techniques, including simulations and games became a part of the educational scene.

Use of simulation and gaming techniques in formal education became common in the 1960s (Rockler, 1978, p. 295), particularly at the elementary and secondary levels (Maidment & Bronstein, 1973, p. 13). At the undergraduate and graduate levels the major use was in political science courses (Maidment & Bronstein, 1973, p. 12). Progressively, the use of simulations and games spread to other areas of higher education, including the various health professions. For example, simulation techniques have been used in education of medical students since the mid-1960s (Barrows, 1968; Hoban, 1978). Nursing educators have also used simulation techniques for many years, although the term, simulation, was not used until recently. Examples include the practice of basic skills using models, such as Mrs. Chase, in skills laboratories, use of simulated nursing stations in a laboratory setting, and the use of role playing to gain insight into the feelings of others and for learning and practicing interpersonal, problem-solving, and crisis intervention skills. More recently, there have been a number of textbooks and articles written by nursing educators that specifically discuss the use of simulation and games. Many of them will be cited throughout this chapter.

This chapter focuses on the application of simulation and games to nursing education. Terms are defined early to distinguish between the two. Simulation and games are then discussed together in the area of potential educational benefits since previous writings often have not made a clear distinction between the two. After this initial common discussion, simulation and games are covered separately. Examples are given, processes identified, and uses established. The chapter ends with a listing of limitations and concerns applicable to both simulation and games.

DEFINITIONS

It is apparent when reading about simulations and games that there is much inconsistency about the use of the two terms. Often the terms are used together, that is, simulation games or simulation/games, although what is being discussed is clearly one or the other but not both, or both are discussed without identifying which is which. Other authors have provided guidance in developing definitions that help to clarify and distinguish between the two terms (Cooper, 1979; Rockler, 1978, pp. 288–289; Thiagarajan & Stolovich, 1978, pp. 8–13). The following are the definitions of these terms as used in this chapter:

SIMULATION: A realistic representation (model) of the structure or dynamics of a real thing or process with which the participant, as an active part of the experience, interacts with persons or things in the environment, applies previously learned knowledge to make responses (decisions and actions) to deal with a problem or situation, and receives feedback about responses without having to be concerned about real-life consequences.

GAME: An activity governed by precise rules that involves varying degrees of chance or luck and one or more players who compete (with self, the game, one another, or a computer) through the use of knowledge or skill in an attempt to reach a specified goal (gain an intrinsic or extrinsic reward).

SIMULATION GAME: An activity that incorporates the characteristics of *both* a simulation and a game; a contest that also replicates some real-life situation or process.

It is apparent, then, that all games are not simulations; all simulations are not games; and an experience may be both a simulation and a game depending on its specific characteristics. With simulation there is a distinct and explicit analogy between the activity and real life, while in a game, which is not also a simulation, that analogy with real life may be a distant abstraction. Many games bear little or no resemblance to actual life processes and situations even though they use social interaction as a mechanism of play and require active participation of the student.

It is helpful to view learning experience on a continuum in relation to its closeness with reality. Table 3-1 reflects levels of learning from the two extremes—concrete and abstract—and is a combination and adaptation of the ideas presented previously by Dale (1969) and Russell (1974, p. 73).

A game may fit at different levels of this continuum, depending on its unique characteristics. Many games are highly abstract, using auditory or visual stimuli only (e.g., word games, spelling games, question-and-answer games, crossword puzzles, and card games). Others are more concrete as they move closer to representing real-life processes and activities, for example, computer or group problem-solving games. Those activities that can be classified as simulations and simulation games fall closer to the level of concrete experiences. However, direct involvement in a contrived experience can itself represent varying degrees of closeness to reality. For example, practicing a skill, such as preparing and starting an intravenous infusion, can be accomplished at varying degrees of "realness." One level is practice without the use of a mannikin; another is practice using a mannikin without simulated veins; another is practice on a simulator with veins; and the next would be practice on a simulated patient (a peer or someone else trained to behave and respond like a patient). Each has certain values in relation to learning and level of anxiety experienced by the student. For example, a beginning student may gain more, initially, by working with a mannikin rather than a simulated patient since level of stress is likely to be increased when practicing on a real person. However, a more advanced student would be likely to gain more from working in a more complex, realistic situation.

Table 3-1
Levels of Experience

Concrete Experiences
  1. Direct participation in real-life events (clinical experience)
  2. Direct involvement in a contrived experience in an environment that is a representation of reality (simulation: role playing, practice of skills, simulation games, clinical simulation)
  3. Direct observation of an actual experience or demonstration (field trips, demonstrations, observer of dramatizations or clinical practice)
  4. Indirect perception of experiences by visual representation (filmstrips, movies, videotape, television, exhibits, photographs)
  5. Indirect perception of experiences by audio representation (records, audiotapes, sound tracks)
  6. Reading descriptions of experiences (printed matter: texts, articles, case studies)
  7. Hearing descriptions of experiences (lectures, audiotape, discussion)
Abstract Experiences

SOURCE: Adapted from Russell, J. D. Figure E, *Modular instruction.* Minneapolis, Burgess Publishing Co., 1974. Used by permission.

POTENTIAL EDUCATIONAL BENEFITS OF USING SIMULATION AND GAMING

Many authors have described the benefits associated with using simulation or games, or both. Those from Greenblat, (1981, pp. 142–143) are summarized below:

1. Motivation and interest in the topic, course, and learning in general are increased.
2. Cognitive learning, including factual information, concepts, principles, and decision-making skills, is improved.
3. Later course work is more meaningful; students are led to more sophisticated and relevant inquiry; and participation in class discussions is increased.
4. Affective learning associated with the subject matter is improved by altering students' attitudes and perceptions of issues and people and increasing their empathy and insight into others different from themselves.
5. General affective learning is improved by increasing each student's self-awareness and sense of personal effectiveness.
6. Classroom structure and interactional patterns are improved by promoting good student-teacher relations, encouraging the free exploration of ideas, decreasing the punitive role of the teacher, increasing student autonomy in the learning situation, and increasing exchange of ideas among different types of students.

Most of the evidence to support these claims is experiential rather than experimental.There is limited empirical evidence to substantiate the superiority of simulations and games over traditional methods for cognitive learning. Bredemeier and Greenblat (1981, pp. 165, 167) summarize the "hard" evidence that is available to support the value of simulations and games in comparison to conventional methods. In the cognitive area they conclude that there is evidence to suggest that "simulations/games are at least as effective as other methods in facilitating subject matter learning and are more effective aids to retention." In the affective area they conclude that "under certain circumstances and for some students, simulation-gaming can be more effective than traditional methods of instruction in facilitating positive attitude change toward the subject and its purposes."

As in other fields, most reports in the nursing literature describe educational uses of simulations and games without providing specific research evidence of their effectiveness. However, there are some studies in nursing education and practice settings that discuss affective and/or cognitive gains from using simulations and games. Examples of recent studies follow:

1. Shaffer and Pfeiffer (1980) compared the use of videotaped simulations of critical incidents in community nursing with printed case studies. They found that the students using the videotaped simulations expressed a preference for this method and participated in discussions at a significantly higher level than those students using written materials only. They also found that there was no significant difference in the amount of cognitive learning between the two methods.

2. In their use of the simulation game "Mental Hospital," Laszlo and McKenzie (1979) found that participating personnel developed greater sensitivity toward patients in mental hospitals. Also, they found that participants who "experienced" being mental hospital patients developed markedly in awareness about patient rights and that they were highly motivated to obtain more information in this area.

3. Godejohn, Taylor, Muhlenkamp, and Blaesser (1975) found that two simulation games produced significant decreases in authoritarianism and social restrictiveness scores on a scale measuring opinions about mental illness, while the scores for the control group remained the same. They conclude that these results provide compelling evidence to support the use of simulation games for changing attitudes toward mental illness.

4. Jeffers and Christensen (1979) demonstrated the value of simula-

tion in the development of clinical observational skills and a smoother transition into an actual leadership experience.

A few studies that attempt to determine the validity of specific simulation techniques are also available. Four examples follow:

1. Holzemer, Schleutermann, Farrand, and Miller (1981) found modest evidence that a written simulation is a valid measure of clinical problem solving.
2. del Bueno (1983) found videotaped simulations to be a useful, reliable method for assessing nurses' ability to make specific clinical decisions. She contends, however, that no conclusions can be drawn about what the participants would do in actual clinical situations.
3. McDowell, Nardini, Negley, and White (1984) found that student nurse practitioners' performance on clinical examinations using simulated patients correlated closely with class standing and ratings by clinical preceptors.
4. McLaughlin, Carr, and Delucchi (1981) found that two clinical simulation tests were both reliable and valid. They contend that the findings suggest the usefulness of such tests in nursing education.

Research findings about the effectiveness of computer simulations are given in Chapter 15.

Continued research regarding the advantages and limitations of simulations and games as educational tools is needed, as is systematic development of simulations and games for specific purposes. An emphasis should be placed on identifying ways to test the unique effectiveness and impact of these strategies as an integral part of the instructional program. Precise knowledge about how and why simulations and games work is needed. It is highly probable that they produce effects that have not yet been specified or measured, particularly considering the current availability of technology through which realism can be greatly enhanced.

SIMULATION

Several factors call for the use of alternative strategies in nursing education, particularly for the clinical component. Critics of nursing education at the college and university levels contend that it is too theoretically based, that students have inadequate clinical experience, and that much of what is taught is inconsistent with the "real" world of nursing. Issues associated with teaching in the clinical area include (1) the need for close supervision especially at the early skill development stage, thus making it more costly and time-consuming; (2) the decreasing availability of clinical facilities for student experience due to an increase in the numbers and varieties of students in the health professions; (3) the unpredictability of clinical experiences, thus an inability at times to plan specific experiences desired for all students; (4) the concern for client safety and comfort; and (5) the difficulty with precise evaluation of performance in the clinical setting.

These factors can be at least partially dealt with through the use of simulation as a strategy for teaching and evaluation. In addition, simulation techniques can be used in an attempt to incorporate accepted principles of learning related to motivation, active participation, relevance and transfer of learning, individual discovery of knowledge, and feedback about performance. The use of simulations and games may be justified by the gains in affective objectives alone in spite of the current absence of proof of their superiority over traditional methods for achievement of cognitive objectives.

Further justification for the use of experiential techniques with nursing students is found in the recognition that most students in nursing programs are of the "sensing-feeling" type (Bradshaw, 1978, p. 33). Bradshaw states:

> One of the major characteristics of this group appears to be their affinity for learning through the use of their senses. These persons are more comfortable and able to perceive their world more clearly through their sense of touch, feel, smell, sight, and taste. They are often categorized as 'concrete' thinkers because they determine the reality of a thing by whether it can be taken in through the senses. 'Experiencing' becomes the key word and a major activity through which an instructor can reach many students without resorting to telling.

Thus, simulation and gaming techniques that increase the extent of concreteness of the learning experience should prove most productive for nursing students.

Types of Simulation

In their writings on the use of simulations in the health professions, Maatsch and Gordan (1978, pp. 127–133) identified five types of simulation. Their classification has been somewhat modified and expanded for use in this chapter and includes (1) written simulations, (2) role played simulations, (3) mediated simulations, (4) physical simulators, (5) live simulated patients, (6) computer simulations, and (7) gamed simulations. These simulation types are not mutually exclusive. One or more may be incorporated into any single activity. However, they will be discussed separately for the sake of simplicity.

Written Simulation.   A written simulation is a paper-and-pencil presentation of actual problems or cases about which the student must make decisions as if performing in the situation. With each decision the student receives feedback about the effects of that action and incorporates that information into the next decision. The progression of events follows that established by the actual situation. The best example of written simulation is the clinical problem-solving technique, patient management problem (PMP).

A PMP is a paper-and-pencil branched programmed activity simulating the decision-making process as if in an actual patient encounter. It was originally developed for use in medical education and licensure (Hubbard, et al., 1965) and was first introduced to nursing education by de Tornyay (1968) with the "simulated clinical nursing problem test." The PMP can be used either for teaching or evaluating problem-solving skills, including making judgments in the clinical area. de Tornyay (1968) stated the belief that they are especially helpful for emphasizing problem-solving skills that cannot be adequately measured by traditional multiple-choice test items and for providing predictions about a student's future clinical performance.

McGuire and Babbott (1967) outline five essential characteristics of a clinical problem which claims to simulate a real patient encounter:

1. The problem must be presented in a realistic manner with the amount and type of information that would be available to the student on the encounter with the client.

2. It must require a series of sequential, interdependent decisions on the part of the participant as would be reflected in the actual resolution of a problem.

3. Each decision must be followed by the receipt of realistic information about the results of the decision, which can then be used in making subsequent decisions.

4. The format must be such that an ineffective or harmful decision cannot be retracted after the results of a decision are known.

5. It must allow for different approaches for dealing with the problem and variable patient responses in relation to each approach.

The key process, then, is receipt of baseline information, decision, feedback about decision (more information), subsequent decision, and so forth. Students have an opportunity to select from among relevant and irrelevant and beneficial and harmful options. Thus, each student can follow a different path to obtain additional information and solve the problem. The mechanism also provides for remediation or termination of the activity (depending on whether the PMP is being used for teaching or for evaluation) should the student select an alternative that is inappropriate or dangerous.

Nursing literature contains descriptions of the use and evaluation of the PMP at various levels of nursing education. One study (Page & Saunders, 1978) describes an experience with a written simulation for teaching and evaluating first year nursing students' use of the assessment and planning phases of the nursing process. They conclude that the technique has value as a teaching/learning tool by complementing existing methods and by dealing with such constraints as client safety when teaching in the actual clinical setting. Available research in nursing literature also supports the continued investigation of the PMP as a tool for the measurement of clinical problem solving/decision making (Dincher & Stidger, 1976; Holzemer et al., 1981; McLaughlin et al., 1981; Sherman, Miller, Farrand, & Holzemer, 1979). Although definitive conclusions cannot yet be drawn regarding the effectiveness of the PMP, it is viewed as having potential for measuring clinical judgment in a variety of practice and educational situations. Future efforts are expected to refine further the design of PMPs and to test their reliability and validity.

Role Played Simulation. Role playing is a simulation technique in which one person assumes the role of another. Therefore, participants who are involved in simulations that call upon them to respond as themselves (such as with PMPs just discussed) are not involved in role playing. It should be pointed out, however, that role played simulations have less fidelity with reality than those in which participants deal with problems as themselves.

A few major points, only, will be made about the use of role playing. For the reader who desires more detail about either the development or use of role playing situations, McKeachie (1978, pp. 136–141) may be useful.

The primary purpose of role playing is to help participants and observers gain new perceptions about human relationships—particularly insights and empathy into the behaviors and feelings of people who are different from themselves. Only willing players should be selected, since they must be able to become involved in the role without being threatened or exposed by it. The technique forces the participant to think about the person whose role is assumed. It has been used for many years in psychiatric nursing in an attempt to provide an essence of reality.

Role played simulation may be partly structured or completely spontaneous once roles have been assigned. Typically, it involves the use of a critical incident or problem situation depicting conflict between persons, such as with a nurse and a noncompliant client, in which participants play specific roles in the way that they visualize each person would react. Usually, a limited number of the members in a group are involved in the role play while the remaining members act as observers. Specific tasks may be assigned to observers in order to focus their attention on desired aspects of the situation.

The length of the role play itself varies but typically lasts from 5 to 15 minutes. Upon termination of the role play, the participants and observers analyze what occurred, what feelings were generated, what insights were gained, why things happened as they did, and how the situation is related to reality. The procedure usually includes asking participants to discuss their feelings about the roles and their observations about interactions before asking observers to enter into the discussion. It is important to focus criticisms on the role played and the problem presented rather than on the person playing the role. Analysis and discussion may be aided by being able to review the role played situation; therefore, videotaping can be used if more precise recall of the incident is desired.

Examples of role played simulations used with undergraduate students are provided in the nursing literature. Daniel, Eigsti, and McGuire (1977), in their desire to minimize reality shock in case load management in community health, used a simulated exercise to familiarize students with roles of various community health personnel. In groups of six, in assigned roles, the students worked on a realistic case load management task. Upon completion of the task each group presented its plan and rationale to another group. The authors felt that this activity was helpful for providing a more complete picture of a community health agency as well as for depicting a more realistic experience with case load management.

Reichman and Weaver-Meyers (1984) used a combination role play and simulated patient technique to help students develop a better understanding of the problems and feelings of the handicapped and design appropriate nursing interventions. The authors conclude that the students were better prepared for the clinical situation as a result of their participation in this activity.

Another example is one used at the graduate level (Keller & Mac-Cormick, 1980). Graduate students learning about curriculum development were placed in faculty roles by random drawing to make up a task group with the responsibility for developing a masters and a doctoral program in nursing. The simulation lasted for the entire semester and culminated with a report about the programs developed to the real faculty in the setting.

Mediated Simulation. A simulation in this category uses audio and/or visual media to present a problem, case, or task; to represent some aspect of an interpersonal encounter; or to provide an avenue for analysis of a role played or other simulated situation. Such mediated situations may be used either for teaching or evaluation. The two types discussed here are videotaped simulations and electronic reproductions.

Videotaped Simulations. Videotapes are often a part of simulation exercises. A common form is that depicting clinical situations or illustrating interpersonal relationships and interviewing techniques. These make use of a problem situation that may be acted by a trained "patient" or taken from a commercial videotape or a prepared videotape of a real patient situation. The student is given verbal and nonverbal cues via the videotape, as well as data in written form sometimes, to which verbal and nonverbal responses are stated or demonstrated or more information is requested. Students may be asked to give original responses or required to select from a list of alternatives. If the latter format is used, videotaped responses to each alternative can be prepared for an ongoing dramatization of the interview situation. In this way, the student receives immediate feedback regarding the effects of actions and can proceed logically through a selected situation. An added benefit is that the videotaped sequences can be interrupted at any point for analysis and discussion, which makes them useful for groups as well as for individuals.

A videotaped depiction of an actual client situation can also be combined with written simulations for teaching and evaluating clinical assessment and decision-making skills. It is possible, using available technology, to prepare interactive programs that will allow a student (1) to go through a complete simulated clinical situation in order to learn various skills before confronting them in an actual clinical setting or (2) to be evaluated on skills previously learned in another situation.

Several examples of the use of videotaped simulations for teaching and evaluation are found in nursing literature. Three previously cited in this chapter include the use of timed videotaped simulations to assess staff nurses' clinical decision-making skills (del Bueno, 1983), videotaped critical incidents to stimulate analysis and discussion by students (Shaffer and Pfeiffer, 1980), and a combination of written and videotaped simulations with nurse practitioners and physicians (McLaughlin et al., 1981).

Examples of use of videotaped simulations for evaluation and testing are provided by Rogers (1976) and Richards, Jones, Nichols, Richardson, Riley, and Swinson (1981). Rogers used videotaped sequences focusing on particular behaviors to validate the competence of registered nurses in interpersonal skills. The students were asked to list verbal and nonverbal responses to each behavior and to state their rationale for each response. Responses were then evaluated as most therapeutic, appropriate, or least therapeutic with students being rated as competent if 75 percent or more of their responses were identified as being in the first two categories.

In the second situation, Richards and associates developed videotapes of situations frequently encountered in an acute care psychiatric setting. Four interview situations were dramatized to which students were asked to respond, write a description of the observed behavior for charting, identify major patient problems and appropriate actions, write a diagnostic label for the behavior, and list common treatment modalities. Student responses were evaluated, and the results made up 50 percent of the clinical grade. The authors conclude that the use of this technique provides a more accurate indication of ability than do the traditional methods of evaluating clinical performance.

Other examples of variations in the use of videotaped simulations include videotaped peer interviews for later analysis and discussion (Rynerson, 1980); videotaping of a dressing change on a "patient" for later evaluation by the student, peers, and teacher (Memmer, 1979); and videotaped illustrations of home health care (Steiner & Rothenberg, 1980).

Electronic Reproductions. This category of mediated simulation includes the audio reproductions of human cardiac and respiratory sounds. Such reproductions can be used to teach and evaluate students who are learning basic and advanced physical assessment skills and to use tools for monitoring various body processes, such as fetal heart tones during pregnancy and labor. One technique for adding realism is to have the student place the stethoscope directly on the playback unit in order to focus attention, increase concentration ability, and remove distractions.

Physical Simulators. This category includes the use of three-dimensional lifelike models of part or all of the human body to teach or evaluate specific clinical skills. They provide the student with a means of learning, practicing, and repracticing. The goal is to increase student confidence and competence in the performance of clinical skills for later application to the clinical setting. Another advantage is increased patient safety and comfort as students become more proficient. When used for evaluation, the student can be either observed directly or the performance videotaped for later viewing by the teacher.

A wide variety of models of the human body is currently available, including some designed to aid in the development of specific skills, such as enema administration, urinary catheterization, breast examination, administration of injections, colostomy care, and cardiopulmonary resuscitation. Their approximation to reality varies from simple models to be practiced on to those that provide some type of response to student actions. The well-known "Mrs. Chase" is an example of the former, allowing students to practice such procedures as bed baths and positioning. A more sophisticated model is the intravenous (IV) injection arm, which is used to do venipunctures, give IV injections, and administer IV fluids. It provides a more realistic experience as there is a "blood" return and an opportunity to actually inject fluids into the simulated veins. Even more sophisticated computerized robots have been used for some time in the education of medical students (Denson & Abrahamson, 1969). Sim-One, a computerized robot developed by the medical school at the University of Southern California, is used to train residents in anesthesia administration. It simulates human reaction—changes in color, respirations, blood pressure, heart action—in response to the administration of drugs and gases, thus providing a risk free mechanism for the practice of complex skills. Another robot, Harvey, is an animated mannikin that can simulate cardiovascular disease states (Hoban, 1978). Harvey can be programmed to exhibit eye grounds, pupillary reactions, aging, stroke, and alterations in blood pressure. Such simulators, besides providing the risk-free setting, also furnish immediate feedback to the student, allow a student to progress at his or her own rate, and permit individual acts to be repeated as often as necessary.

There are numerous reports in the nursing literature about the settings in which less sophisticated physical simulators are used. Representative of these are the Skills Laboratory at San Jose State University (Rochin & Thompson, 1975); the college laboratory at the University of Wisconsin (Haukenes & Halloran, 1984); and the practice laboratory at the University of Connecticut (Infante, 1981). There have been no reports in the nursing literature about the use of robots like Sim-One and

Harvey, perhaps because of the high costs of these innovations. Should funding be available, such robots offer the same advantages to nursing education, especially in the area of nurse practitioner training, as they do for medical education.

Live Simulated Patients. This type of simulation, useful for either teaching or evaluating, involves the use of persons trained to act in the role of the patient (Hoban, 1978). It is a technique that has been used for some time in medical education (Barrows, 1968). The person playing the role of the patient is directed to exhibit certain clinical behaviors, provide a specific history, respond in certain interpersonal ways during an encounter with a student, and, at times, give students feedback about performance of skills. The episode may also be videotaped or attended by an objective observer for the purpose of providing further feedback about student behaviors.

The "patient" may be played by a peer, drama student, paid actor, or faculty member. Rochin & Thompson (1975) described the use of peers acting as the patient for the practice of psychomotor skills. Peers also served as patients during a 2-day workshop that simulated a hospital day and was intended to improve the transition from the practice lab to the actual setting (Sullivan et al., 1977). Actors were used to prepare videotapes for simulated nursing rounds intended to sharpen observational skills (Jeffers & Christensen, 1979) and to provide students with practice in interviewing and learning about heart and respiratory sounds (Lincoln, Layton, & Holdman, 1978). The sequence of events identified in the latter situation was observation of a videotape demonstrating assessment, lecture-discussion, supervised practice with a peer, practice with a simulated patient, and, finally, assessment of real patients. The result of decreased fear of making mistakes or harming the patient supports the use of this technique for initial skill development.

Reports on the use of simulated patients for evaluation are also found in the nursing literature. McBride (1979) reported on their use for evaluation of clinical psychomotor skills in the learning laboratory. McDowell and associates (1984) reported on their use for the evaluation of student nurse practitioners' performance. McDowell and associates state: "We have found that the use of simulated patients in performance evaluation increases objectivity, allows for the comparison of each student's performance to identical criterion measures, and provides for feedback which students can use to strengthen their clinical skills" (p. 37). They go on to say that this activity was rated highly by both faculty and students and that all students perceived the experience to be similar to an actual patient encounter.

Computer Simulation. Simulations of this type use a computer to present cases, provide information requested by the student, incorporate decisions made, and provide feedback to the student about the effects of decisions. Both psychomotor and cognitive decisions can be incorporated into computer simulations. For example, the computerized robots discussed in the section on physical simulators can be programmed to respond in certain ways to specific student actions. However, most computer simulations in medical and nursing education involve the simulation of patient care problems similar to the PMPs discussed in the section on written simulations. Typically, the computer presents a patient situation to the student who requests additional information, makes responses, intervenes, and receives feedback about the consequences of decisions made. Thus, the student gains practice in clinical decision making and judgment without the fear of doing something wrong or harming a patient. In computer simulations involving a high degree of interaction between the program and the learner, such as that which can be accomplished with computer-assisted interactive video using videotape or videodisc, specific audio or visual segments can be triggered in response to a learner's decision. Thus, the closeness to reality is enhanced, and the opportunities for individualization of learning are limitless. (See Chapter 15 for further discussions of computer simulations.)

Gamed Simulation. This category of simulation includes those activities that have the characteristics of both a game and a simulation, as defined at the beginning of this chapter. Thus, a gamed simulation (or a simulation game) must be active and interactive in a problem situation, operated according to set rules, and involve an element of competition in reaching the specified goal. It usually involves winners and losers; however, the gamed simulation can be designed so that everyone who is involved in the activity wins if the specified goal is achieved. Simulation activities that require game boards, dice, cards, and so forth are also referred to as simulation games, although they may not have other gamelike characteristics, since they do contain some element of chance characteristic of games.

Simulation games appropriate for use in nursing education can be found in guides (Horn & Cleaves, 1980; Stadsklev, 1979), catalogues (Sim-Ed, 1978), individual publications (Wolf & Duffy, 1979), and articles in professional journals (De Bella-Baldigo, 1984; Farley & Fay, 1983; Kaye, Linhares, Breault, Norris, Stamoulis, & Kahn, 1981; Kolb, 1983; Laszlo & McKenzie, 1979; Plasterer & Mills, 1983; Ulione, 1983; Woodbery & Hamric, 1981). Some deal with theoretical content, others with attitude change, and others with clinical processes, systems, or sit-

Table 3-2

Examples of Gamed Simulations Suitable for Nursing Education

Title of Gamed Simulation	Availability	Number of Players	Playing Time	Objectives and Description of Activity
Bafá bafá	Simile II P.O. Box 910 Del Mar, CA 92014	12–40	1½ h plus 30 min to discuss	Participants live and cope in a "foreign" culture and are both perpetrators and victims of stereotyping. Demonstrates the phenomenon of culture shock, negative effects of stereotyping, and the development of understanding of reasons behind behaviors.
Synoptics	See Dearth and McKenzie (1975) for complete description	12	40 min play plus 15 min for decision	Deals with role bias and selective perception and the importance of being aware of the perspectives of others. Designed to help health professionals view the delivery of health care from various perspectives. Uses roles of nurse, doctor, and administrator. Observers act as the jury for decisions.
Mental hospital	See Laszlo and McKenzie (1979) for complete description	Varies	Varies	Health personnel participants play the roles of patients in a mental hospital and attempt to earn their discharge and get a job. The goal is to change the attitudes of hospital employees toward increased sensitivity and to increase knowledge about patient rights.
3-North	See Kolb (1983) for complete description	2–4 individuals or teams (max. 10–12 players)	1 to 1½ h	Simulates a general pediatric unit and patient situations. Participants use a problem-solving approach to collect data, identify problems, and plan care related to patients with fluid and electrolyte problems. Patient situation cards, data cards, planning sheets, and score sheets are used. Played in phases reflecting the nursing process.
Into aging	See Farley and Fay (1983) for complete description. Available from Chas. B. Slack, Thorofare, NJ 08086	5–15 players, 1 director, 3 facilitators	Approx. 40 min plus debriefing	Stresses the psychosocial aspects of aging. Allows participants to experience positive and negative events associated with aging. Requires props to simulate various professions as well as conditions of the elderly. 3 levels of elderly living are depicted: independent, semidependent, and dependent.

uations. A sampling of what is available is presented in Table 3-2. A sample of a complete simulation game is given in Appendix 1.

USING SIMULATION FOR INSTRUCTION

A simulation experience includes those elements identified as critical in an actual situation and omits nonessential elements. Presentation and complexity of data can be controlled. Elements of a real situation can be experienced without risk to clients. A consistent experience can be provided for different students. An experience can be repeated as often as desired or can be interrupted for discussion or feedback. Simulations provide the student with direct, active experiences, which decrease the need for clinical facilities at the unskilled practice level and increase the student's readiness for application of knowledge and skills to the actual situation. The quality of learning is improved when the student has had previous experience with a situation before confronting it in the work environment. Furthermore, the use of simulations provides desired experiences to all students without having to depend on their availability in the clinical arena.

Simulations deal with systems and processes and the development of complex skills associated with them. Thus, they prepare individuals to make decisions and to judge decisions made by others. Simulation is particularly useful when the components of a task are complex and difficult to analyze. It provides the essence of those real-life situations about which strategies must be learned. Ideas are developed and tested in a safe environment without fear of doing something wrong or harming a client. Creative behavior and divergent thinking are encouraged rather than having one "right" answer projected. Decisions and their consequences are studied. The intent is to increase the student's awareness of what the real-life situation will be like and increase the chance for successful performance when the student is in the actual situation. In addition, students may increase their personal sense of competence and confidence in dealing with new situations; gain an awareness that there are many ways to deal with a problem; achieve insight into the behaviors of self and others; increase their tolerance for different points of view; and increase their skill for working with others to solve a problem.

Hoban and Casberque (1978, p. 148) identify four properties that simulations should have in order to be of instructional value. They are:

1. The student should respond sensitively to the stimulus in the simulation. . . .

2. The spatial, tactile, chromatic, mobile, auditory, and/or temporal relationships found in the simulation should be analogous to real life. . . .
3. The fidelity of the critical properties and actual sequence of the activities in the simulation should be sufficient enough to assure that the activity being practiced transfers to real situations. . . .
4. Feedback to the students should provide them with information about the consequences of their actions. . . .

Although each of these properties may be variable in different simulations, all should be present to some degree in every simulation activity. The first property requires that students actively participate in the activity. Simulation is an experiential strategy since it involves a high degree of involvement between the participant and elements in the environment. These elements can be other people, computerized or non-computerized mannikins, equipment, models, or a computer program. The participation may be through hands-on involvement (as in the use of models for practice of pelvic or breast examination and colostomy care) or through intellectual involvement (as in the use of written or computerized patient problems to practice decision-making skills). Either way the student is not the passive participant in learning that is often the case with traditional methods.

The second and third properties deal with proximity to reality in relation to physical characteristics, critical elements, and sequence of events. The models used should be as realistic as possible. For example, those models most closely approximating reality, such as computerized robots, provide experiences that give the student a sense of involvement in the actual situation and increase the ability to transfer learning to the real setting. Traditional classroom techniques often deal with what *might* be; on the other hand, simulations deal with what *is* since students are required to respond as if they were in the real situation.

The fourth property deals with feedback to the student about behaviors during the simulation. Primarily, this involves the student becoming aware of the consequences of actions taken. Hoban and Casberque (1978, p. 148) identify three types of feedback: sensory, direct instructional intervention, and critique. With sensory feedback the students use their own senses to determine the appropriateness of their actions. For example, breast examination models simulate various types of nodules. By examining the breasts, the students receive sensory feedback by locating the nodules and differentiating among the types. With direct feedback, students are given information about appropriateness of their actions via a written or mediated instructional package, the instructor, or a person who is playing the role of a patient. For example, the student in a simulated interview situation can receive feedback about verbal or nonverbal behaviors, or the student using a computerized or written patient problem can receive feedback about each action taken. In critique the feedback is given at the end of the simulation. In this way, the student can compare what has been done with what experts in the field or other objective observers would recommend.

The Process of Using Simulation for Instruction

As stated in the definition given previously, an activity is a simulation when it is a realistic representation of an actual situation. It must incorporate the roles, events, and consequences of a real situation or process. It allows a "slice of life" to be discussed, managed, manipulated, and repeated within a condensed time frame for the learning benefit of the participant.

Preliminaries. Simulation activities are best incorporated as one strategy among several as an integral part of an instructional program. Simulation should not be used simply for the sake of using a different approach. As with any other strategy, simulation exercises must be selected and developed because they are expected to provide the most useful mechanism for reaching specific objectives.

Once it is decided that simulation is best to use for certain objectives, the teacher has several tasks to complete. The first, of course, is either to select a simulation activity that is already available or to design one for the purposes desired. A discussion of design is beyond the scope of this chapter; however, other resources are available that provide guidelines. Greenblat and Duke (1981) include seven chapters on the elements of design and construction of gaming-simulation, and Maidment and Bronstein (1973, pp. 29–57) and Stonewater (1978) provide very helpful, brief descriptions of the design process in a single chapter and an article. Recent articles in nursing journals that specifically address the developmental process for simulations or games include Kolb and Shugart (1984), Walljasper (1982), and Wolf and Coggins (1981).

Simulations that are commercially available can be located by referring to guides and catalogs already mentioned (see page 39). Simulations in a variety of subject areas, including health and medicine, are available. Although those specifically designed for nursing are limited, some that are designed for other related areas may be useful for specific objectives that are common to several health care fields.

Any educational tool is only as effective as the teacher who employs it. Since simulation techniques require specialized skills that are not usually included in the graduate preparation of nursing educators, it is necessary to develop them through practice, workshops, reading, and supplementary courses. Bevis (1982, p. 217) provides helpful ideas about how the teacher can prepare for a class using experientially based learning:

1. Formulate the student objectives (desired behavioral outcomes); make explicit the processes and information expected to be learned and the behaviors that will be outcomes.
2. Design (a) the teaching strategies, (b) possible teaching tactics, and (c) the evaluation tool.
3. Make preparatory assignment to students.
4. Require evidence of completion of assignment.
5. Write a description of the learning activity for the class (if problem solving, write the problem situation).
6. Do the activity prior to requiring it of students.
7. Have a list of principles that pertain to the subject and are available for reference to ensure that appropriate content is used in the process as well as provide for comments on student activities.

Before and at the time of the simulation, students need information about what they are expected to accomplish; the constraints, if any, under which they must operate; and what roles and responsibilities they will have to assume. Orientation about learning outcomes directs the student's attention to what is required, thus creating a positive *set,* and motivates the student by making the relationship between the activity and learning needs explicit.

Background knowledge is important to productive involvement in simulation activities and is one factor that differentiates simulations from nonsimulation activities. With simulations, application of previously learned knowledge is required. Assignments are needed that will provide the students with guidance in obtaining necessary knowledge. Resources may include listening to lectures, completing independent learning packages, using audiovisual materials, attending workshops, and so forth. Variety is helpful so that the student can select those resources most conducive to personal learning styles. Guidelines for what information is crucial can also be helpful in focusing the students' attention, thus making preparation more productive.

During the Simulation Activity.   The basic process for use of simulation is that participants are placed in a situation that involves the key variables of real-life roles, conditions, and processes in which the participants must make decisions as if they were in the actual situation. As each decision is made, consequences become known and, thus, must be considered in subsequent decisions.

If the simulation is designed as an independent activity, the teacher participates as an observer to provide feedback about behaviors or as an expert to provide clues about appropriate action. The teacher's involvement may be direct (as with one-to-one observation of a student practicing psychomotor skills), or indirect (as with a videotaped sequence of a student's performance or through the interaction offered via a computer program).

Common group techniques used in simulation activities are role playing and small group discussion. Typically, a case study or problem situation is used for student analysis, consideration of alternatives and consequences, and evaluation of outcomes. The simulation may be introduced by identifying a problem related to a particular topic in order to focus the discussion in the direction desired. Common techniques used to introduce the problem situation include printed situations or videotaped sequences.

Ending the Simulation. One of the critical elements of simulation is that the student gains a sense of closure (i.e., completion of the learning experience). Thiagarajan and Stolovich (1978, pp. 41–42) outline four devices for achieving closure: (1) completion of a time period—establishing a time limit for the activity ahead of time; (2) achievement of a goal—making a decision; (3) completion of a task—development of a teaching plan; and (4) elimination of the competition.

The first three apply to all types of simulations, while the fourth applies to simulation games only since someone is declared a winner according to the rules of play. The authors also state that alternate devices for ending may be used. For example, the simulation can end either when a particular period of time has expired or when a specific goal or task has been accomplished. In situations where students are practicing problem-solving or manipulative skills, it is often helpful to stop the action at different points to discuss key factors, principles, or techniques of problem solving.

Postsimulation Discussion. That part of a simulation activity which helps to surface the learning by discussing what happened during the experience is referred to as *debriefing*. It is recognized as an essential part of simulation activities (Bevis, 1982, p. 218; Bredemeier & Greenblat, 1981, p. 157; Farley & Fay, 1983; Wolf & Coggins, 1981). Central themes in the process include helping students to summarize and reflect on the experience, apply knowledge, and "externalize" the problem-solving methods used throughout the activity. During the summarization of the experience, students need to be given the opportunity to vent and discuss their feelings about the activity before being asked to analyze the experience itself (Joos, 1984). During the analysis of the experience, students must be helped to become consciously aware of any processes and strategies used for problem solving. As a result, the student will be better able to apply what has been learned to varied, future situations.

Although debriefing generally takes place at the end of the simulation, certain aspects can also occur throughout the activity. Action can be stopped for discussion at critical points; questions can be asked; attention can be directed to the objectives; or students can be asked to identify ways that the material can be applied to nursing practice. When used at the end of an activity, the debriefing helps to provide closure and helps students to bring what has been learned to a conscious awareness.

One technique that is recommended for helping students integrate and apply knowledge is asking questions. Questions specific to the objectives of an activity should be planned ahead of time. They can be asked orally during a discussion, in written form for use during a group discussion, or in written form as part of an independent learning package or computer program. The questions used depend, of course, on the situation and the objectives. A few examples that can apply to various situations are given here:

1. What were your feelings at a particular moment?
2. How do values and perceptions affect decisions?
3. How does the experience relate to the objectives?
4. How can the assigned reading, etc. be applied to the experience?
5. How does the experience relate to concepts and skills to be learned?
6. How does the experience apply to other situations you have been involved in or read about?
7. What decisions were made and what were their effects?
8. What influenced the choices made?
9. What was the rationale for decisions made?
10. Did you alter your approach during the activity? If yes, why?
11. To what extent do the results reflect reality?
12. How can what happened be applied to real-life problems?

Finally, an important part of providing closure is a summary of major points and principles. This can be done by the teacher, the group, or individuals. As part of the summary, the student may be offered or asked to think of follow-up activities that will provide a bridge between the experience and future learning. Follow-up activities can include seeing a film, reading an article, attending a group session, interviewing someone, or writing a paper.

Performance in the Actual Setting.   Relevance of the simulation to real-life experiences is important. A simulation that is closely followed by some real-life activity allows for application and validation of what has been learned and an integration of new skills into one's repertoire. The absence of a timely real-life experience in an area closely related to a simulation activity is likely to lessen the learning benefits of the activity.

USING SIMULATION FOR EVALUATION

Any nursing educator will probably admit that evaluation of clinical performance is often a complex and difficult process. The use of simulations for evaluation in nursing education has been discussed by McDowell and associates (1984) and Kolb and Shugart (1984). Simulations for evaluation of clinical decision making are easier to administer than a test experience in the actual clinical setting and help to control extraneous factors that are unrelated to the test situation. Evaluation using simulation is also obviously preferable to standard paper-and-pencil tests when concentrating on psychomotor skills.

Hoban and Casberque (1978, pp. 149–150) discuss four principles that should be applied when using simulation for clinical evaluation. They are:

1. The performance (knowledge, skill, or attitude) that is expected of the student at the end of training should be specified along with the minimal acceptable level of performance the student is required to demonstrate. . . .

2. The simulation should represent reality with enough fidelity to assure face validity of the test of the student's performance. . . .

3. The simulation being used to evaluate student performance should be standardized: the simulation should produce the same kind of responses from a variety of students and provide the same feedback to students when they engage in similar activities. . . .

4. Decisions regarding the purpose of the evaluation should be made before a simulation is used. . . .

Using simulation as a diagnostic tool versus its use as a tool for certification represents the difference between formative and summative evaluation and places teacher and student roles on two entirely different levels. For example, when using simulation as a diagnostic tool, the teacher functions in a supportive role in helping a student identify the direction that future work should take. This function of simulation applies particularly at the skill development stage so that students become aware of performance expectations and ways to achieve the competence needed for practice in the actual setting. On the other hand, when simulation is used for certification, the role of the teacher becomes judgmental in deciding if the student has achieved the desired level of mastery. This function applies to the evaluation/testing of skills performance that is part of a course or certification procedure or to determine the level of performance of students desiring advanced placement in an educational program.

GAMES

Another technique related to simulations and simulation games in purpose and justification, but different in structure and process, is that of games, that is, games that are nonsimulation activities. The term "game" is defined as presented at the beginning of this chapter. Thus, it would involve some type of competition and a "reward" when the goal is reached. The competition may be with one's self, the game, a computer, or other people. It may not, therefore, be competition in the usual sense of the word. Many games also encourage cooperation for the achievement of group goals for a team at the same time that they include the element of competition with others. As with simulation games, nonsimulation games can involve winners and losers, but the game can also be designed so that all participants "win" with the achievement of the stated goal, achievement of new learning, or demonstration of past learning.

Games change the traditional learning situation into one that is active and motivating. By their nature, games actively involve the learner in selecting cards, rolling dice, answering questions, moving game pieces, and so forth. Any involvement in a game precludes passivity. As with any other strategy, they should be selected because it is thought that they are best for reaching course objectives. Games can be used with individuals, pairs, or groups. They often, but not always, require peer interaction and cooperation. They allow learning to take place in a nonthreatening, nonjudgmental atmosphere in which the student maintains more active control (Crancer & Maury-Hess, 1980).

Games can be relatively simple in design, as with many card games, question and answer games, and board games. Others are much more complex, with intricate rules and procedures of play. A key factor in their success in a learning situation is that the rules are understandable and easily communicated to other people. In many instances, however, all rules do not have to be understood before the game begins, since rules and procedures can be clarified during the process of game play.

Purposes of Educational Games

The times when games are appropriate for use in business and industry (Tansey & Unwin, 1969, p. 23) are also applicable to their use in nursing education. Games are appropriate for teaching/learning when the task to be learned is complex, when equipment needed is costly or easily damaged, when the behavior to be learned has a potential for injury or discomfort, or when a real-life situation is unattainable or inconvenient. Further, since games turn learning into a participatory activity, they are also appropriate when active involvement of the learner is desired.

Educational games can be used to introduce a topic or concept, set up group learning situations, provide a higher degree of enjoyment with learning, serve as a medium to demonstrate knowledge and skill, provide relaxation, and serve as an alternative mechanism for evaluation and remedial work. For example, simple games involving matching items, arranging cards, or filling in crossword puzzles can be easily incorporated into an independent study package as part of the learning activity itself, for self-evaluation, or for testing. Such would be particularly appropriate to use with terminology and definitions.

In group situations, games offer an opportunity to demonstrate and surface knowledge and skills. For example, in a team game in which members accrue points by answering specific questions, a student can gain greater self-esteem by knowing the answers and helping the team to win. It is possible, however, that self-esteem could be lowered if the student is unable to answer questions. Other learning gains may still occur, however, as a result of hearing questions and answers that stimulate recall and reinforce learning. There may be a few students who dislike competition and may not enjoy educational games that emphasize the competitive element. If this is the case, other games that focus on cooperation rather than on competition to achieve goals can be used.

Educational Games for Nursing

Nursing literature contains many references to the use of games for specific learning tasks. The tendency by some to use the term *simulation game* even when the activity described is clearly a game with no apparent similarity to true simulation (as defined in this chapter) and to use the term *game* when the activity does, in fact, involve simulation reflects the lack of a clear differentiation between these terms in previous years. Games that are also simulations have been listed earlier in this chapter. In this section, activities that are distinctly games without the use of simulation as a central focus will be included. Examples of games given below are from both educational and practice settings and represent varied content and purposes.

> *Spot On!*, a board game to evaluate knowledge about nursing problems (Pullan & Plant, 1978).
>
> *Disaster Game*, to increase earthquake disaster preparedness of hospital personnel (Haggard, 1984).
>
> *Orientation Game*, to orient to hospital policies and procedures (Heatwole, 1984).
>
> *The Response is Right: A Communication Game Show*, for selecting interpersonal responses sensitive to client's feelings (Eakes & Finnen, 1985).
>
> *What Happened?*, to motivate staff nurses to consistently write nursing care plans (Walljasper, 1982).
>
> *T.E.A.C.H.*, for students learning to assess and teach patients with neurological deficits (Engelke, 1983).
>
> Six games, *It's a G.A.S.* (General Adaptation Syndrome), *The Pluses and Minuses of Life* (Fluid and electrolyte and acid-base balance), *How Sweet it Isn't* (Diabetes mellitus), *Positive Pressure* (Respiratory), *K.I.S.S.* (Cardiovascular problems and blood dyscrasias), and *Vertigo* (Neurological), to teach theoretical content in pathophysiology (Crancer & Maury-Hess, 1980).
>
> *Navigating the Inner Sea*, to teach about renal system pathophysiology (Marcus, 1983).
>
> *Closing*, to help participants identify breaks in operating room sterile technique (McClean, 1983).

Most of these games can serve as examples for those who are interested in developing games for educational purposes. Also, the resources cited previously for design of simulations are equally helpful for the design of games (see page 43).

A complete game is provided as an example in Appendix 2. A more detailed description of several games is presented in Table 3-3. No effort has been made to evaluate quality or appropriateness for purposes stated. There has been an attempt, rather, to include some variety in type and subject. Commercial games can be located by referring to the catalogs and guides cited on page 39.

LIMITATIONS AND CONCERNS

Although simulation and games have many positive features that are thought to facilitate certain types of learning, it must be stressed that they are not a cure for all problems in education. It is, therefore, important to be aware of some of the potential limitations or problems that can be associated with simulation and games. The following points have been synthesized from several resources (Pearson, 1975; Seidl & Dresen, 1978; Thiagarajan & Stolovich, 1978, pp. 59–65; Wolf & Duffy, 1979, pp. 30–31).

1. When too much emphasis is placed on the details of the activity rather than on the process, when too much emphasis is placed on competition, or when students do not associate enjoyable activities with learning, students can be left with a lack of sense of learning.
2. When there is oversimplification of reality, students can be led into improper learning or a mistaken illusion of understanding.
3. When activities are performed exclusively in a group or exclusively alone, the needs of all students will not be met.
4. When there is inadequate debriefing to externalize learning, when there is a lack of follow-up application, or when students are distracted by unrelated events or personal frustrations, learning will be incomplete.
5. When the model for reality is biased, there can be an improper manipulation of attitudes and values.
6. When emotions are involved, some students can become overly intense or anxious.
7. The amount of time and effort required to develop simulations and games reduces their likelihood of cost-effectiveness in comparison with traditional methods.
8. Teachers who are tradition bound may have difficulty in dealing with the loss of control over students, the stringent requirements

Table 3-3

Examples of Nonsimulation Games Suitable for Nursing Education

Title of Game	Availability	Number of Players	Playing Time	Objectives and Description of Process of Game
I.D.-C.C.D.	Sim-Ed College of Education University of Arizona Tucson, AZ 85721	3–5 per group; as many groups as desired	1–2 h	Assists students in identifying five common communicable diseases of childhood in relation to common and medical terminology, incubation periods, communicability periods, symptomatology. Prior preparation is required. Positive and negative reinforcement are used (Sim-Ed, 1978).
Bingo I and Bingo II	John Wiley & Sons 605 Third Avenue New York, NY 10158	3–9	Varies	Competitive games that emphasize rapid thinking and re-call. Focus is on reinforcement and retention of learning. Bingo I requires knowledge of drug classifications. Bingo II requires knowledge of diagnostic tests and respiratory drugs (Wolf & Duffy, 1979).
Nutrition game	Graphics Co. P.O. Box 331 Urbana, IL 61801	2–6	1–2 h	Designed to increase knowledge about nutrients, food costs, and health. Uses cards with common foods as well as penalty cards, bonus cards, and play money.
Social security	Available from the Ungame Co., 1440 So. State College Blvd., Anaheim, CA 92806	3–6	1 h plus 15 min prep.	A noncompetitive board game using cards, a die, and a spinner. Purpose is to facilitate openness and commu-nication and increase insight and understanding among par-ticipants. Intended to improve self-expression of feelings and ideas.
Clot	Ortho Diagnostics, Inc., Raritan, NJ 08869	1–4, or 2–4 teams of up to 4 players each	30 min	Designed to teach and reinforce knowledge of hemostasis and the blood coagulation process. Uses a playing board and tokens. Winning is achieved by reaching a designated point on the playing board (Horn & Cleaves, 1980, p. 413).

of process teaching, the increased level of activity in the classroom, and the use of seemingly "frivolous" methods for serious purposes.

These limitations and problems can be dealt with somewhat by the systematic development of the activity, careful selection and use of simulation and games for specific purposes, thorough preplanning by the teacher, and adequate inservice and teacher training in the use of nontraditional methods.

SUMMARY

This chapter has dealt with the use of simulation and games in nursing. There has been a particular attempt to clarify definitions of terms. Types of simulations, purposes, and procedural elements have been discussed. Many examples of both games and simulations from the nursing literature have been cited. It is clear that there are many educational benefits that can be derived from the use of simulations and games if they are used appropriately. Claims about the potential learning benefits of these strategies have been discussed, and a summary of the available empirical evidence about effectiveness has been included. Although research evidence of effectiveness is somewhat limited and incomplete, various learning theories justify the use of simulations and games along with other strategies. Ongoing research is needed to determine the unique values of these strategies and the circumstances under which they best achieve those values.

APPENDIX 1
SAMPLE SIMULATION GAME: HERE COMES THE JUDGE*

Purpose

To facilitate participation in a group endeavor to solve simulated nursing problems.

*From Bevis, E. O. (1982). *Curriculum building in nursing* (3rd ed.). St. Louis: Mosby, pp. 215–216. Used by permission.

Description

A game called "Here Comes the Judge" employs the team concept and inter-group cooperation to beat the other team. Each group solves a specific given problem about a topic selected by the teacher. The groups go through all phases of the problem-solving process; they carefully document each alternative that might be an acceptable intervention, select an intervention, and justify the intervention selection with sound documentation. One team presents the problem as they solved it going through each stage. The challengers must catch them out—find and prove the flaws. In cases of impasse a group of judges makes decisions about who wins the point.

Points accumulate, and the winning group is rewarded.

Objectives

This game is contrived so that to reach the established goal the participant will:

1. Gather, organize, document, and assimilate information collected by the participants.
2. Critically choose the information and predictive principles appropriate to specific problems.
3. Utilize data in the appropriate facets of problem solving.
4. Participate in a mutually accountable way in a group problem-solving endeavor.
5. Use other members of the group for information, validation, feedback, negotiation, and judgment.
6. Encourage communications, peer support, evaluation, and critiquing of the authoritative resources cited and question validity of resources by citing authoritative opposing views.
7. Utilize the problem-solving strengths of all members of the group by varying player roles and group composition.

Rules

The class is divided into three basic groups:

1. The group presenting (usually 3 to 5 students).
2. The group who have the first right of challenge (usually 3 to 5 students).
3. The group of judges who arbitrate challenges and rebuttals and award the decision to the group who best substantiate their statements. The awards are made in points, and the judges keep score. If the groups wish to award prizes, they may determine what these are to be—losers buy Cokes, and so forth.
4. If the class is larger than 15 to 18 students, the students not immediately involved in one of the three groups have the privilege of challenging any

decision after it has been made and before the next phase of problem solving continues; however, their challenge must be substantiated as above. If in the opinion of the judges this group makes their challenge, they collect the point.

Procedure of Play

The game may be used for the solving of a whole problem or for any selected part of problem solving, that is, problem identification phase, problem data phase, or decision phase. The game can be spread over several class periods or contained in one period. Several class periods permit additional research by enthusiastic players. Books and so forth are permitted in class.

1. Statements on transparencies or on butcher paper may be prepared ahead of time or as part of the class.
2. A member of the presenting group is chosen by that group to act as moderator for the group. However, it is the responsibility of all the presenting members to coach and strengthen the group's presentation, that is, to assume responsibility for making as valid and strong a case as possible for their portion of solving a problem.
3. The presenting group presents the whole problem briefly. This gives the players an overview and prevents challenging material that is covered later. During this overall presentation, challenge groups can take notes on incorrect, omitted, or extraneous material for use during the challenge part of the game.
4. Points are awarded by the judges as follows:
   a. The presenting group gets 1 point for correct and accepted presented material.
   b. The group citing data or material omitted by the presenting group collects 1 point for each concept area accepted by the judges as essential omitted material.
   c. Challenged material is arbitrated by the judges, and the group who are adjudged as correct win 1 point. If the presenting group are deemed correct they are awarded 1 point for being incorrectly challenged; if the challenge group are deemed correct, they are awarded 1 point for being proper in their challenge.
   d. Material that is included by the presenting group that is challenged for being extraneous, inappropriate, tangential, or unnecessary to the solution of the problem can be awarded a point for the winning group in the same way.

APPENDIX 2
SAMPLE NONSIMULATION GAME: CLOTHESPIN GAME TO LEARN ABOUT LEARNING*

Objectives

At the end of this activity you will be able to:

1. State the difference in discovery learning and modeling.
2. Compare the differences in time needed to learn a task among (a) those using exploration and discovery learning techniques, (b) those using modeling techniques, and (c) those who have the benefit of practice.
3. Identify the role of reinforcement in learning and name some of the forms that reinforcement takes.
4. List learning propositions that can be derived from this activity.

Directions

1. Divide into groups of three players.
2. Designate one person as discovery learner, one person as modeling learner, and one person as timer-recorder.
3. Take six wooden pieces and three metal pieces from the clothespin box.
4. Give two wooden pieces and one metal piece to both the discovery learner and the modeling learner.
5. The discovery learner must put the clothespin together without prompting or guidance from the other members of the group.
6. The timer times, in seconds, how long it takes the discovery learner to complete the task.
7. The timer and the modeling learner smile, nod, encourage, clap, cheer, or do anything else they think will encourage and reinforce the discovery learner while he is doing his task as long as they think he is moving in the direction that will lead to success. They may not offer him any advice or directions.
8. The timer marks down the time used by the discovery learner in completing his task.
9. The modeling learner places the clothespin that is now back together in front of him. Using it as a model and having observed the discovery learner complete the task, the modeling learner proceeds to put the second clothespin together.

*From Bevis, E. O. (1982). *Curriculum building in nursing* (3rd ed.). St. Louis: Mosby, pp. 216–217. Used by permission.

10. The timer again times the operation and records the time in seconds. The difference in the two times is calculated.

11. The discovery learner and the timer use the same reinforcing tactics listed in item 7 to encourage and reinforce the modeling learner.

12. The discovery learner takes the remaining two pieces of wood and one wire and puts the clothespin together. He can look at the clothespins that are put together, if he chooses. Reinforcing behaviors are again used by the other group members.

13. The timer again times the discovery learner and records the time as "practice number 2."

14. Someone collects the times, averages them, and puts the findings on the blackboard.

15. Each group uses assigned texts, class notes, any other available resources and experiences, feelings and observations made during the activity to list learning propositions they saw enacted or experienced while participating.

16. The class may or may not wish to award a prize to the group identifying the most nearly complete and accurate list of learning propositions that they saw in actual operation during the activity.

4

Developing
Psychomotor Skills

Astronauts are rocketed into space and sent on journeys around the earth only after they have mastered all the skills essential for successful flight. Many of these skills are complex psychomotor skills that require hours of practice and rehearsal to ensure mastery. Each planned movement is carried out with accuracy and efficiency, because there is no place for human error or hesitancy at the controls of a spacecraft. In other words, only those who have reached complete mastery of the art and science of space flight are sent aloft.

In basic nursing education programs, students are prepared to enter the profession with many beginning skills. The novice is not expected to have mastered all of the skills embodied in practice before embarking into the work setting.

The acquisition of skills has long been the primary desire of nursing students during their educational programs (Paynich, 1971). Recently, strong interest in this area has been displayed by new graduates, nursing service employers, and faculties of nursing schools (Collins & Joel, 1971; Benner & Benner, 1979). Nursing service settings have developed programs that focus on the skill development and practice needs of the beginning nurse (Atwood, 1979).

This chapter was written by Sharon Eaton, R.N., Ed. D., Assistant Professor of Nursing, California State University, San Francisco and Grace Davis, R.N., M.A., Director, Department of Educational Services, Children's Hospital, San Francisco, California.

LEVELS OF PERFORMANCE

Psychomotor skills are often a major component of procedure or skill lists used to determine levels of performance of the recent graduate. Skills lists are commonly used as guides for planning experiences that offer practice in those nursing procedures essential to patient care. The level of competence of students or novice nurses is often judged by the degree to which they can smoothly and efficiently perform nursing procedures. Teachers of nurses play a vital role in helping learners acquire the skills needed for practice. This chapter discusses the area of psychomotor skill learning, its importance in the practice of nursing, and implications for teachers.

Psychomotor skills are described by Richardson (1969) as manipulative skills that require the learner to perceive and coordinate sensory stimuli to complete purposeful movements. Children learn many psychomotor skills essential to the development of independence and survival in the world around them. Adults continue to learn and develop psychomotor skills to help them adapt to the demands of the reality-based work world.

Nursing schools graduate students who are beginning practitioners. Practice and experience are required before the beginner can be expected to reach a high level of competence in the art and science of nursing. According to Benner (1984), nurses graduate from educational programs at the level of an advanced beginner or what she terms a competent level of performance. Advancing levels of expertise are developed as clinical experience enables nurses to incorporate their background of understanding into their performance. The nursing literature (Lewis, 1971; Gudmundsen, 1975) is filled with pleas for a return of the "art" to nursing. One component of this art is the smooth performance of procedures and the dexterous handling of equipment.

COMPONENTS OF PSYCHOMOTOR LEARNING

To understand the nature of psychomotor learning, a brief review of the theories that guide this area of learning is in order.

Bloom (1956) described the importance of the psychomotor area of learning as one of the three learning domains—cognitive, affective, and psychomotor. He stated that teachers had responsibilities for writing objectives and planning learning activities to meet the objectives of each of the three domains. Nursing school curricula reflect the attention given to each of these domains as teachers plan learning goals for their students.

Because psychomotor performance involves observable behavior, it has been especially appealing to behaviorists. Robert Gagné focused on the stimulus-response (S-R) theory to outline the conditions for chaining that occurred in the carrying out of a skill. The six conditions he (Gagné, 1965; Gagné & Briggs, 1974) identified are:

1. Each S-R connection must have been previously learned (e.g., to open a locked door a person must be able to identify the upright position of the key, insert it in the lock, turn it, and push the door open).
2. The steps, or links, in the chain must be performed in the proper order. This could be taught either by demonstrating the proper sequence and then inviting the learner to perform, or by using verbal instructions as prompts (e.g., "All right, now that you have the key in the lock, turn it, and then push the door open").
3. The individual steps must be performed in close succession to establish the chain.
4. Repetition is usually necessary if the act is to be performed easily and efficiently, since it often takes several tries to smooth out clumsy and superfluous movements.
5. The terminal step, or link, must result in success, which provides reinforcement (e.g., the door must open).
6. Once a motor skill has been learned, it can be generalized (e.g., the technique for opening one lock can be applied to opening a slightly different one). However, it may be necessary to teach the student to discriminate if there is a significant difference in the second act (e.g., opening a lock by turning the key counterclockwise).

To develop teaching methods for learning complex psychomotor skills, the teacher analyzes the skill and divides it into its parts or subskills. The subskills are placed in logical order. The learner sees the total psychomotor skill demonstrated, then each subskill is identified and demonstrated in sequence.

Supervised practice periods are provided immediately following the demonstration. As learners practice, the teacher provides verbal guidance and reinforcement. Learners carry out the complete skill unassisted. The teacher might identify similarities between skills that learners had previously mastered and new psychomotor skills. The teacher needs to be alert for any conditions within the practice setting that might interfere with learning (fatigue of learner, noisy environment, etc.).

Skinner (1968) used the phrase "movement duplication" to describe learning motor skills. He said that modeling was the first and vital step in the learning of a motor skill. The aim of modeling was to make the behaviors conspicuous to the learner. Later, the learner might practice in front of a mirror or be recorded on videotape to become his own model. Practice was a necessary component of duplication as Skinner described it.

Simpson (1966) described another dimension in the acquisition of a psychomotor skill. She described the following mental aspects of skill acquisition:

> *Perception* is a crucial beginning step in performing a motor act. It is the process of sensory input, cue selection, and translation. The learner places, in priority order, sensory stimulation and environmental cues and relates these to the action in performing a motor act. For example, when a nurse changes a child's bottle of intravenous solution, the process of perception occurs. The nurse observes and handles the bottle and tubing, is sensitive to the child's needs for reassurance and the parents' needs for information, and recalls the principles of aseptic technique learned in the past.
>
> *Readiness,* or *set,* occurs when the learner has developed mental, physical, and emotional readiness to perform the actions. In other words, learners are able to call upon mental pictures of themselves beginning the action, having the physical and physiological capabilities to complete the action, and are psychologically ready to try. Simpson's taxonomy (1966) continues with descriptions of performance responses.
>
> *Guided response* is discussed as an early step in skill development. During this phase, learners imitate actions they have seen demonstrated. With the cueing of the teacher and by trial and error, learners achieve appropriate responses.
>
> *Mechanism* includes learned responses that become habitual. Learners now have confidence and some skill in performing procedures.
>
> *Complex overt response* is described as the final level in psychomotor skill acquisition. Uncertainty has been resolved; performance is smooth, precise, free from hesitancy, and has become automatic.

The Dreyfus (1981) model of skill acquisition has been used by Benner (1984) to describe the process of competency development in nurses. First-year nursing students are described as being in the novice stage of skill development. They follow procedural steps and rules rigidly. At graduation nurses are viewed as being in the advanced beginner stage. They demonstrate acceptable performance and recognize aspects of situations that need consideration in practice. Practicing nurses who have incorporated experiences and mastered skills are seen as experts. They are able to attend to unusual patient problems and make provisions for the unusual. The expert's performance is fluid, flexible, and highly proficient.

In addition to the process of teaching psychomotor skills as described by these theorists, attention needs to be focused on other aspects of the teaching-learning process. Richardson (1969) has described in detail the use of visualization as an important factor in improving skills performance. He described how learners were able to improve their skills in dart throwing, high jumping, and hooping baskets by simply carrying out those motions in their mind's eye. Students simply sat in the classroom, closed their eyes, and "saw" themselves performing these acts successfully. Athletic coaches emphasize and assist their students in developing skills of visualization to improve skill performance and develop internal readiness.

Kieffer (1984) reported that the administration of injections is one of the most important skills that nursing programs should teach for competency. Eaton (1984) incorporated visualization experiences while teaching nursing students to prepare and give injections, in addition to the traditional practice. Although she found no significant differences in performance of the students who were exposed to visualization experiences, the students reported that they felt more confident.

TEACHING PSYCHOMOTOR SKILLS

To apply the above theories to nursing education, the teacher starts by describing why and how each specific psychomotor skill fits into the total practice of art of nursing. The needs for safety of practice and assurance of quality care for people are among the most important reasons. This explanation forms the basis on which the teacher then plans experiences for the learner.

The *demonstration phase* of teaching deserves careful attention. The initial demonstration should be smooth, skilled, and successful. All learners should be able to see and hear clearly. In a large group when intricate hand movements are being demonstrated, a video camera might be focused on the demonstration with monitors placed throughout the room so that learners are able to watch movements on a television screen.

It is during the step-by-step demonstration that Skinner's (1968) suggestions of exaggerating movement and slowing down action are helpful. To illustrate this process, a skill foreign to many but an enjoyable one—that of a basic tap dance step—could be chosen. The dance step is demonstrated on a tabletop where all learners can hear the count and see the foot tapping out each of the five components of the step. The demonstration is repeated several times, starting with one foot and then the other foot, until all the learners in the room are tapping in time. At the end of 5 minutes, all learners are able to imitate the five components of the step. Smooth, skilled imitation or mastery is not the aim of this exercise, but some learners with prior dance experience may be able to perform skillfully. This exercise combines the phases of demonstration and guided practice. Learners receive positive verbal reinforcement as they imitate each component of the exercise. As is often the case, those who learn quickly help others until the whole group learns the tap step.

The same principles are applied in teaching the skill of preparing and giving a medication by injection. The skill is performed in its entirety by a skilled practitioner in order that students view a smooth and proficient demonstration. This skill is then divided into short progressive steps with each step shown separately. The parts of the equipment are identified by name and function. Students practice each step independently until the entire performance is complete and the skill can be demonstrated at the level of expected competence.

The expert practitioner is not always the best person to demonstrate complex psychomotor skills. Learners may feel overwhelmed, put down, and hestiant to try a new procedure if teachers are tempted to "show off" expert skills in the demonstration phase. Another cautionary note about the use of experts to demonstrate skills is offered by Dreyfus and Dreyfus (1981). They describe "experts" as those who have incorporated each of the factors (steps) of the skill into their performance to the extent that they can no longer identify the factors or steps. In the demonstration phase, it is important that the steps be identified clearly for the learner.

The next phase in learning psychomotor skills is *guided practice*. Some helpful hints for teachers to consider during this phase are:

1. Learners need to explore and manipulate equipment as soon as possible after the demonstration. They need the tactile experience in order to diffuse anxiety that might be generated about handling equipment. Learners are encouraged to explore materials using

all their senses and to handle equipment with their eyes shut so that kinesthetic feelings are aroused. Many adult learners are self-conscious about trying new psychomotor skills. They worry about looking foolish and making errors. It is crucial that the learning environment be made warm and accepting, inviting the learners to try things, take risks, and experiment.

2. Individual differences are important variables in learning psychomotor skills. Some of the differences might be related to manual dexterity, attitude, motivation, confidence, kinesthetic awareness, intelligence, or age of the learners. In planning learning experiences, these factors must be considered.

3. Practice periods vary for individual learners and take a variety of forms. Complexity of the psychomotor skill determines the amount and type of practice required to learn the skill. Such activities as knitting or needlework have been used to develop fine motor movements and finger flexibility.

4. Feedback on performance during the practice phase is vital to reinforce correct behaviors and eliminate errors. Peer groups are useful for analyzing performance and providing immediate feedback. Videotaping can be used effectively by learners to critique their own performance during this stage.

5. When a learner is stuck at one step of the performance and consistently errs, it may be helpful to have the learner repeat the error over and over to make it very visual and bring awareness of the error to a conscious level. The teacher may, if done with good humor, demonstrate and exaggerate the error so that the learner sees and acknowledges it. It is wise to remember that an adult learner is fragile when frustrated. In this self-centered state, the learner may overreact to less-then-tender methods of correction.

6. Teachers should be aware of left-handed learners and make provisions for them. These learners may find it helpful to face the teacher and mirror the movements. Right handed learners may prefer to imitate the teacher's movements by standing beside the teacher and facing in the same direction.

7. Teachers should remain silent except to offer positive cues and give encouragement to learners as they perform each step. Beginners who have no basis on which to evaluate their own performance need feedback when they complete each step. Teachers must avoid the temptation to take the learners' hands and guide the performance, because learners need to perform movements independently. If teachers point out similarities between new and

previously learned skills, it helps learners transfer information to new situations. For example, there are similarities between handling a bulb syringe to perform an irrigation and the manipulation of a disposable syringe to administer a medication.

8. It may be helpful if teachers share personal examples of their own ineptitude as they initially learned skills. It may comfort struggling learners to know that others had problems in the beginning. However, learners tend to be self-centered in skill acquisition, so references to the experiences of others should be limited.

Simulation experiences are frequently used during the guided practice phase. Pilots who are learning to fly an airplane are taught in a simulated environment. They learn flight maneuvers in a model long before they enter the cockpit of the actual aircraft. Similarly, nursing programs have simulated environments in which learners can manipulate models and equipment free from the pressures of the actual situation (Infante, 1981).

Some educators question the value of simulated experiences. Thorndike warned in the 1930s (Bugelski, 1971) that there might not be such a thing as transfer learning. Skills are learned strictly in the situational context presented and need to be relearned in any other context. Montag (1951) also questioned the transfer value of simulated experiences and placed nursing students directly in the clinical area to learn basic skills. Whether or not simulated experiences accelerate skill acquisition may be still in question, but learners report feeling more adept when they practice in a skills laboratory. If they perceive themselves to be more skilled, perhaps this perception enables them to perform with more confidence, less hesitancy, and increased skill.

The final stage in the development of a psychomotor skill is *mastery*. Mastery performance is skilled, smooth, dexterous, efficient, and is adapted to incorporate cues from the current situation. Mastery is rarely accomplished in the student phase of learning and is the accomplishment of very few. Acceptable levels of performance of psychomotor skills are most often not at a mastery level.

Once attained, the maintenance of mastery level of achievement requires continued practice. One component of practice at this level is mental rehearsal. For example, musicians, golfers, athletes, and others prepare themselves for performances by first visualizing themselves in action and performing at peak level. To use a nursing example, nurses who have mastered the dialysis procedure report the value of time spent rehearsing the procedure verbally and visually before they begin the procedure with a patient.

SUMMARY

Improving the performance of psychomotor skills is one of the solutions to returning the "art" to nursing. The development of psychomotor skills is complex, and examples from the fields of art, aviation, athletics, and nursing can illustrate the process of skill acquisition. Consideration of the developmental process should be a guide for those involved in teaching skills and evaluating performance.

Teaching methods, such as visualization, cueing, and other techniques, facilitate skill acquisition.

5

Asking Questions

Teachers ask students questions for a variety of reasons. They may wish to find out what a student already knows about a given subject or situation, or they may wish to stimulate interest in a new topic. Teachers may use questions as a stimulus variation from lecturing. Or, teachers may utilize questions as feedback to determine if students have already grasped the major points under consideration. Questions, when skillfully asked, help students to see relationships and link the unknown to the known. In addition, questioning permits student and teacher to explore ideas together. The art of questioning, more than any other single teaching skill, can assist teachers in conveying their interest, enthusiasm, and continued pursuit of learning.

What teachers need to give and what they need to ask form an important facet of teaching strategies. If the development of students' autonomy in thinking is an important objective, the "seeking" functions of teaching assume greater importance than those of "giving." In order for students to develop concepts by their own efforts, teachers must become guiders of the questioning process.

Basically, there are three kinds of questions—factual or descriptive, clarifying, and higher order.

FACTUAL OR DESCRIPTIVE QUESTIONS

Factual questions include those that can be answered from either memory or by description. Factual questions are elicited by such words as:

who, what, when, or *where.* For a factual question, the student is asked to recall information previously acquired. Many facts are important because they provide the building blocks for concepts and generalizations. The following are examples of factual questions:

1. "What is the normal white blood cell count?"
2. "What is the normal range of blood pressure?"
3. "Who is eligible for welfare in our country?"

Descriptive questions, although more complicated than factual questions, require that students respond from either memory or simple descriptive statements. They, too, deal mostly with facts. Descriptive questions differ from factual questions in that the student is required to organize thoughts in a logical relationship and to respond with a longer answer than the straight-forward response of the factual question. Examples of descriptive questions are:

1. "What are differences in the symptoms of a patient in diabetic coma and in insulin shock?"
2. "Who is eligible for medicare and medicaid?"
3. "What does Satir mean when she calls one member of the family the 'identified patient'?"

CLARIFYING QUESTIONS

The second type of question is the clarifying question. Clarifying requires that teachers ask questions that help students to go beyond a superficial response. This can be done in five ways (Far Western Laboratory for Educational Research and Development, 1969):

1. *Asking questions for more information and/or more meaning*
   The teacher seeks additional clarification from the student. Examples of questions that might be asked are:
   A. "I don't quite understand what you mean."
   B. "Tell us more about the point you just made."
   C. "What do you mean by the term _____?"
2. *Requiring student to justify response*
   Here the teacher wants to be certain the student really understands the point just made in order to increase the student's critical awareness. Such questions designed to assist the student are:

A. "What are the assumptions you are making?"

B. "What are your reasons for thinking this is so?"

C. "Suppose you were debating your point of view with an opponent. What points might your opponent bring out?"

3. *Refocusing the student's attention on a related issue*

The teacher may wish to assist students to clarify a different, but related, issue in order to foster transfer. Examples of refocusing questions include:

A. "What are the implications of this discussion for patients who are not hospitalized?"

B. "How does this relate to . . . ?"

C. "How does John's response relate to Joan's?"

4. *Prompting the student*

If the students are unable to determine relationships for themselves, a hint from the teacher may assist them. Examples of prompting questions include:

TEACHER: "Mary, you have stated that your nursing care plan for Mrs. Smith included special skin care. What is the reason?"

MARY: "Her skin is edematous. This requires special care."

TEACHER: "That's very true. What are some of the complications that can occur when excess fluid is retained in the tissue?"

MARY: "Edema predisposes to infection."

TEACHER: "Right! Any special reason why this happens?"

MARY: "Well, I don't know."

TEACHER: "What might there be about edema that predisposes to infection?"

MARY: "Oh, I see. It probably is a good culture media for infection."

TEACHER: "And what might some other complications be?"

5. *Redirecting the question*

This is a technique designed to broaden the participation of other students in a clarifying session by changing the interaction from the teacher and one student to the teacher and other students. An example of redirecting is:

TEACHER: "Mary, you have stated that Mrs. Smith complained of thirst following her surgery. What might be the reason for this symptom?"

MARY: "She was given preoperative medications that decreased her fluid production."

TEACHER: "That's one possible reason. Paul, what might be other plausible reasons?"

Other techniques could include asking other students why they agreed or disagreed with a student's response.

HIGHER-ORDER QUESTIONS

The third type of question is called higher-order questions. These include those questions that cannot be answered simply from memory or perception. Higher-order questions prod students to think beyond the facts, sequences, descriptions, or set of circumstances. They help students to establish relationships, compare and contrast concepts and principles, make inferences, see causes and effects, and find rules and principles rather than merely define them. Furthermore, they help students to use ideas freely and critically.

The word "why" is frequently used in higher-order questions. "Why" questions frequently require the student to go beyond the factual or descriptive answer by generalizing, inferring, classifying, or concluding. However, the mere use of the word "why" in a question does not necessarily guarantee that such a question is a higher-order question. For example, asking a student "Why does blood pressure elevate when blood vessels are constricted?" is a straightforward factual question if the student need only repeat what has been read in a textbook or previously learned. Were the student required to figure out the answer, it would be a higher-order question. Depending on the student's previous experiences, what may be a factual question for one student may be a higher-order question for the other.

Higher-order questions perform three specific functions:

1. *Seeking evaluation*
   Evaluative questions have no "right" answer but deal with matters of judgment, value, and choice. In order to arrive at an answer, students must set up standards and measure the idea at hand against such a standard. An example of such a question would be: "Should every family have a guaranteed minimum income?"

2. *Seeking inferences*
   An inference is an idea or conclusion following from a set of facts or a premise. These questions may be used when the teacher wishes students to relate something newly learned to something previously learned. They may be used to derive a reason or motive

from a set of circumstances. An example of a question designed to foster inference is:

"Why must a surgery consent form be signed before the patient has preoperative medications?"

Inferences involve either deduction or induction. Deduction occurs when students reason from a generalization or principle to the specific situation. An example of a deductive question is:

"Individuals react differently to painful stimuli. What are some of the ways that your patients have exhibited they were in pain?"

Induction, on the other hand, requires that the student extract the generalization from a collection of examples or specifics. Nursing instructors would be utilizing an inductive strategy were they to assign a group of students to patients with a specific nursing problem—for example, immobility. By assigning students to hospitalized patients who are immobilized for a variety of conditions (patient in a cast, patient on complete bedrest, depressed patient, etc.), the teacher would be helping students to identify the patients' nursing needs. The inductive type of question to assist students in forming generalizations would be:

"What can you generalize about the nursing needs of all of these patients?"

3. *Seeking comparisons*

Comparison questions help students to establish whether ideas are contradictory to one another, similar or dissimilar, and related or unrelated. The key words for these questions are *compare* and/or *contrast*. Examples of this type of question are:

A. "Compare the symptoms of drunkenness and diabetes."
B. "Is there a connection between stress and grand mal seizures?"
C. "What is the relationship between poverty and illness?"

CONVERGENT AND DIVERGENT QUESTIONS

In an environment arranged to encourage student participation, the instructor can encourage either "intellectually divergent" or "intellectually convergent" participation. In a convergent climate, students ask questions closely related to the immediate situation, such as lecture presentation, laboratory experiences, demonstration, and so forth. A convergent climate for interaction aids the students' comprehension of whatever tasks or knowledge is germane to the immediate learning environment.

In the intellectually divergent climate, the student is reinforced for stating ideas and making intellectual discoveries. The instructor implementing this climate is not threatened by questions to which there are no ready answers and which may be only tangentially related to the planned sequence for the class period. This kind of climate rewards such student behaviors as application, synthesis, perception of relationships, and creative problem solving.

RESEARCH ON TEACHERS' USE OF HIGHER-ORDER QUESTIONS

Higher-order questions have no right or wrong answers but are designed to help students to problem solve and think abstractly. Included in higher-order questions are the questions designed to foster divergent thinking. They are questions that generally have no known answer, as they are predictive and reach to the unknown. Some examples of divergent questions are:

1. What would happen if all health professionals who had received federal support during their training were to be required to practice in an underserved area?
2. What would the effect be on the public, the employer, and the individual nurse if a national credentialing center for nursing were to be developed?
3. What are the consequences for the public and the nursing profession of implementing two levels for nursing practice: professional and associate?

In an attempt to determine the types of questions most frequently initiated, Scholdra and Quiring (1973) analyzed the level of questions asked by faculty in a baccalaureate school of nursing. They were interested in finding out if the questions posed by instructors were consistent with the higher-level objectives from Bloom's *Taxonomy of Educational Objectives* (1956) involving analysis, synthesis, and evaluation. They analyzed the kinds of questions asked by nursing instructors and students in the clinical conferences and related the questions to the terminal objectives for the respective clinical courses. Out of a total of 617 questions asked by 16 instructors during 22 conferences, only six higher-level questions were asked, even though the stated objectives in three of the six clinical areas surveyed specified that higher cognitive level thinking was the desired learning outcome. Lower-level questions comprised 98.9 percent of the total number of questions asked by the teachers and students during these conferences. Based on their findings, these investigators pose an important question to all nursing faculty: are nursing instructors who ask low level questions justified in expecting their students to develop high level skills, such as those involved in the processes of analyzing, synthesizing, or evaluating?

In another study, Craig and Page (1981) were interested in finding out if the level of questions asked by nursing instructors could be improved by the use of a teaching module specifically developed to provide the information and practice necessary to classify, generate, and evaluate questions in terms of Bloom's (1956) work. Learning activities designed to meet these higher objectives included the classification, generation, and analysis of questions asked during an instructor's recorded postclinical conference with students. Using a pretest-posttest control group design, these investigators found that the experimental group exposed to the self-instructional module asked a greater percentage of higher-level questions than did the control group. These investigators believe that their study supports the conclusion that nursing faculty can increase the percentage of higher-level questions asked when they have inservice education in the instructional skills needed to conduct postclinical conferences. They also concluded from their study that whereas the nursing knowledge and expertise of the instructors were evident, many conferences consisted of a student recital of the tasks performed during the clinical experiences as well as a description of a patient's diagnosis, medications, and treatment. They point out that such enumeration of data really does little to foster the cognitive processes required for effective problem solving needed for the practice of nursing.

Gall (1970) raises some important questions about teacher behaviors in regard to questioning strategies. Essentially, he points out that given the importance of questions in teaching, researchers still do not know much about them. He asks two exceedingly important questions: (1) What educational objectives can questions help students to achieve? and (2) What are the criteria of an effective question and how can effective questions be identified? He also cautions that questions asked by an instructor should not be viewed as an end in themselves, but rather as a means to an end—producing desired changes in student behavior.

In his discussion about questioning behaviors, Gall (1970) raises another issue of great importance to nursing instructors. He states that the types of questions that students ask should be of great interest to instructors. For example, in introducing a new topic, students should be asked what they believe they need to know. This is of utmost importance for nursing students as they prepare for clinical experiences. The instructor who desires to develop inquiry attitudes in students will foster question-asking skills in students and then will provide reinforcement for such behaviors.

The educational use of questioning was viewed critically by Wenk and Menges (1985). They draw reference to a large, cross-institutional post-secondary study (Barnes, 1983) that revealed that only a small portion of class time was spent in teacher's questioning of students or in students asking questions. It was pointed out that about one-third of all questioning did not elicit a response from the students. Other studies led these investigators to the conclusion that the portion of class time spent in questioning is low, that questions are predominantly in the area of stabilized knowledge requiring memory skills, and that the research on questioning has not demonstrated significant relationships between questioning behaviors and student outcomes. However, the studies are few in number and tend not to be focused on higher-order questioning.

Higher-order questions are difficult for the teacher as well as for the student. They require an excellent grasp of the objectives to be achieved and knowledge beyond the given facts for both teacher and student. However, the positive reinforcement from students who are stimulated beyond the usual responses should help the teacher to become motivated to practice this technique.

SEQUENCING QUESTIONS

The sequencing of questions is of specific importance in planning a questioning strategy. If higher-order questions are asked before students have the specific information or recall required to respond to the questions, they, or the teacher, may become frustrated and discouraged. The following represents a specific questioning strategy utilizing all types of questions previously discussed:

1. *Eliciting facts or conditions*
   "What is happening?"
   "How does it happen?"
   "When does it happen?"
   "Where does it happen?"

2. *Eliciting explanations or comparisons*
   "Why does this happen?"

"What are the variations? Why?"
"Why do you find it so?"

3. *Clarifying for generalizations and consequences*
"What does this mean?"
"What does it accomplish?"
"How do you explain it?"
"In what other situations would it apply?"

It is not necessary to follow the above sequence in order. Teachers may begin asking questions at the second, or even the third, level. Should students not be able to respond to a higher-level question, the teacher may find it desirable to ask questions to elicit lower-level response and then ask the higher-level type of questions.

Prior to a questioning strategy, it is necessary that the teacher *set the focus*. This establishes both the topic to be discussed and the particular cognitive operation to be performed. If this is not clearly done, the students will tend to indulge in associative thinking and branch off to some word or phrase and elaborate tangentially, which can lead to topics not relevant to the discussion. Focused questions can be open-ended, permitting alternative answers, or closed, limiting responses to one "right" answer. Asking, for example, what is the daily requirement of calcium leads to one right answer. However, if the teacher asks for the reasons some persons have a calcium deficiency, this will lead to a variety of speculations and additional use of knowledge.

Questions such as "What constitutes good care of a patient in traction?" will foster training in the arbitrary evaluation of information and may develop unproductive modes of thinking in students. Such a question assumes that one can judge without a criterion. Students have two alternatives. They can guess what the teacher wants or they can try to remember what the book says. A focused question would include the criteria. For example: "How would you provide countertraction for a patient in Buck's traction?"

The impact of questioning lies not in its single acts, but in the manner in which the skilled teacher is able to combine the types of questions into a pattern. These include the particular combination of focusing, extending, and lifting from one level to another; the length of time spent on a particular operation; how the functions of giving and seeking are distributed; and the way in which the intake of information is alternated with the processing, transforming, and synthesizing of information.

One final word about questioning. Note how attorneys phrase questions. They ask one question at a time. Saying to a student in the clinical area, "What medication are you giving; what is its dose; for what is it given; and what are the side effects?" is an overloaded question, to put it mildly. It is difficult to think and listen at the same time. Therefore, by asking one part of a question at one time, it helps the student to sort out parts of a question.

SUMMARY

Questioning techniques are used for a variety of reasons. These include finding out what a student already knows about a subject or situation, as a feedback mechanism, or to develop autonomy in thinking. Questioning permits students and teachers to explore ideas together.

6

Creating Set

The term *set* refers to the response system that predisposes an individual to view and approach a problem in a predetermined manner. Hyman (1964) defines set as an attitude of mind and an organizer of information. Those actions leading to the stimulation or evoking of a set in a learner are referred to as *set induction* in learning psychology. The concept of preinstructional procedures, or set induction, comes from the research on learning indicating that activities preceding a learning task will influence the outcome of that task. Some instructional sets promote learning superior to others for certain specified learning goals.

Set induction provides a motivational aspect to learning. De Cecco and Crawford (1974) have identified three concepts—arousal, expectancy, and incentives—as major factors that account for motivation. These three concepts also point the way toward helping the instructor develop techniques to guide the student toward being motivated to learn.

AROUSAL

The arousal function is the instructor's effort toward maintaining the student's interest in learning. It involves the continuing responsibility to guard against boredom during learning. It involves actively involving the student in the learning process. By providing a certain measure of freedom to wander from one aspect to another in order to allow students to discover relationships and meanings, the instructor creates an environment that fosters excitement. In such an environment, curiosity, exploration, and discovery will prevail. This is the environment in which the students find it fun and invigorating to learn and safe to make mistakes.

Capturing an audience's attention is the first thing required of any performer. This category includes school of nursing teachers. Most students will pay attention to the instructor, at least for a few minutes, but they will not continue to listen actively to a mediocre lecturer or discussion leader. Lowman (1984) makes the point that college teachers need to stimulate emotion, but their reason for doing so differs from entertainers. The entertainer's goal is to stimulate emotion for its own sake, while the classroom instructor uses emotion to engage students' attention fully on the content selected for presentation and to transfer to them his or her own passionate interest in the subject.

In addition to positive emotions, skilled instructors avoid stimulating negative emotions, such as anger, anxiety, or boredom. The best way to keep students from being bored by a subject is to show them that *you* are not bored by it. Students respect and respond to genuine enthusiasm that a teacher has for a subject. However, it must be cautioned that students are able to spot the shallow or even fraudulent instructor who relies on emotional appeals to gloss over a superficial understanding of the content or to present material in a slipshod manner, no matter how enthusiastically.

EXPECTANCY

The expectancy function of the teacher requires that learning objectives be described specifically for the student in terms of what the student will be able to do and know when a particular class, unit, project, or experience has been completed. Statements of instructional objectives should be concrete enough for the student to know the outcome that the teacher expects. A specific objective focuses the learner and gives promise that something new will be achieved. Unfortunately, students become accustomed to abstract statements of instructional goals and have learned from past experiences that they can ignore them without harmful consequences. An example of a concrete statement to guide the learner is, "At the completion of today's class on the concept of *anxiety* you will be able to identify several differing behaviors of clients who exhibit anxiety." The instructor should continue by giving several contrasting examples of behaviors, such as the client who talks incessantly and asks for the nurse constantly and the client who is withdrawn and emotionally immobilized. By asking the students which example illustrates the concept *anxiety* more fully, the students can grasp the full range of the behaviors that illustrate the concept, and they are also set toward the learning goal.

INCENTIVE

The incentive factor closely relates to positive reinforcement as discussed in Chapter 1. Promising to provide feedback to students and developing checkpoints and standards for assessing their own achievement, and a positive approach toward the learning process all provide reassurance to students.

Set induction also helps students to build a cognitive bridge from what preceded to what will follow in the instructional sequence. The creative use of set induction provides the teacher with tools to help students to see the relevance of the learning experience. The activities for which set induction is particularly appropriate are:

1. *At the beginning of a course*
   The first introduction can help students to become excited about the learning experience to follow, interact readily and enthusiastically with the teacher, and explore the literature and other resources with meaningful purpose.

2. *Before classroom discussion*
   Precueing students about the expectations of the discussion will frequently prevent the wasting of time caused when students do not really understand the purpose of the discussion.

3. *Preceding a new clinical experience*
   Here the relieving of the anxiety of the unknown, the reassurance that the experience to follow is one for which the student has been prepared, and the linking of this experience with previous experiences are essential.

4. *Making an assignment*
   A set designed to increase attention to the task tends to increase the desire of the student to complete the assignment for intrinsic motivation and curiosity rather than completion merely to meet requirements to achieve a grade.

INFLUENCE OF SET

Every person has experienced set. If we are told that a given speaker is an expert, we tend to regard what the speaker says with more credibility. If we are led to believe that a given task is difficult, then we will find it so. If we are helped to see the relevance of a task, we will find the learning more meaningful and will be motivated to learn.

Set, then, predisposes us to view and approach a situation in a given way. An example of the influence of set in solving problems was experimentally illustrated by Luchins (1942). He gave his subjects, who ranged from elementary school pupils to graduate students, jars of differing sizes and instructed them to obtain a specified amount of water by using only the measures of the jars available. He substituted both different jars and amounts of water to be obtained for a series of problems. For the first problem he asked the subjects to obtain 20 quarts of water by using a 29-quart jar and a 3-quart jar. He showed the subjects how this could be accomplished by filling the 29-quart jar and then filling the 3-quart jar three times. Similarly, in order to get 100 quarts from a 127-quart jar, a 21-quart jar and a 3-quart jar, the subjects would need to fill the 127-quart jar, pour off 21 quarts, leaving 106 quarts and then pour off 3 quarts two times to achieve 100 quarts. After several such examples involving three different sizes of jars, Luchins asked his subjects to obtain 20 quarts from a 23-quart jar, a 49-quart jar and a 3-quart jar. A significant number of his subjects continued to utilize the three jar technique, even when the simple solution involved merely pouring off three quarts into the 3-quart jar from the 23-quart jar. Thus, Luchins concluded that the subjects were under the influence of a predisposing way of solving the problem.

Another simple example of how set influences us is to ask persons to draw four lines connecting all of the nine dots below without tracing back or lifting the pencil from the paper.

•   •   •

•   •   •

•   •   •

It is interesting to note that most individuals attempt to solve the problem by drawing lines *within* the confines of the nine dots. The solution lies in going beyond the dots, as below:

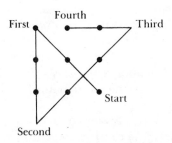

Predisposition tends to tell us to confine our solutions to previously learned tasks rather than find new or creative solutions. Both of the examples just discussed demonstrate what is referred to as "functional fixedness." The problem solver has been using information from one situation to the next when it will not operate successfully for the new situation. One simple example of "functional fixedness" is using an item for a single purpose when it may have several. A rubber ball is something to be thrown, and it also may provide excellent squeezing exercise for the hand.

The principles of the two examples just discussed are well illustrated in a study by Tuckman, Henkelman, O'Shaughnessy, and Cole (1967). They wanted to find out the effects of appropriate and inappropriate practice experiences on students' approaches to arithmetic problems.

Three short experiments were undertaken, each with from 30 to 50 college students as subjects. Each involved a sequence of three practice problems without feedback followed by a criterion problem. The problems involved a matrix of numbers to be added. The investigators found that when the practice problems and the criterion problems were structurally similar, those subjects who had had problem-solving experience tended to find shortcuts that helped them find a solution more often than did those subjects not having had problem-solving experience. However, when the practice problems and criterion problems differed considerably, those subjects having had experience tended to search for a shortcut unsuccessfully and thus required a longer time to find the solution than those subjects not having problem experiences.

The above study emphasizes the need for teachers to provide purposeful clarification of the goals of instruction and to be aware of the impact that the introduction to a given topic will have on future learnings.

SET AND CREATIVITY

Kramer, Tegan, and Knauber (1970) assessed the effect of informational pre-sets on baccalaureate nursing students. Their study focused on the creative use of library resources by students. "Creative" was defined as an uncommon or novel response reported to be workable. Their investigation was a replication of Hyman's (1964) study in which it was demonstrated that informational pre-sets affect the solving of a given task and enhance or hinder the formation of creative or uncommon solutions.

A bibliography was considered to be a limiting type of "advance organizer" or pre-set, because it structures material to be learned according to topics and prominent authors. Students were given the explanation that, in order to allow freedom of choice, a bibliography would not be given for the child area of nursing. Four experimental groups were presented with both common and uncommon ways of obtaining information. For example, reading a pediatrics textbook and using the bibliography at the end of each chapter, if additional source material was needed, was deemed common. In contrast, forming an informational reading and discussion group in which other students would report and critique what they had read was considered uncommon. Critical pre-sets were given to two of the experimental groups. One group was asked to list the disadvantages of the common solutions; the other was asked to list the disadvantages of the uncommon solutions. The remaining two experimental groups were given constructive presets: one group was asked to list the advantages of the common solutions; the other was asked to list the advantages of the uncommon solutions. A control group of students was given no pre-set but was asked to list all solutions considered to be effective, as well as stating the advantages and disadvantages of each. Six weeks later all students were asked to list the solutions they had *actually used* in obtaining information.

It was found that there were significant differences in the occurrence of the uncommon responses in the group receiving the pre-set of being asked to list the disadvantages of common solutions. This group came up with many more unusual responses than the other three experimental groups but not significantly more than the control group, which had no informational input in terms of suggested solutions at all. This led the investigators to suggest that the general information given to *all* students—that of freedom to select material for themselves—was *in fact* a pre-set in itself.

This study lends support to the notion that teachers do affect student creative problem-solving behavior through the use of specific sets or directions. It further indicated that specific pre-sets tend to lose their power over time. The results suggest that specific pre-sets can transfer to other common or uncommon solutions to problems. It is interesting to note that the students stated far more unusual solutions than the faculty had anticipated!

von Oech (1983), a creative thinking consultant, illustrates the power that a creative mind has to transform one thing into another. He points out that by changing perspective and playing with knowledge and experience, the ordinary can become extraordinary and the unusual commonplace. He states (p. 7) that:

DISCOVERY CONSISTS OF LOOKING AT THE SAME THING AS EVERYONE ELSE AND THINKING SOMETHING DIFFERENT

The major reason, according to von Oech (1983, p.9) that people are not able to "think something different" is because they have mental blocks. He gives ten mental blocks that get in the way and are hazardous to thinking in new ways. These blocks, that are well elaborated in his book, are:

1. The right answer
2. That's not logical
3. Follow the rules
4. Be practical
5. Avoid ambiguity
6. To err is wrong
7. Play is frivolous
8. That's not my area
9. Don't be foolish
10. I'm not creative

Two stories illustrate von Oech's (1983, p. 10) approach to opening mental locks. They bear repeating here:

A Zen master invited one of his students over to his house for afternoon tea. They talked for a while, and then the time came for tea. The teacher poured the tea into the student's cup. Even after the cup was full, he continued to pour. The cup overflowed and tea was spilled onto the floor.

Finally, the student said, "Master, you must stop pouring: the tea is overflowing—it is not going into the cup."

The teacher replied, "That's very observant of you. And the same is true with you. If you are to receive any of my teachings, you must first empty out what you have in your mental cup.

Moral: We need the ability to unlearn what we know.

Without the ability to temporarily forget what we know, our minds remain cluttered with ready-made answers, and opportunities for new directions are decreased. The opening of the mind is not easy. How does von Oech (1983, p. 11) suggest this be done? Again, he turns to a story:

At another lesson the teacher and the student are discussing a problem. Despite lengthy discussion, the student doesn't seem to understand the point that the teacher is making. Finally, the teacher picks up a stick and gives him a whack on the side of his head with it. Suddenly, the student begins to grasp the situation and "think of something different."

Moral: Sometimes, nothing short of "a whack on the side of the head" can dislodge the assumptions that keep us thinking "more of the same."

Anything that helps students to discover an opportunity that wasn't previously apparent can help to generate new ideas. A great deal of the educational system is designed to help students to accept the ten mental locks previously given. It is not easy to break out of patterns, particularly those that have been so carefully instilled. von Oech (1983) points out that innovators constantly have challenged rules. He gives many excellent exercises for those who wish to give themselves and others a "whack on the head" to unlock their minds for innovations and creativity.

SUMMARY

Preinstructional set can vary in length and elaborateness. Its purpose is to clarify the goals of instruction, motivate students to learn, and help students to see the relevance of the learning task. Set assists in organizing information by providing a common frame of reference. Set gives students an attitude of mind that helps them to accept or reject learning experiences. Because learning is a sequential process in which past learning forms the foundation for future learning, set helps students toward a cognitive bridge from one topic to another.

7

Achieving Closure

Closure is achieved when the major purposes and principles of a class, a course, or a program have been completed. Closure is complementary to set induction. It links the new knowledge to past knowledge and acts as a cognitive link to future learnings. Closure is of importance before going on to a new topic. It should provide more than a summary or review of what has been said.

EFFECT OF CLOSURE

Johnson (1965) draws a distinction between instructional closure and cognitive closure. He differentiates between the two by stating that instructional closure is reached when the class is completed and the *teacher* has shown the link between past knowledge and new knowledge. On the other hand, cognitive closure is reached when the *student* has reached closure and made the association between the old and new learnings. It can readily be seen that it is the latter—cognitive closure—that provides the more relevant learning goal.

The concept of organization and meaning in learning can be described in the principle as stated by Blair (1948): learning proceeds more rapidly and is retained longer when that which is learned possesses meaning, organization, and structure. After all, the major purpose for education is that it should serve us in the future. Transfer cannot occur by itself. It needs to be fostered by teaching behaviors. Closure is one teaching behavior that can assist the student in drawing meaningful relationships and forming an organization for transfer.

In testing the effects of cognitive closure on the achievement of ninth grade students, a study by Johnson (1965) indicated that cognitive closure as perceived by the student was positively associated with both immediate and delayed performance on tests of achievement. His findings give further support to the notion that learner achievement is significantly affected by the way in which the learner perceives the learning set as well as whether or not the set is perceived to be fulfilled by the student. In brief, both perceived learner set and perceived cognitive closure affect learner achievement. In addition to content achievement, it was found that students with perceived cognitive closure participated with greater willingness in subsequent learning experiences.

HELPING STUDENTS TOWARD CLOSURE

Allen and Ryan (1969) suggest three useful approaches to assist students toward closure, as well as to help the teacher ascertain whether closure has been achieved. These are:

1. *Review and summary*

   During a discussion with students, many different situations can be described, and students may respond in a variety of ways to the topic under discussion. While exploring a topic, it is not unusual for students to stray from the topic to tangential points or unfruitful paths. In order to give meaning, thrust, and organization to a free discussion, it is necessary for the teacher to listen to the meaning of what is being said, inventory comments, and abstract the ideas in order to summarize succinctly and help give the students a capsule summary of the salient points made by the group.

2. *Application of what has been learned to similar examples*

   Comparing the summarized ideas with a model of the structure of the content under consideration assists students in organizing the new information. For example, if students were discussing the care of immobile patients, a general discussion of the specific problems presented by each of the student's patients would bring forth much data. The teacher might, then, compare the summarized problems of these patients to a model of the problems of immobilization as generalized from groups of patients. By reinforcing the main points brought out by the students, and tying these points to previous learnings, the teacher can assist the students to extract generalizations from the specific aspects of the topic.

3. *Extend what has been learned to new situations*
   This teaching behavior helps students toward transfer of knowledge from one situation to another. For example, following a discussion emphasizing the need to protect patients with debilitating conditions from external infections, asking students about other situations in which patients should be especially protected will help them to gain understanding that any patient with suppressed immunity factors is particularly susceptible to infection.

CLOSURE AND FEELING OF ACHIEVEMENT

In addition to pulling together the major points and acting as a cognitive link between past knowledge and new knowledge, closure provides students with a needed feeling of achievement. By providing closure the teacher can use students' contributions and fit them into a meaningful whole in order to help students to incorporate new ideas into their cognitive structure. Everyone has had the experience of being involved in a group that seemingly has failed in its decision-making process. The skillful leader who can order all the comments, point out areas of agreement and disagreement, and help the group toward defining next steps is achieving closure.

CLOSURE AND TRANSFER OF LEARNING

As previously stated, in addition to providing a sense of accomplishment, closure should provide value for the student. Transfer is perhaps the most significant criterion of learning. It refers to the extent to which knowledge and abilities learned in one situation will apply to a new and different situation. There are two major principles pertaining to transfer that are relevant to closure. The first is that transfer occurs when there is a recognized similarity between the learning situation and the transfer situation. The key word here is *recognized,* which implies that it is recognized by the learner. By pointing out other situations in which the generalizations under consideration will apply, transfer is being reinforced. This principle has been supported by experimental evidence, and the theory underlying transfer is that learning experiences with "identical elements" help students to generalize to new situations.

The second general principle of transfer applicable to closure is that transfer will occur to the extent that students expect it to occur. It is not sufficient for new situations to have identical elements with the learning ones for students to know generalizations. In addition, students must perceive the identical elements in the new situation or recognize that the generalizations apply to the new situation. The study of organizational theory may lead to an understanding of the way complex organizations are structured, but it will not necessarily help a nursing student to understand the hospital as a complex organization unless the knowledge is applied to several types of organizations with the expectation that such knowledge is both usable and will assist the learner in the future.

USE OF CLOSURE

Closure is an appropriate activity to perform before going on to any new concept, idea, or problem. Because it is complementary to set induction, closure can be combined with establishing set. There are times, however, when closure is particularly relevant, such as at the end of a class session. Teachers often do not allow sufficient time for closure. Rather, they wait until the last minute of the class and become aware of the time because students are shuffling in their seats and the classroom door is being opened by the next group of students. With this interference, the closure may consist of a hurried one sentence summary followed by "That's it for today" with students scarcely listening at all.

The opposite can also occur. The students may achieve closure before the teacher! In this case, the teacher is dragging out points that are obvious and is taking a longer time to summarize than it took the group to bring forth the ideas in the first place. Under these circumstances, the teacher is belaboring the point in an unfruitful way. When a class is finished, it is finished; attempting to keep students to the appointed hour will only mean that they are physically present.

Closure is suitable for the completion of a unit of study or a course. Ways of achieving closure might include a case study; reading a poem that draws together the ideas to be conveyed; or presenting an analogy or short story that is read or distributed. The major idea that the instructor wishes to leave with the student can frequently be dramatically illustrated.

SUMMARY

Closure, as a teaching technique, helps students to abstract the very major ideas presented in a class, a teaching unit, or a course. It provides a link between what has been learned to the application of the knowledge. Closure is important because organization and meaningful learning assist in transfer in forming relationships. Furthermore, closure helps to give students a feeling of accomplishment and satisfaction in what they have learned. Closure should aid in leaving students with an "itch" or desire to test and incorporate what has been learned and to include the newly acquired knowledge and skills into their own behavior set—and still be eager to learn.

PART 2

STRATEGIES FOR TEACHING GROUPS OF STUDENTS

8

Teaching by Lecture

The lecture is perhaps the oldest teaching strategy for large group teaching. Long before the invention of the printing press, groups of scholars sat with their tutor, listened, and took notes on his wise words. Because books remained expensive for some time following the invention of printing, the only way that a person could become educated was by the transmission of information through the teacher. As textbooks became more readily available, the lecture in the college and university was employed to reinforce and supplement written reference materials. Suffice it to say that the lecture should never be used for reading aloud from the textbook!

A deductive strategy is most commonly used in teaching by lecture. The teacher begins with a definition of the concepts or principles, illustrates them with examples, unfolds their implications, and provides closure by helping the students incorporate the new ideas into their schemes of cognitive structure. This type of teaching provides immediate reinforcement of the rule or principle being discussed. Presenting rules first can be effective because it can be more useful to the nursing student to remember a general statement; for example, that an increase in tissue or fluid in the cranium will lead to increased intracranial pressure rather than remembering that a cerebral vascular accident, a tumor, or trauma will all lead to increased intracranial pressure.

THE FORMAL LECTURE

A formal lecture is one in which the lecturer does all of the talking. It is organized for the participants, and decisions are made in advance of the presentation. The disadvantages to this type of teaching strategy are that the "telling" technique is often an indication of subject matter domination in the learning process. Too much emphasis is put on certain facts and materials to be learned and too little on the learning process itself, and on the desired results. In this way it may encourage the retention of facts as an end in itself. Furthermore, exposition as an approach to teaching tends to emphasize the wants and desires of the lecturer to the exclusion of the students' needs. It fosters dependence on the teacher as the final authority, thus inhibiting the exploratory aspect of learning. Most important, the formal lecture creates a passive type of learning that tends not to be retained.

The lecture as a teaching method has been denounced mostly as a reaction against its long years of misuse and overuse. Its misuse occurs when it is used when other strategies would achieve the particular learning objectives, as active learning is preferable to passive learning. College students often state that they enjoy lectures, but it should be borne in mind that when the instructor capsulizes all the pertinent information, students are saved a trip to the library to dig it out for themselves. Every problem solved by the teacher is one less problem for the student to solve. Attitudes, skills, and feelings cannot be learned through pure "show and tell" procedures.

There are reasons that lectures are not uniformly excellent in higher education. Satterfield (1978) estimates that the average lecturer speaks at the rate of 150 words per minute. This means that a 50-minute lecture produces 7,500 words! He also points out that very few writers could be as prolific, and at the same time exercise all the careful revisions required to produce an excellent treatise, using the number of words that lecturers must use during a given course that employs the lecture as the only teaching method. In view of all of the criticisms lodged against the college lecture, Satterfield (1978) summarizes the situation with a resigned statement. He points out that lecturing is likely to remain the most prevalent practice of college teaching. If this is so, and we have no reason to challenge this statement based on our own observations of teaching in schools of nursing, it behooves those who lecture to learn to do it with a moderate (at least) degree of skill.

ADVANTAGES OF THE LECTURE

In spite of the criticisms of the lecture method of teaching, there obviously must be many advantages to it, or this widespread teaching technique would not have survived for so many generations of college students. The specific advantages of the lecture method of teaching include:

1. It can help to emphasize and clarify important points and thus channel the thinking of a group of students in the given direction.
2. The lecture can enliven facts and ideas that might seem tedious on the pages of a book.
3. Lectures can expose large groups of students to authorities in order to share first-hand experiences. It is indeed inspirational for students to experience the enthusiasm and excitement that a nursing leader feels for our profession. This excitement can be transmitted to large numbers of students when such a person is invited to speak to and with students on campus. A nurse returning from another country can share perceptions of a different culture, as well as add a fresh way of viewing nursing problems in our nation, with groups of students by lecture.
4. An individual who is testing a nursing theory can share ideas before publication and thus give students the advantage of hearing truly original ideas.
5. The teacher's experience, enthusiasm, and special way of organizing materials, presented with masterful delivery, can serve as a motivation and inspiring experience for students. For introducing a new topic or concept, explaining a process, telling how something is done, giving perspective to the work of the class, or summarizing what has been learned, the lecture has no equal.

Research suggests that a first-rate lecture is better than written material at emphasizing conceptual organizations, clarifying issues, reiterating critical points, and inspiring students to appreciate the importance of key information. The clarity of an excellent lecture aids understanding and creates a state of intellectual excitement. The lecture is probably most effective for motivating students to learn more about a topic. Good lectures that engage the listener are very difficult to ignore.

Lecturing to Large Classes

It is safe to state that most teachers prefer small sections to larger ones. However, given the budgetary constraints of our current times, practical considerations require that large classes be taught, and it is important to consider ways in which the objectives, methods of presentation, interpersonal atmosphere, and administrative problems of the large class differ from a small one. For purposes of definition, a small class is one in which there are fewer than 35 students, a moderate size class has fewer than 60 students, and a large class is one in which there are fewer than 100 students (Lowman, 1984, p. 153). Student achievement and satisfaction have been compared in small and large classes. Research suggests that college teachers can achieve many educational objectives in large classes just as well as in smaller classes. For example, McKeachie (1978) found that scores on final exams do not differ because of class size. However, large classes cannot meet objectives best approached through discussion, such as retention, critical thinking, or attitude change. Furthermore, large classes are less effective than small ones for students who need interpersonal attention from teachers in order to do their best. Highly dependent, less academically able, and poorly motivated students do not do as well in large sections. Be that as it may, skillful lecturers can offer exciting and meaningful educational experiences and can compensate for the liabilities associated with large class size. The lecture, therefore, becomes the major teaching strategy, and the lectures must be dynamic and engaging.

Southin (1984) points out that large class size is not itself an impediment to learning. In fact, he says, students may be far better off sitting in an auditorium with hundreds of other students listening to a well-prepared lecturer in command of the subject who communicates the excitement of the discipline than they are in a small group plagued by a rambling bore who communicates nothing but mediocrity. Large audiences actually tend to bring out the best in a lecturer because of their responsiveness and the sense of responsibility that such an audience fosters. The temptation to improvise, or to come to class unprepared, is always present when the class is small. We have all wasted the time of a few people by thinking out loud, and doing so in front of a handful of students seems no different. In contrast, a large class is less forgiving.

The greatest objection that students have to a large class is that it doesn't give them the opportunity to know their professor. This is a major risk. Lowman (1984, p. 154) offers some excellent suggestions for maximizing opportunities for personal contacts with students during class. He suggests that the instructor come to class 5 to 10 minutes early, stroll around the room, and chat informally with students. Occasional personal disclosures also add intimacy to large lecture classes. Staying after class is another way to encourage interaction. However, in the last analysis, the initiative rests with the students, and those who really want to get to know their professor can do so. Furthermore, in nursing classes, the closeness between student and faculty member comes through the clinical exposures.

Teachers of large classes may, at times, have to resort to special techniques to get feedback from students. Not all students feel comfortable asking questions or coming to the instructor. Therefore, asking for written feedback during the course is essential. Most colleges and universities ask for course and faculty evaluations at the end of the course, but that doesn't help the student currently taking the course. Midquarter evaluations are of help to the faculty member for changing or keeping the course as is. A simple device, such as handing out cards approximately every fourth class period inviting students to write questions, or comments, which can be answered in writing by the instructor, can be of help in letting students know the instructor's interest in them.

Lowman (1984, p. 117–118) makes the following ten important points about lecturing:

1. Fit the material you present to the time you have available.
2. Seek concise ways to present and illustrate content. Express concepts in the simplest terms possible and define technical terms when using them.
3. Begin each course and class by pricking the students' interest, expressing positive expectations, and sharing the objectives you have with them.
4. Follow a prepared outline but include improvised material or illustrations. Appear spontaneous even when you are following the outline closely.
5. Break up the monotony of lectures by varying methods of presentation.
6. Use a wide range of voices, gestures, and physical movements, but be yourself. Develop a varied and interesting style consistent with your values and personality.
7. Give students time now and then to catch their breath, and ask questions.
8. End each lecture with a conclusion that connects what has happened today to what will be covered during the next meeting.
9. Be guided by your students during your lectures. Continually observe their reactions, acknowledge them, and modify your approach when indicated.
10. Remember in your relationships with students that all of you are persons first, and students and teacher second.

LECTURE-DISCUSSION

The informal lecture, or lecture-discussion as it is frequently called, is perhaps the most common teaching strategy used in classroom teaching in colleges. With this method the presentation is supplemented by audiovisual aids, and students are encouraged to interrupt for questions, comments, and clarification.

McKeachie (1963) states that the use of both, lectures and discussions, is a logical and popular choice in courses in which the instructors wish not only to give information but also to develop concepts. The lecture can effectively present new research findings; the discussion can give students opportunities to analyze the studies, find relationships, and develop generalizations. By participating actively in discussion, students not only learn the generalization but also develop skill in critical thinking as well.

As with all teaching strategies, it is imperative that the teacher have a clear-cut purpose for what is to be accomplished. In organizing a class around a lecture and lecture-discussion method, the teacher plans the class so that it will progress in an orderly manner. A short overview helps students to focus on the topic; a creative way of producing set helps students to enter into the class both cognitively and affectively. The teacher plans for the supporting data needed to substantiate views and has additional material ready if further clarification is necessary. However, merely because the teacher has the examples does not constitute rationale for using all of them. Repetition beyond that needed to assure understanding tends to be boring.

ORGANIZING THE LECTURE

Foley and Smilansky (1980) offer some excellent advice for organizing a lecture. Essentially, a lecture should be organized into three parts: an introduction, body, and conclusion. It adheres to the old teaching adage of "tell them what you are going to tell them, tell them; and then tell them what you told them."

The Introduction

The component of set induction in Chapter 6 applies to the introduction of a lecture. All too often lecturers begin by merely stating the topic (e.g.,

"Today we will discuss the care of the patient who is anxious") and then proceed immediately to the body of the lecture. An effective introduction to a lecture delineates the specific topics that will be covered and states the order in which they will be discussed. In introducing the topic of caring for clients who are anxious the lecturer could say: "Today we are going to discuss anxiety and the ways in which your clients may manifest it. We will define anxiety, discuss its prevalence, its origins in terms of psychoanalytic and other theories, the precipitating factors, and the major ways in which anxiety can be alleviated." Sometimes opening a lecture with a series of questions may peak the interest of students.

In order to assist students in following the organization of the lecture, an outline is helpful. This can be written on a chalkboard or shown on an overhead projector. The entire outline can be presented at once to allow students to view the total lecture organization before its beginning, or the teacher may wish to vary this by presenting points one by one and adding to the outline as each new idea is presented. For the latter plan, an overhead projector provides an excellent means for adding points, while allowing students to keep the preceding ones in view. Either using overlays to build up the outline, or covering up on the transparency the ideas yet to be discussed using a piece of opaque paper, can be effective. Such an outline helps the teacher follow with the planned sequence, as well as allowing students to contribute in a focused manner. It assists the teacher in avoiding unnecessary repetition or gaps in presentation.

The ground rules for the lecture should be stated. For example, the lecturer may not wish to interrupt the presentation with questions from students. In that case, it is important to state that a specified period of time at the conclusion of the lecture will be reserved for questions. Or the lecturer may prefer to have students ask questions at the conclusion of each segment of the lecture. In either case, it is essential that the lecturer repeat the student's questions so that all in the room have heard the question before the lecturer launches into the answer or discussion.

Body of Lecture

The body of the lecture should be organized so that information flows logically from one point to another. It should not deviate from the boundaries established in the introduction. Poor planning, or to be more precise, inadequate planning, results in rambling presentations and frequent digressions that make it difficult for the audience to pay attention to what is being said. Some lecturers are overly enthusiastic in their approach and attempt to include too much material in the lecture. As a matter of fact, too much material is frequently the result of inadequate preparation. It takes longer to prepare carefully for a short lecture (or a short article) than to allow oneself the luxury of going on and on.

During a lecture, the teacher should be sensitive to feedback from the students, particularly the nonverbal cues that can indicate lack of understanding, boredom, or daydreaming. It is important to emphasize that although such cues as yawning, whispering, or sleeping may indicate that the material or its presentation is not stimulating to students, the teacher should take into account other reasons, such as poor ventilation, inadequate lighting, or the time of the day, as other possible causes of inattentive behavior from students. A droning voice on a warm summer day following lunch does lull students to sleep! Note how an information-giving television program, such as a news commentary, is paced. Short bits of information are given, interspersed with a videotaped "on the scene" report, still pictures, or illustrations of the event. Remember the reason Hayden suddenly raised the volume on his *Surprise Symphony.* It was to awaken the slumberers during a chamber music concert! Varying the stimuli by these means and such others as shifting from expository teaching to discussion become essential to maintain or regain the active involvement of the learner.

Eye contact with the audience is also important. Beginning, or insecure, lecturers sometimes keep their eyes glued to the back of the room instead of scanning the entire group. Moving about provides a changing focus for the audience and varies the stimuli. However, too much moving can be distracting. Although there really are no hard and fast rules for improving presentation styles, because each person has a unique personality and should develop his or her own style, some ideas are discussed later in this chapter. Summaries of research on teaching effectiveness consistently cite qualities such as warmth, enthusiasm, and motivation as features of the effective lecturer and instructor (Foley & Smilansky, 1980). How does one demonstrate these elusive characteristics? Unfortunately, no magic formula exists. It has been suggested that one ask for help from colleagues who can give specific and constructive feedback after attending a lecture. Videotaping a lecture and reviewing the tape repeatedly has helped many novice (or experienced) lecturers to improve their presentation styles.

The Conclusion

The principles discussed in Chapter 7 on achieving closure relate to this part of the lecture. All too often lecturers simply run out of time and hastily conclude what they want to say. The salient points should be repeated, and if the lecture will continue on the same topic or one closely related, the content of the summary can provide the bridge to the next lecture. Sometimes questions are effective. For example, in discussing the concept *anxiety* students could be asked to identify symptoms of anxiety in each client they care for during their next clinical experience.

Lecturing Style

The enthusiasm of the lecturer is probably the most important aspect of style. After all, if he or she finds the subject dull, so will the students. However, given that fact, there are certain techniques and pointers that can help a teacher to deliver a lecture with force and style.

Beginning lecturers often ask if lectures should be written out in their entirety, sketched in outline, or delivered off-the-cuff. It can be said that as long as the results are the same—seeming spontaneity—it really makes little difference. Whatever works best for the lecturer is the answer. It is wise, however, to remember that prose written to be spoken is different than prose that has been written to be read. Many experts suggest that what has been written should be scored for delivery, with pauses marked and particular words and phrases singled out for emphasis or inflection. Many lecturers recommend that it is important to practice reading a lecture out loud (provided that the wall between colleagues' offices can buffer the noise). These are techniques followed by every excellent speech deliverer, and teachers should pay as much attention to their students as they do to other audiences they may have.

Fuhrmann and Grasha (1983, p. 155) give some practical points for varying the stimuli during a lecture. They include the following points:

Create Movement. Standing in the same place and presenting information can become monotonous for students. Move about the room, including up and down the aisles. Students, also, get tired of sitting in the same place for a long period of time. Change the pace by setting up small discussions, buzz groups, or allowing students a "stretch" break every 45 minutes.

Use novelty. Vary the teaching method through audiovisual aides, small group discussions, guest speakers, or using colored chalk to direct attention. These means will be more fully described in the next section.

Vary intensity. Vary the rate, tone, and inflection of voice. Listing major points on a chalkboard or handout also helps ensure that people will notice them.

There are few aspects to lecturing more important than the speaking voice of a lecturer. Poor enunciation, harsh or nasal voice quality, and distracting speech mannerisms distract students, sometimes to the point of not paying attention to what is being said. Beginning a sentence with "uh," "well," or "okay" is annoying to those who must listen to this voice warm-up.

Pitch is an important voice quality. Lowman (1984, p. 76) points out that a voice ranging melodically between high and low tones is much more likely to keep listeners' attention than a monotonous voice that merely uses one or two notes. The way in which a lecturer uses inflection also contributes to audience interest. Speech with little or no emphasis is unlikely to engage and maintain someone's attention. Although it is more difficult to pin down than other characteristics, the degree to which speech sounds relaxed or tense may contribute significantly to its overall effect on listeners. When speakers have a relaxed style, their speech seems to be fluent. Hesitant, jerky, or piercing speech can create tension in the listeners.

The best way to improve voice presentation is to listen to oneself critically and note if meaningless vocalizations are used. Lowman (1984, p. 78) offers some helpful suggestions to lecturers, which bear repeating here. He suggests that faculty enlist the aid of a colleague and first record a simple conversation. Next, he suggests waiting a few days to listen to the recording and then setting aside an hour or so to do the following:

1. Listen to each recording completely without stopping to take notes.
2. After listening, record your initial reaction to hearing yourself speak. What are your feelings (defensive, critical, pessimistic, puzzled, ashamed?) Try hard to listen to yourself as if you have never heard it before.
3. Listen to the recording a second time, jotting on a piece of paper the words that seem to best describe your voice. Again, try to think of it as a voice you have never heard before.
4. Within 24 hours of listening to the taped conversation, have one of your lectures tape recorded. Listen to it and note if there are differences between your conversational voice and the voice used for lecture.

Lowman (1984) has devised a Speech Assessment Rating Form, which can be found at the end of Chapter 4 in his book. He also offers a number of helpful hints on voice improvement.

In addition to voice quality, many teachers speak too quietly. This is a particular problem with women who may speak in a weak and timid voice. Projecting the voice to the back row of the classroom is essential and requires a combination of volume and energy. It requires much practice to learn to speak loudly, enunciate clearly, and develop a pleasant tonal quality. Masterful lecturing is a result of more than an engaging speaking voice, but the skill with which a teacher uses this oral bridge to students will strongly influence the effectiveness of his or her presentation.

In addition to voice quality, the gestures used by a lecturer can increase attention greatly and emphasize relationships with content. As with other teaching techniques, the personality of the teacher is relevant to how gestures are used. Some teachers remain relatively stationary standing next to the lectern or moving beside it occasionally. Others gallop about the room, including up and down the aisles. Regardless of the way in which the individual instructor is comfortable, body language can convey a message. Slumping over the lectern or slouching while pacing back and forth, can convey a lack of energy or enthusiasm or lack of self-confidence.

One effective technique is to use different sides of the room to play different roles in expressing differing sides of an argument, displaying differences in age (for example, answering a question as a ten-year-old on one side of the room and as a four-year-old on the other), or role playing in general.

Lecturing style comes from practice, from feedback, and from showmanship. Instructors who win major teaching awards in universities usually do so because of their lecturing skills and styles. Like "Masterpiece Theatre," excellent lectures seem to satisfy the students' need for a dramatic spectacle and offer an interpersonal arena in which important psychological needs are met.

AUDIOVISUAL AIDS

Audiovisual aids are adjuncts to the teaching process. In order not to limit communication with students to voice and gesture alone, they should be used. Teachers have been using illustrations as long as they have been teaching. Such great teachers as Socrates and Archimedes drew pictures and diagrams in the sand to illustrate their points. Because it is thought we remember only 10 percent of what we hear and 20 percent of what we see, retention is increased by using illustrations. The chalkboard is one of the oldest and most used of audiovisual aids. It needs no explanation, except to point out that its use for drawing illustrations greatly enhances the clarity of some materials. For some inexplicable reason, when teachers draw on the board they usually feel compelled to apologize for their lack of artistic ability before or immediately following completion of their masterpiece. In addition to drawing attention to the very aspect they wish to avoid, this remark can become somewhat disconcerting to students who hear the same apology from teacher after teacher. Remember that no student expects a nursing teacher to be a van Gogh or a medical illustrator. Nursing instructors who are unduly sensitive about their lack of artistry might wish to carefully draw their pictures on the board before class. One effective use of the chalkboard involves drawing on the board, erasing the board leaving the outline (not discernible to the class) and whipping up the picture by tracing the outline in front of the class! Another idea is to use the artistic skills of students. In addition to receiving a clear illustration, this can serve as a way to recognize special talents of students.

The advantages of using colored chalk in illustrating a lecture are dramatically told by Eleanor Clark, the 1981 Council for Advancement and Support of Education's "Professor of the Year" (Ingalls, 1981). She states that slides, overhead transparencies, and material presented by means of opaque projectors all present students with a whole picture, whereas drawing on the chalkboard allows the students' minds to follow what the teacher is doing rather than wandering to other topics.

Overhead Projector

The overhead projector is perhaps the easiest of all of the audiovisual aids to use. This optical instrument enlarges a 10-inch transparency to viewing size on a projection screen within a distance of a few feet. Because it is operated from the front of the class, the teacher controls the management rather than relying on a technical aid. The teacher thus avoids distracting instructions and can integrate the material from the transparency with the presentation naturally and without losing eye contact with the class. The transparency can be a diagram or written or pictorial illustration. Reed (1968) lists several pertinent points for the teacher to observe when operating the overhead projector in order to increase the effectiveness of the material presented. The placement of the projector and screen in relation to the class is of importance. Both the teacher and the head of the projector can obstruct the view of material for the student unless the screen is carefully placed. If the head of the projector is not placed at a right angle to the screen, distortion of the image, known as "keystoning," will occur. This creates an image larger at the top than bottom. To gain better visibility in the classroom, placing the screen higher and slanting the screen will prevent the "keystone" effect. Because the light of the overhead projector tends to draw students' eyes to it, it should be turned off when not specifically in use. Also, while changing the transparencies, the light should be turned off to avoid the phenomenon of visual confusion.

Transparencies for the overhead projector can be easily made by the instructor by writing with a waxed pencil or special felt-tipped pen. Duplicating illustrations or prepared materials can be done by using a specially treated transparency and a thermal duplicator. The materials are either color sensitive or color can be added by special overlay material or colored pens or pencils. It takes but a few moments to make an attractive transparency. The most dramatic transparency illustrates a single thought or comparison. Too much detail in a transparency can confuse viewers and lessen the impact of the visual image as a communications tool. A good transparency contains one idea, visual identification, legible writing (at least ¼" high), and imaginative design. Color should be used for emphasis of a particular part of the transparency. Overuse of color will detract from its value. Commercially prepared transparencies are available for purchase from textbook companies. These transparencies are prepared in color with overlays, which assist in giving added dimension to the material. In addition to the anatomical charts, to which this material readily lends itself, nursing examples include such lessons as preparing and calculating solutions, the patient and circulatory disorders, and the patient and fluid balance.

The addition of an attachment, which polarizes light on specially treated overlay materials or materials laminated onto the transparency, gives the effect of movement. This is particularly effective when motion adds to the learning experience, as with the circulatory system. It also serves as a stimulus variation.

Slides and Film Strips

Slides that are well produced provide the clearest and most accurate images of all audiovisual aids. They can be changed with ease, and modern classrooms include equipment that enables the lecturer to control the pace at which the slides are changed. The lecturer does not have to lose eye contact with the audience, and slides can be easily integrated into the lecture with a minimum of distraction to the audience.

Foley and Smilansky (1980) offer four points for use with instructional media that are particularly applicable to the use of slides. First, they should be carefully incorporated into the verbal presentation, with the objective of illustrating and clarifying particular ideas, rather than provide a major focus. Second, media should only be used when they enhance understanding of the subject matter. Third, audiovisual aids should be clearly visible and audible. Too much information on a slide detracts rather than clarifies. Finally, preview all of the slides before presentation to be certain that they are in order, right side up, and that the screen can be lowered at the appropriate time.

Slides and film strips are commonly used to illustrate a real-life situation. For example, in helping nursing students to describe the appearance of a patient, color slides of patients who are cyanotic, or who have skin rashes, could be used as illustrations. Commercially prepared film strips illustrate basic nursing procedures.

MOTION PICTURES AND TELEVISION

When sound and motion are added to pictures, their usefulness as a teaching aid is multiplied by both learning retention and transfer, because more senses are brought into play by the student. Both motion pictures and television are very useful tools for the teaching-learning process.

Motion pictures and television can be employed as media to present more complex and lifelike stimuli in the classroom. By means of closed-circuit television or videotape, clinical situations can be brought to the classroom for discussion and critique. Time-lapsed videotapes can telescope time and permit students to understand the problems of chronic disabilities and their effects on patients, for example, without waiting the several years for the process to unfold. Edited tapes provide teachers with a tool that can specifically suit their own purposes. Commercially produced motion pictures provide the teacher with the advantage of having a readymade teaching aid. In some locales, schools of nursing are pooling their faculty resources by videotaping expert lectures and thus bringing master teachers to other schools of nursing when it fits into the borrower's course plan. This plan could be offered, either through videotape recordings or educational broadcast television to bring nursing's leaders to every school of nursing in much the same way as, several decades ago, Dr. Harvey White and seven Nobel prize winners and other distinguished scientists brought an excellent basic college physics course to many universities—an array of talent virtually impossible for any one university to gather for itself.

An old, but still relevant, study designed to compare student achievement and attitudes under three conditions: off campus television instruction, on-campus television instruction, and instructor-present, no television instruction, Dreher and Beatty (1958) found few significant differences in achievement for any of the conditions or subject matters. The subjects taught were psychology, economics, basic communications, and creative arts. Students with low grade-point averages did significantly better with televised instruction in both psychology and economics. The off-campus television students tended to favor television instruction, while the on-campus television group tended to be more disapproving than off-campus students. The nontelevision, instructor-present group tended to be least critical of their courses of all. It is, of course, important to add that the variables included more than television or lack of it. Those faculty who prepared classes for the television presentations had at their disposal innumerable resources, including graphic arts specialists, technical advisors, and colleagues. Seldom does an individual college teacher have such resources. Therefore, because television teaching is more public in both resources and critique, it helps the teacher to present material in varying ways, which in themselves lead to more effective teaching.

All of the aforementioned teaching aids require some degree of hardware. Every teacher has had the disconcerting experience of having difficulty with the equipment or having a film arrive too late to be of use in planned learning sequence. Although most of the newer equipment is easier and handier to use, it is important to advise that the machines should be tried out before class. Films or videotapes that are difficult to see or hear detract from the learning situation. Problems can and do occur.

Handouts

Handouts provide organization and a reminder of what the students have heard (or will hear) in the lecture. Although they are no substitute for a clear and engaging lecture from which the student generates actively a personal set of notes, one can, at least, be certain that all students will carry away the same partial notes. In addition, they provide the student with a useful souvenir of the class. Students like "freebies," and handouts seem to provide a sense of getting something useful.

Although it is perfectly true that varying the stimuli within a class period is necessary in order to increase the attention span and receptivity of students, random selection of materials for the sake of their use alone leads to unproductive results. Audiovisual materials should not be used for their own sake but rather for their ability to communicate more fully to students.

RESEARCH ON TEACHING BY LECTURE

The research studies focusing on teaching by lecture compare it with teaching by group discussion. The results are largely inconclusive, very possibly because of the lack of differentiation of the desired outcomes. When one asks whether lecture is better than discussion, the appropriate counter is "For what goals?"

McKeachie (1963) summarizes the role of the lecture in higher education by pointing out that research results provide little basis for a supportable answer. The research results do not contradict, and sometimes support, the notion that the lecture is an effective way of communicating information. However, there is evidence that other methods of teaching may be more effective than expository techniques when achieving higher cognitive and attitudinal objectives.

SUMMARY

Many teachers favor lecturing because it is efficient and takes less time than helping students to discover principles for themselves. Lecturing gives the teacher control over the learning process. It assists in giving students an organized view of nursing as a discipline because the experienced nurse who teaches is a more effective organizer of nursing than the novice nursing student. However, if a teacher lectures, it is important that the lecture be well organized and delivered.

9

Teaching by Seminar

Anytime more than two persons gather together to discuss an idea, debate a point, analyze an issue, or work together to gain consensus, it becomes a group discussion. Discussion may be defined as the free and unhampered consideration of a problem by a cooperative group of persons talking together under the guidance of one of its members.

The small group discussion allows students to interact with one another and with their instructor, to give as well as take, and to develop confidence in their own ideas and their abilities to express themselves with clarity and logic. Discussions bring about divergent views and help students toward a more creative approach to problem solving.

Small group instruction can be employed in several ways in the nursing school curriculum. Patterned after a common procedure in universities, large classes may be sectioned to allow students adequate opportunity for discussion. A large number of students may have been presented with the same ideas through expository teaching. Because of the size of the class, interaction between students and between student and teacher is limited. Following immediately, or later during the week, students in smaller groups meet with their own section instructor to exchange ideas. The instructor, in order to perform a consultant role, would need to have firsthand knowledge of the expository session. Students are provided the opportunity to raise questions about points not clear to them and test their own thoughts.

Group conferences, following clinical experiences, provide the opportunities for group problem solving and comparing and contrasting patients' nursing problems. It is in the postclinical nursing conference that a great deal of discovery or inductive teaching-learning can take place. For example, if the nursing problem under discussion is nursing interventions in caring for patients with long-term disabilities, the students may have cared for patients with such problems as sensory deprivation, locomotor difficulties, or chronic pulmonary problems. In addition to the subject-matter sampling that can take place in this way, students also may seek assistance from peers to help them identify alternative ways of solving nursing care problems. In addition to the one patient each student may have cared for, vicarious experiences are multiplied by the number of students in the group.

SEMINAR TEACHING

Not all small groups can be considered seminars. It is a misuse of the term when it is used to indicate a course with small enrollment, or an undirected, unfocused discussion by instructor or students or both. The seminar is guided discussion with the student taking the intellectual initiative. The teacher is a member of the group, sometimes acting as leader, other times as consultant. Discussion involves the sharing of ideas and information, the give and take of opinions and exploration of problems and questions.

Discussion assumes that desirable learning outcomes are possible when students can argue, judge data, draw conclusions, compare, and contrast. The group experiences center on the learning activity rather than the teacher or subject matter as determined by the teacher. The value of discussion is in its provision for student involvement and the practice it affords students in assessing, relating, summarizing, and applying ideas. Discussion techniques can promote deeper understanding of learnings as well as affect attitudes, interests, and develop desirable interpersonal relationships. In the words of Lowman (1984, p. 119):

> A useful classroom discussion, unlike a dormitory bull session, consists of student comments separated by frequent probes and clarifications by the teacher that facilitate involvement and development of thinking by the whole group. Dynamic lecturers captivate a class by the virtuosity of their individual performances. Master discussion leaders accomplish the same end by skillful guidance of the group's collective thinking processes.

Discussion, like the lecture, produces strong positive or negative attitudes in both instructors and students. These attitudes are based more on philosophical values than on experience. For some, discussion seems desirable because using it implies that students have important thoughts and experiences to contribute. Discussions recognize students as active participants in their own learning. Students frequently value discussions because they view their teacher as more egalitarian or democratic during discussion exchanges than during lectures.

However, faculty members who view education as the acquisition of information rather than as the development of thinking skills or critical perspectives may find discussion of little immediate value. The educational objectives must always be considered. For example, discussion is not effective for presenting new information that the student is already motivated to learn.

As with other teaching strategies, discussions must be well planned in order to be effective. The quality of discussions is dependent upon how well the instructor performs. Stage presence, leadership, and force are just as important in leading a discussion as in presenting a lecture. In addition, more interpersonal understanding and communication skills are needed. It has been stated that leading an outstanding discussion is more difficult than giving a lecture of comparable quality. Leading a discussion well requires energy, creativity, and spontaneity.

Student-Teacher Interactions

Fruitful discussions require two-way communication. The flow of information is among and between individuals. Two-way communication is sometimes difficult to achieve because there may be status differences between the people communicating. Fuhrmann and Grasha (1983) use the term *psychological size* in discussing the impact one person has on another. This impact is viewed as the potential that one person has for helping or hurting others. People who are perceived as psychologically big have a great potential for influencing and controlling other individuals. This perception interferes with an open dialogue when one party is seen as psychologically bigger than the other. Obviously, this often happens within the classroom.

Psychological size has consequences other than interfering with two-way communication. When someone is perceived as psychologically big, students expect that individual to solve problems, to see that all goes well, to take care of them, and to tell them what things to do and how. This dependence can lead to apathy and lack of initiative.

Fuhrmann and Grasha (1983, p. 143) suggest several negative factors that can contribute to an instructor's psychological size and have implications for teacher-student interactions. These factors include:

1. *Use of high status and titles*
   It is too easy for faculty members to forget the effects that status and titles can have on others. Consistently using *doctor* or *professor* presents an image of a person who is more competent, somewhat distant, more intelligent, and certainly more powerful. This may cause students to feel less free and open in discussing or contributing their thoughts and ideas.

2. *Use of terminal statements permitting no disagreement*
   The examples in the section titled "Discussion Stoppers," later in this chapter, include many of the statements that contribute to psychological size. Such statements as "There is nothing to be gained from further discussion" has the effect of stopping it.

3. *Use of a very formal manner*
   Some teachers come across in a very formal manner to their students. Their body posture is not relaxed, they stand in front of a seated discussion class, they have a harsh look, and they sound like authorities. They often interrupt their students. Whether they mean it or not, the impression they create is that they are solidly "in charge." Given this picture, students will hesitate during their discussions or will have difficulty initiating or feeling free and unhampered during them.

4. *Use of punishing remarks*
   Making such statements to students as "that is illogical," or "how could you possibly believe that?" may be perceived by students as punishment. It creates an environment in which students will keep their thoughts to themselves.

5. *Displaying large amounts of detailed knowledge*
   A discussion should not disintegrate into a lecture. Furthermore, giving large amounts of information creates the image of the teacher as the expert and can destroy a discussion.

6. *Use of language that is too complicated for the learner*
   Although it is important for students to learn the concepts and terminology of nursing and the health sciences, care must be taken to avoid overdoing the use of jargon and technical terminology. It is always better to bring the words to the level that students can understand, or they will turn away from the discussion in frustration.

7. *Failure to use the student's name*
   In small discussion groups it is important that the instructor know the students and call them by name. It puts students at ease and reinforces the fact that they are important.

8. *Overemphasis on grades and grading*

   Instructors who stress the importance of material for the examinations are constantly placing themselves in the role of an authority who gives or withholds rewards. Some students will resent these actions and interpret them as attempts to control their behavior. The resultant lack of involvement may be a symptom of such feelings on the part of students.

RESEARCH ON SEMINAR LEARNING

The research pertaining to student-centered versus instructor-centered teaching is relevant to seminar teaching and learning. A wide variety of teaching methods are described by such labels as "student-centered," "nondirective," "group-centered," or "democratic" discussions. All these techniques have in common the breaking away from the traditional instructor dominated classroom in order to encourage greater student responsibility and participation.

As we discussed previously, a major reason that it is difficult to gather evidence about the superiority of one teaching method over another is because it is difficult to delineate the teaching method that is most productive when one deals with "learning" in global terms. Moreover, the standard of measure for most studies on teaching methods in higher education is the traditional achievement test of knowledge acquisition rather than tests of application or problem-solving skills.

Although scores on objective examinations are little affected by teaching method, other factors indicate that student behavior apart from the usual testing situation may be influenced in the direction of educational goals by student-centered teaching. McKeachie (1966) summarizes the results of research on student-centered teaching methods as not impressive, but supporting of the theory that student-centered methods are effective in achieving higher-order cognitive objectives and in producing noncognitive changes, such as role flexibility and insight.

ADVANTAGES OF SEMINAR LEARNING

An understanding of the group process is an important objective of the school of nursing curriculum. Nurses, as well as other health professionals, work together in every aspect of the helping endeavor. We work as team leaders and team members in providing direct patient care services; we collaborate with other health professionals in the planning of health care; we work with clients and their families; and we serve as members of committees, boards, and commissions both in the community and in our educational institutions. The seminar method of teaching provides first-hand experience in group decision making and group problem solving.

An important contribution of the group problem-solving process is the effect it has in modifying an individual's own style of solving problems through exposure to how others solve problems. Individual solutions are built one upon the other, thus giving the student many more alternative solutions than might have been possible previously.

The usual process followed in group problem solving is that group members exchange information relevant to the problem, one or more solutions based on the information are proposed, and, finally, agreement is reached. In the early phase, that of exchanging information relevant to the problem, students have the opportunity to review knowledge pertaining to the problem. Resources, such as reference materials and consultants, can be brought in or sought by the group.

VARIABLES IN GROUP PRODUCTIVITY AND GROUP SATISFACTION

There is a rich body of research on small groups. We will limit our discussions in this chapter to groups formed for the purpose of meeting educational objectives—task-oriented groups. It must be noted that students may or may not select the group they are in, or may or may not have the option of attending group meetings. In schools of nursing where students progress together throughout their nursing school experiences, a small group of classmates may well take on the characteristics of what Cooley (1909) terms the "primary group." These characteristics include a strong sense of individual identity to the group. It involves a great feeling of sympathy and mutual identification with other members of the group. Group members consistently use the word "we" when referring to their group. Such groups cannot tolerate antagonism because the primary relationship entails a positive valuing of one another, a sense of "we-ness," of belonging together and sharing a common identity. An example of such primary group behavior is demonstrated when a delegation of nursing students is selected to protest such action as one of their members failing a course.

Three of the most important variables pertaining to group productivity and group satisfaction are group leadership, group size, and the communication structure. We will consider each of these factors next.

Group Leadership

Much has been written about group leadership. Many small groups have two different leadership needs. The first is a task leader who supplies ideas and guides the group toward problem solution. The other leadership need is the social-emotional role to help boost group morale.

Some groups experience difficulty maintaining a balance between the task orientation and the social-emotional functions of the group. Bales and Slater (1955) explain the events leading to hostility toward a task-oriented leader. Initially the group members feel satisfied with the progress they are making toward the task. If the group leader utilizes prestige given to the leader to talk a large proportion of the time, eventually hostility will be aroused from some group members. They will eventually transfer some of their initially positive feelings toward the leader to another person who is less active but who expresses their own negative feelings. This latter person becomes the social-emotional leader in representing the values and attitudes that have been disturbed, deemphasized, threatened, or repressed by the task-oriented leader. It is when this occurs that true differentiation of the leadership role occurs.

Groups vary in the extent to which they emphasize task and social-emotional abilities as criteria for leadership. Bales and Slater (1955) suggest that the degree of role differentiation varies directly with the extent to which task functions are unrewarded or costly to group members. When a group experiences little satisfaction in working together toward a goal, the social-emotional functions and task functions tend to be centered on different persons. These conditions tend to occur in a group where there is lack of consensus on the goal, where communication skills are underdeveloped, and where there is little consensus on values and activities.

The implications for teachers indicate that any set of circumstances that reduces the need for differentiation of leadership roles will tend to keep the balance between the task accomplishment and the emotional needs of the group members. Thibaut and Kelley (1959) point out that hostility toward the leader and role differentiation are reduced when the leadership style encourages a wide distribution of directive acts so that no one person becomes the sole target of hostility. Thus, the democratic leader who encourages division of responsibility and participation in decisions may well be able to carry on both task and social-emotional roles.

An investigation conducted in a classroom situation indicates that arousal of hostility toward an instructor is a direct function of the extent to which the instructor violates the legitimate expectations of the students by following his or her own inclinations rather than the students' wishes (Horwitz, 1963). In this study, instructions were given in college ROTC classes too rapidly for the students to grasp them thoroughly. It was agreed that votes would be taken to determine if the instructions should be repeated before going on to the next task. In one group, called the teacher-centered condition, students were informed that the instructor's vote would have twice the weight of the students' combined vote. In the second group, called the student-centered condition, students were told that the instructor's vote would be weighted only one-fourth that of the student group. The actual votes were disregarded and the prearranged experimental conditions were substituted. It was announced to the teacher-centered group that the instructor favored going on to the next topic while slightly more than half of the students had voted to repeat the instructions. With these ratings it was legitimate to go on to another topic because the group had been told that extra weight would be given to the instructor's vote. When the same announcement was made to the student-centered group, the action was perceived as illegitimate because the instructor was arbitrarily reducing the weight given to the student's votes. Considerably more hostility toward the instructor was generated in the student-centered group.

Group Size

As anyone who has experienced the group process will attest, the larger a group becomes the less it is able to accomplish. Gibb (1951) suggests that idea productivity is a *negatively accelerated* increasing function of the size of a group. Much of this appears to be related to need satisfaction. If a group is very large, obviously the individual's needs cannot be met often, as each person must wait his or her turn. As is frequently observed, the rate of participation in small groups tends to be fairly equal among members, but in large groups the majority of the talking is done by the same few persons. Although the increase in size, theoretically, means that each individual will have the opportunity to learn from more persons, this advantage is counteracted by the factors just mentioned. Although the literature does not cite an optimum number for group productivity, many nursing schools vary the number of students for seminars between 10 and 20.

Communication Structure

The well-known phrase "let's sit in a circle" is frequently heard in teaching. Although many students complain that this seating arrangement is overdone, there is research evidence supporting this plan to facilitate communications. Individuals find it more satisfying to communicate directly with one another rather than receiving communications through a third party. This includes nonverbal communications as well as verbal. In fact, nonverbal communications depend on sight and, hence, are completely impossible if the individuals cannot view one another. Leavitt (1951) found that when he placed his subjects in a circle they communicated more freely with one another and expressed more need satisfaction. Face-to-face contact facilitates feedback.

ROLE OF INSTRUCTOR IN FACILITATING GROUP GOAL

Although the group leadership will change, depending on the objective of the group setting, the instructor is generally perceived as a leader by students because of the position. As such, it is the instructor's role to be knowledgeable in the subject under discussion in order to be a resource person. It is also the instructor's role to keep the group from floundering in an unproductive way. There are ways in which teachers can facilitate group discussions.

First, no matter what the objective of the small group discussion is, one common aspect is that it is the members of the group whose opinion, comments, or questions are being sought—not the teacher's. Speaking tends to be an occupational disease among college teachers. It takes much practice and soul-searching to reach the degree of teaching maturity that allows for patience with students and to not tell students either a solution or idea until they have had the opportunity to explore the issue thoroughly by themselves.

Because individuals tend to speak more when they know one another, instructors facilitate communications when encouraging a friendly environment, by helping students to know one another. In a large school it cannot be assumed that everyone knows one another. The introductory phase of the group process cannot be rushed or ignored. Experience teaches us that it generally takes several meetings.

Instructors can facilitate the group's goals by outlining what needs to be accomplished or the topic for discussion. They can do this themselves, or they can help the group do it for itself, depending on the objectives of the group meeting. This lends support to one of Hilgard's (1956, p. 486) learning theories—individuals need practice in setting realistic goals for themselves. If goals are set too low, little effort will be elicited; if too high, they may predetermine failure. Realistic goal setting leads to more satisfactory improvement than unrealistic goal setting.

In addition to knowing the structure of the subject to be discussed, instructors can help to create a climate for a free and unthreatening discussion. Knowing the students, instructors can draw out timid students by giving them opportunities to express themselves and reinforcing them for speaking. A somewhat shy student may not be able to discuss ideas simply because she or he is not aggressive enough to cut in on classmates' discussions. The teacher who is sensitive to nonverbal cues may facilitate this student's speaking by merely stating, "Mary, you look like you wish to add to this last statement." The instructor can help over-eager students gain self-understanding of their need to be heard or dominate a conversation to the exclusion of others. The instructor, likewise, can assist the student who becomes unduly uneasy when verbally challenged. Faculty members often ask how one deals with the student who is aggressive, sensitive, or retiring. Because individuals differ so much, it is virtually impossible and extremely dangerous to suggest any approach without knowing all of the variables involved. Every approach to a student, as to a patient, is a hypothesis about human behavior. The sensitive instructor is alert to opportunities to try different approaches, seeks and accepts feedback, and attempts many alternatives to assist each student in the group.

CONDUCTING A DISCUSSION

Conducting a class discussion requires on-the-spot decisions, diagnoses, and formulating questions. In developing the skill of leading a class discussion, bear in mind that there is no such thing as a perfect discussion. However, some discussions are more effective than others in terms of student learnings and outcomes.

One of the first tasks the instructor must perform is to "get the ball rolling." When the teacher runs out of ideas, brainstorming is a technique that can get the group started thinking toward a solution to a problem. "Brainstorming" was first used in the business world. The rules of brainstorming are that group members give whatever idea occurs to them about a problem. Other members of the group are prohibited from evaluating the idea as presented but are encouraged to free associate and contribute their own ideas. De Cecco (1968) has summarized the studies made of the usefulness of this technique as follows: (1) training in brainstorming increases creative problem solving; (2) brainstorming produces more problem solutions than do methods that penalize bad ideas in some way; (3) more good ideas are produced with brainstorming than with conventional techniques; (4) extended efforts to produce ideas lead to an increased number of ideas and proportion of good ideas; and (5) students in creative problem-solving courses (which include brainstorming) obtain higher scores on tests of creative abilities than do students who have not had these courses. Although students do not evaluate ideas submitted immediately, there is a need to return later to determine the probable significance and worthiness of each idea. If not, it may turn out to be the kind of solution attributed to Will Rogers when he suggested that the best way to capture the enemy's submarines during the war was to heat the ocean to a sufficient degree to cause them to float to the surface. When asked how this could be accomplished, he replied "Don't bother me with the details. I'm an idea man!"

Once the group discussion is started, there are ways to keep the discussion on the track. There are four discussion leadership skills: focusing, refocusing, changing the focus, and recapping what has been said. Each will be discussed.

Focusing

People tend to indulge in associative thinking. They branch off from one idea to another. Providing that the group returns to the original task, associative thinking can be tolerated. But, unless brainstorming is the objective, it is the role of the discussion leader to ask a question that specifically sets the focus. Focusing questions may be open-ended, such as "Why do you think patients miss clinic appointments?", or they may be such that a single answer is appropriate to gather information.

Refocusing

Refocusing is necessary when the group has strayed from the original topic, and the discussion leader wishes the group to return to it. At times this is done directly such as saying "Let's go back to the topic at hand."

It can be done more subtly when the teacher shifts the angle by repeating what a student has said and asks a question that prompts students back to the subject.

Changing the Focus

When a group has obviously discussed a topic sufficiently, and no new ideas or information are forthcoming, then it is usually time to change the focus. An example of this might be "Now that we have listed all the physiological changes occurring with advancing age we can think of, what other changes occur?"

Recapping

The recap is a brief version of a summary of what a group has said. Its purpose is to lift out ideas that have been offered in order to make them more understandable to the group and to set a clearer perspective. Recaps help students to see relationships and make conclusions.

DISCUSSION STOPPERS

Eaton, Davis, and Benner (1977) identified 11 teacher behaviors that inhibit student participation during discussions. They point to the necessity for teacher understanding of the reasons that classroom or conference discussions can fizzle out. They suggest that the teacher, often inadvertently, causes sluggish discussions that result in more teacher-talk than discussion from students. The discussion stoppers they have identified are as follows:

1. *Insufficient "wait-time"*
   This occurs when teachers hasten to answer a question themselves, rephrase the question, or add further information to the question instead of allowing time for thoughtful responses from the students.

2. *The rapid reward*
   Rapid acceptance of a correct answer favors the faster thinker or speaker, whereas those in midthought are cut off prematurely. Although positive reinforcement is an important factor, too

rapid or too forceful a reinforcement can prevent further extension of an idea by other students.

3. *The programmed answer*

Examples within this group include questions that are really not questions and serve to irritate students and block further discussion. The following illustrates this point, "Do you think it would be important to learn about different cultural patterns before doing community health nursing?" The teacher obviously has the answer in mind and is asking for students to confirm it. It is such an obvious question that few students would be willing to dignify it with a response.

4. *Nonspecific feedback questions*

Within this group of questions are the global questions that are asked to determine if students have understood something that they just heard. With specific feedback questions the teacher can find out what is or is not understood rather than asking a diffuse question that does not diagnose the problem and does not foster discussion.

5. *Teacher's ego-stroking*

Teachers who tend to talk a great deal, and, more importantly, put themselves in the role of the ultimate authority, can inhibit classroom discussions. These are the teachers who do not allow students to expand on their ideas or who do not place value on student observations and thoughts. Although the teacher may not intend to enhance his or her own power, prestige, or control, the outcome of presenting oneself as the authority is the disruption or squelching of thoughtful, risk-taking discussions in the classroom.

6. *Low-level questions*

Questions designed to elicit factual or informational level answers tend to end a discussion. Questions of a higher level, designed toward more synthesis, analysis, or evaluation, foster discussion because they encourage creative and critical problem solving.

7. *Intrusive questioning*

Included in this group are questions that go beyond the level of trust or sense of privacy felt by another person. Personal questions, questions that a student is reluctant to answer, and failure to share feelings are all included in this group. A sensitive teacher should avoid such questions when it is evident that a student is uncomfortable responding to them.

8. *Judgmental response to student answers*
   This occurs when the teacher appraises the student's response in a value-laden way and makes personal judgments about the student's response. Students are reluctant to make contributions to a discussion when they feel they might be criticized or embarrassed. The hazard of making judgmental responses increases when the teacher does not know the social and cultural context of the learner.

9. *Cutting students off*
   Instead of refocusing the discussion, at times teachers cut off their students by pointing out that a question will be answered later in the course, or there isn't time to consider a specific aspect at this time. Refocusing a discussion in a positive and nonthreatening manner that does not end a discussion is a skill to be achieved.

10. *Creating a powerful emotional atmosphere and then ignoring feelings and responses*
    This occurs when a highly charged environment is created, and the teacher is insensitive to the degree of emotions generated. For example, if students are discussing death and dying and a student wants to express a personal example, if the teacher continues with the theoretical content without acknowledging the emotional aspect, discussion can be stopped.

11. *Hiding behind the role of teacher*
    This is a subtle and elusive characteristic of some teachers that prevents students from seeing their teacher as a genuine human being interested in and responsive to them. The mental image the teacher has of herself/himself should be examined and clarified. Teachers who are sensitive to the feedback their students give them can be helped to break their preconceived notion of how teachers should perform with their students.

Careful review of the discussion stoppers described above may well give teachers additional insight into how their behavior can inhibit discussion and is suggested as a departure point for self-analysis as well as examination of one's own discussion techniques.

A FEW CAUTIONS ABOUT DISCUSSIONS

As with any teaching strategy, discussions must be directed toward the learning objective. If a discussion is pointless, then students are wasting time. If a discussion is dominated by one or a minority of persons, either teacher or students, it becomes a lecture. If students are not prepared for a discussion, they will flounder and pool their ignorance. Students sometimes have negative feelings about seminars because they have had previous unsuccessful experiences with them. The expression, We've been grouped until we're pooped, is heard by students who have experienced unproductive discussions. Seminar leaders can err in two ways— they can be so permissive that the discussion never becomes focused and meaningful, or they can dominate the conversation with their own ideas, thus inhibiting their students.

SUMMARY

In order for a discussion to be a meaningful and valuable learning activity, it must have some guidance. Keeping the contributions germane to the topic is important if the group is to avoid pursuing tangents that are not productive. The instructor's role includes facilitating communications of all the group members, challenging students, identifying when the group needs information to keep it from floundering, creating a climate for free discussion, and summarizing to keep the group to the task.

Above all, it is important for the instructor to be a sensitive observer of the group process and to avoid domination of the group by some students and withdrawal from the group by others. Unfortunately, once a discussion has deteriorated, it is more difficult to renew it than to have attempted preventive measures earlier.

By seeking clarification of issues and allowing minority viewpoints to be expressed, each member's contribution can be appreciated. An environment in which healthy disagreement is permitted helps to bring out divergent opinions. Because the goal is to seek individual students' ideas, the fact that the student has spoken is what should be reinforced, not necessarily what the student has said.

Instructors who are skilled seminar leaders receive rewards. They know the satisfaction to be gained from successful task accomplishment—helping students solve problems together. As with others who are in leadership roles, instructors may suffer anxiety imposed by the possibility of failure, rebuffs in their attempts to lead students, and guilt when students do not achieve to the degree anticipated. It takes much practice to become skilled in the group process. It is an effort well worth making in terms of student outcomes.

10

Teaching with Guided Design

Cognitive learning theories suggest that challenges presented by the problems and issues faced by students are important factors in motivating students to learn (Fuhrmann & Grasha, 1983). Without an understanding of the larger questions and problems of a field, students may do no more than commit to short-term memory the unassimilated data that are part of the field. Memorizing pre-established answers cannot help students to deal with the complex problems they will face as professionals. Students need to learn to link learned facts, concepts, and principles with new knowledge in order to be able to make the sound decisions required for dealing with the variety of problems they will encounter. Wales and Nardi (1984) pointed out that one of the reasons many people have great difficulty in making decisions is that the process itself may not be formally taught in school. A specific teaching strategy designed to help students become more adept at problem solving and decision making aids in this process. Although developing decision-making skills is discussed in the later chapters on the use of technological aids to help students in clinical decision making, in this chapter a way that decision-making skills can be fostered in the classroom through a teaching technique called *Guided Design* will be explored.

GUIDED DESIGN TEACHING DEFINED

Guided Design was originally developed for engineering students by Wales and Stager (1977). It employs an organized problem-solving format prepared by the instructor. This educational strategy makes it possible for teachers to simultaneously accomplish two goals that its authors claim have resisted integration: (1) teaching subject matter and (2) developing the decision-making skills required to apply what has been learned to the solution of real-world problems. With Guided Design, professional reasoning is modeled, and students have the opportunity to use and apply the material they study to professional decision making. Furthermore, it is believed that the increased motivation helps students to improve retention of the subject matter. The objective of Guided Design is to help students learn how to define problems, generate alternative solutions, defer judgments when necessary, and select final responses after considering criteria for a solution.

ROLE OF THE TEACHER IN A GUIDED DESIGN CLASS

The concept of Guided Design is based on the belief that teachers have more to share than information with their students. This additional factor is how people make decisions. The developers of Guided Design believe strongly that subject matter is important in a Guided Design course; however, it is the way that the student learns the relevant material that is different. For example, in the traditional class, content tends to be given to the student, either through lecture or through a lecture-discussion format. In the Guided Design class, projects provide the focus for the study of subject matter as it is applied to professional work.

Developing a Guided Design Project

The Guided Design project provides students with a model of the way in which some person or group might use key subject matter concepts to solve open-ended problems. Wales and Stager (1977) give 11 steps to assist instructors in developing a Guided Design project. The material below presents a slightly modified version of their guide.

Situation

Describe the setting and the open-ended problem that must be solved. If new concepts are to be learned in conjunction with this project, the situation should provide an appropriate setting for their use.

Goal of the Project Work

State the goal of this decision-making project. When the project is completed, what will be the result?

Gather Information

What information is needed to proceed with the problem solution and where can it be obtained? This step may require additional study, or it could simply mean organizing the background information available for the project.

Component Analysis

Answer the question, "What can be changed?" and list the major factors involved in the situation.

Possible Solutions

Answer the question, "How can each component be changed?" and list possible solutions for each component.

Constraints and Assumptions

List the factors that limit what can be done. In some cases the constraints serve as the criteria for evaluating possible solutions.

Choose

Using identified criteria, evaluate and rank the possible solutions. Before a solution is chosen for further work it should be tested for positive and negative consequences.

Analysis

Dissect the chosen solution, and identify the important factors that must be considered when a detailed solution is developed in the Synthesis step.

Synthesis

Combine the factors identified or the answers to the questions asked in the Analysis step and produce a detailed solution. Note that in the Feedback section of the specific Guided Design project a model solution could be used, or the solution could be left incomplete or omitted for students to learn on their own.

Evaluation

Describe either the evaluation of the solution or the way in which an evaluation could be performed.

Recommendations

Recommend an appropriate course of action.

For detailed information on developing a Guided Design project, the reader is directed to Wales and Stager's workbook (1977).

ORGANIZATION OF A GUIDED DESIGN CLASS

As with all classes, students must be oriented to the goals of the class and the method that will be used. It is important that students understand that the *process* is important and that they will be working closely with others. Depending on whether the instructor plans to develop the entire course around this teaching strategy or use it for several specific classes, the method for evaluating and grading students must be discussed. Wales and Stager (1977) use an exercise called "The Fishing Trip" to introduce their students to the method used in Guided Design learning. This exercise can be found in their workbook and provides a fun and interesting way to give students the opportunity to experience firsthand this problem-solving approach to learning. Regardless of whether or not an exercise is used, students should be urged to read carefully the introduction accompanying the Guided Design exercise, an example of which is provided at the end of this chapter.

To provide for the systematic development of decision-making skills, Guided Design course activities are organized around a series of structured projects, which students work through in small groups during class hours. Giving students the opportunity to find the solutions to a series of open-ended problems is substituted for the traditional linear development of class material. Each problem is designed in such a way that to arrive at a solution the students must apply the subject matter they are learning. The decision-making practice is guided by printed materials prepared by the teacher, designed to provide students with a "slow-motion" experience with the solution for each problem.

In a Guided Design class, students are divided into teams of four to eight students. Although the size of the group is flexible, it is important to remember that too small a group will not allow for the breadth of views of peers, and a group larger than eight may prevent students from sharing information with one another.

Each activity starts with a written instruction that describes a problem situation and specifies the role that the students are to play. They are then asked to identify the problem and set the goal for their work. Following discussion of the question, and after they have agreed on their response, the students give the instructor their written answer. The instructor reviews the students' response immediately. At that time, the instructor may suggest that the students continue to work on the specific part of the problem or may give the group the written feedback to that part of the problem. The students then have the opportunity to compare their result with the printed feedback page immediately, which shows how others who have studied the problem responded. Students are not asked to agree with the answer but rather to examine and consider other viewpoints. This pattern of question-response continues until the students complete their solution of the open-ended problem. The students are free to disagree with the feedback provided and may even develop a better solution. The students read from texts and journal articles to expand their understanding of the problem and the decisions to be made. It is not the actual solution to the problem that is the objective, but the process the students have learned in solving problems that is important. Guided Design combines concept learning and the development of decision-making skills needed to deal with complex problems. A sample of a Guided Design problem, and feedback used to introduce this process to beginning nursing students, will be found at the end of this chapter.

SIMILARITIES OF GUIDED DESIGN AND NURSING PROCESS

Building on the Guided Design systems approach for engineering students, Wales and Hageman (1979) developed this technique as a teaching strategy for nursing education. They described Guided Design as a trilevel system in which the lowest level is the learning of fundamental concepts, principles, and skills. The intermediate level is learning on

Figure 10-1
A Conceptual Model of Guided Design

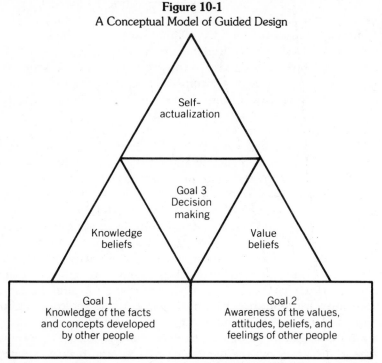

Reprinted from the JOURNAL OF NURSING EDUCATION, March 1979, vol. 18, No. 3, pp. 38–45.
Published by SLACK, Incorporated, Medical Publishers, copyright 1979.

closed problems, and the top level is problem solving on open-ended problems. The basic premise of Guided Design is that education should produce a whole or self-actualized person. This, according to these authors, includes the ability to make decisions based on personal knowledge and value beliefs. The model developed for Guided Design is shown in Figure 10–1.

Learning Objectives

The learning objectives for Guided Design include three major goals:

1. acquisition of knowledge
2. awareness of values
3. ability to make decisions

Wales and Hageman (1979) reinforce the notion that sound decision making requires both knowledge and values. Because one of the major

Table 10–1

	Guided Design	Nursing Process
Steps	1. Identify the problem	1. Assessing
	2. State the problem	
	3. Gather information (can occur here or with any of the other steps)	2. Planning
	4. List the constraints, assumptions, facts	
	5. List possible solutions	
	6. Choose the best solution	
	7. Analyze	
	8. Synthesize	
	9. Evaluate the plan	
	10. Implement the plan	3. Implementation
	11. Check the results	4. Evaluation

Reprinted from the JOURNAL OF NURSING EDUCATION, March 1979, Vol. 18, No. 3, pp. 38–45. Published by SLACK, Incorporated, Medical Publishers, copyright 1979.

goals of nursing education is to help students make decisions based both on knowledge and values, they believe that this approach will help to meet this curriculum goal.

Guided Design presents a challenge to each student's personal value system because every problem presented involves value judgments. Students are encouraged to make free choices from several alternatives after weighing various consequences. The instructor's values are not forced on students, but, rather, values are considered by the students themselves.

Comparison of Guided Design Steps and Nursing Process

In presenting the problem situation, the teacher selects a model problem for helping students learn to perform each individual step and deal with the complete sequence of steps involved in solving the problem. Wales and Hageman (1979) compare the 11 steps used in Guided Design problem solving and the four steps commonly used in the nursing process. These are shown in Table 10–1.

ADVANTAGES OF USING GUIDED DESIGN

Guided Design has been used by teachers in a number of disciplines in addition to engineering and nursing. Its proponents are enthusiastic about the results of using this teaching strategy. Student enthusiasm, motivation and excitement about learning, and increased retention of information are the most frequently cited advantages. Also, students develop more confidence in themselves and their leadership abilities. Perhaps most important, however, is that students recognize that real problems usually do not have a "neat" solution.

Applying the Guided Design technique in a course in nursing research at the master's degree level, Selby and Tuttle (1985) wanted to compare the attitudes of students in their course with student's learning research in a more traditional mode. They found that students who were exposed to Guided Design were significantly more positive in their attitudes toward research. Although their pilot group of students numbered only 25, they found that 71 percent of these students showed a positive change in attitude in respect to importance of research, 75 percent showed a positive attitude in respect to interest in research, and 92 percent stated that they had more confidence in their own ability to conduct supervised research. In addition, improvement in research knowledge as based on pre- and posttest scores was also significantly higher with these students. They also stress that in-class practice of research skills is important and that students are prevented from straying because they receive regular feedback from the written materials and their instructor, the study guide provided with the model, and the other group members.

DISADVANTAGES OF GUIDED DESIGN

As with all teaching strategies, there are disadvantages to the Guided Design model. Some students feel boxed in by the specific situation given to them. Others have difficulty with the intense group activities. From the instructor's viewpoint, developing a Guided Design problem and study guide is time consuming. Each problem must be tested before its use with a pilot group of students.

SUMMARY

As a teaching strategy, Guided Design utilizes many learning theories. Students are actively involved in their own learning; they receive immediate feedback; and both cognitive and process skills are simultaneously developed. Learning is organized around a problem situation, and, although there is no single correct answer to any of the problems, each requires the students to organize their knowledge and examine their attitudes and values toward alternate solutions. In the words of one beginning nursing student, "I am beginning to feel like a real nurse, and I haven't even seen a patient yet."

EXAMPLE OF A GUIDED DESIGN EXERCISE

Introduction

The example you are about to use is concerned with decision making, a basic intellectual process that makes it possible for you to face and solve new problems. The material is organized in an "Instruction-Feedback" pattern for you to participate in the solution of the problem. The purpose is to help you to become aware of the steps you go through in making a decision.

Each member of your group should read each Instruction, then you should discuss it as a team, decide on a group response, and compare your group's decision with the printed Feedback your instructor will then give you. The purpose of the printed Feedback is to allow your group, and each of you, to compare your reasoning with that of others who have worked with this problem. No one should feel that he/she has to accept any of these decisions or that these are the only decisions possible.

Each group should appoint a secretary to record the decisions made by his or her teammates. When the members of the group feel they have completed their answer, ask the instructor to come to the group to check the work or have the secretary take the record to the instructor. If the instructor feels the work has been completed, the secretary will receive copies of the Feedback and next Instruction to give to the group. The instructor may ask your group questions to stimulate further thinking.

INSTRUCTION A:

George P. is a junior in college. He fractured his right leg while skiing during the middle of the winter semester. He sustained no other physical injuries. He was treated by immobilizing his leg and he is now ambulatory.

You are the nurse at the Student Health Service.

What are some of the problems you might consider that George has?

FEEDBACK A:

You might have considered problems in mobility and in bathing. Although these two aspects of his life will undoubtedly be affected, these are general areas and others need to be specified.

INSTRUCTION B: Identify the Problem

At this time you may have some general hunches about the types of problems George is likely to have, but you need additional information in order to determine what specific problems he will have. Then you can decide what might be done about these problems.

What kind of information do you need to substantiate the existence of specific problems and the nature of those problems?

FEEDBACK B:

In order to know how George's mobility is affected you need to know:

1. What kind of a cast he has—above the knee or below the knee? Plaster or fiberglass (can he get it wet)?
2. Does he have a walking cast, or does he need crutches?
3. What are his living arrangements—does he live in a dorm? Apartment? House? Does he live alone? Are there steps?
4. How does he transport himself to school? Does he have others who can help him?
5. What does he do about meals?
6. Besides skiing, what does he do for recreation?

Depending on the answers to these questions, the nature of the problems will vary considerably.

INSTRUCTION C: Identify the Problem

You find out that George has an above-the-knee plaster cast, which cannot get wet, and he must use crutches. He lives on the second floor of a fraternity house near the university. He usually walked to school. He eats his meals at the fraternity house. Besides skiing, George usually jogged every day for exercise. He likes to go to movies and dance. He has had a steady girlfriend for about 1 year. All of his classes are in buildings with elevators.

Now, given the details of George's situation, what problems or potential problems do you think exist?

FEEDBACK C:

1. Mobility seems likely to be a significant problem:
   a. Getting to and from school.
   b. Getting around on crutches on campus and up and down the stairs at the fraternity house.
2. Sitting comfortably for any length of time may be a problem.
3. Sleep may be disrupted until he gets used to the cast.
4. Bathing may be a problem, and he is likely to need help in washing his hair.
5. His leisure activities will be disrupted—no jogging or dancing.
6. He may have a problem feeling dependent on others, since he will need help getting around and in personal hygiene.
7. He may worry about the intimate aspects of his relationship with his girlfriend.

INSTRUCTION D: Setting Goals:

George needs to make decisions about what to do with the problems that have been delineated. You need first to decide what goals you should set with George. What might be his short-term goals? What long-term goals would you establish with him?

FEEDBACK D:

The following are some possible short- and long-term goals.
Short term: George wants to:

1. keep up with his school work.
2. get around as much as possible on crutches.
3. be comfortable and sleep well.
4. continue socializing.

Long term: George's long-term goals might be to:

1. have his leg heal well and completely.
2. not get himself too much out of shape.
3. become independent again.

INSTRUCTION E: Interventions (what to do)

Based on George's goals, what might he do in order to meet these
goals?

FEEDBACK E:

George needs to identify who is willing and can help him to get around in school. He may need help learning to use crutches properly, carrying his books, and getting references from the library.

He also needs help washing his hair and, maybe, with bathing.

He needs to learn to arrange pillows so his sleeping positions are as comfortable as possible.

He needs to identify activities he can do comfortably. He might talk to his girlfriend about his fears about their relationship.

He needs to find out what exercises he can do to keep the rest of his body in shape without compromising the healing of his leg.

He needs to increase gradually his adeptness so that he can depend more on himself and less on others.

INSTRUCTION F: Evaluation

After 2 weeks, with the help of his girlfriend and two other friends, George is able to get around school and the fraternity house. He has made improvements in his ability to use crutches, but he finds that he is too exhausted in the evening to study or socialize or do any of the exercises he is allowed to do. He feels depressed.

How would you evaluate the effectiveness of George's plan?

FEEDBACK F:

Look back at George's goals and see which ones he was able to accomplish. You may find that he was able to achieve some, but not all, of his goals. There are three possible reasons for this: His goals were not realistic; his plan was not adequate to meet all of his goals, and it needs revision; or new information was introduced that required revision of goals and plans.

CONCLUSION

This decision-making process is a step-by-step process in which you need:

1. Information to identify the problem correctly.
2. Identification of the problem.
3. Setting of realistic goals and objectives (which are specific and can be measured and evaluated).
4. Interventions—a plan for achieving goals.
5. Evaluation—have the goals and objectives been met? If not, why?

The Nursing Process is a decision-making process that parallels this process and is the basis for clinical decision making in nursing.

1. *Assessment*—includes data collection based on a physical, psychosocial, and cultural assessment of a client, family, or community.
2. *Planning*—identification of problems, long- and short-term goals, and nursing diagnosis.
3. *Interventions*—what you do.
4. *Evaluation*—ongoing until all goals have been reached.

11

Teaching in the Clinical Setting

Nursing is a practice profession; therefore, experiences in the clinical setting are an integral part of the total educational process for nursing students. The primary purpose of clinical teaching is to provide students with opportunities to have contact with actual clients* in various situations and to use those theories, processes, and skills learned in other courses and settings. The clinical setting is where validation of previously learned principles and concepts occurs and where the use of skills learned in simulated environments takes place. Ideal clinical experiences are those which are closely relevant and timely to what is being taught in concurrent courses and which allow continued reinforcement and practice of what has been learned. Such experiences are vital to a student's developing both competence and self-confidence and the ability to use what has been learned in new, unfamiliar situations.

Those responsible for student learning in the clinical setting need to make sure that what takes place in that setting cannot be accomplished elsewhere. Those things that can be learned in a classroom or nonclinical laboratory should be learned at those sites. Client safety and constraints of time demand that the student be as well grounded as possible in necessary theories, processes, and skills before working with clients.

While the major emphasis of clinical experiences should be application of what has been learned in other settings, the clinical situation

*Since much of clinical teaching occurs outside a hospital setting, we have chosen to use the term *client* unless the discussion relates specifically to teaching in a hospital setting, where the term *patient* is used.

cannot be controlled. There will be times when students are confronted by situations with which they have had no prior experience. Consequently, teachers of nursing students must make an effort to focus clearly on specific objectives for the course and provide support and guidance in those situations for which the students cannot possibly be prepared. On the other hand, there will also be times when desired experiences are not available on a particular day or at a particular time. Again, teachers will need to focus clearly on course objectives in order to make each learning experience as productive as possible.

Topics that are particularly pertinent to setting up and implementing clinical learning experiences for students will be discussed here. Specific areas to be included are selection of clinical agencies for student experiences, planning for specific clinical experiences, implementation of the plan, and evaluation of student learning and performance.

SELECTION OF CLINICAL AGENCIES FOR STUDENT EXPERIENCES

With the decline in the number of diploma programs and the expansion of college- and university-based nursing education, most educational institutions no longer have direct access to clinical facilities. As a result, it is necessary to contract with various agencies in the community to provide student contact with clients.

Selection of agencies for clinical experience depends primarily on the objectives for the specific course; other important aspects directly associated with the course objectives are the type of desired experiences and the level of the student. If objectives indicate that the student is expected to provide direct care to clients and families, the agency selected must allow such activities. If the course is at the beginning level in the curriculum, the agency selected must provide the desired basic experiences for practice of beginning skills and processes being learned in other settings.

Thorough assessment of each agency before student placement must be completed so that the best possible match can be made. Faculty members teaching in the clinical laboratory are the ones who can provide much of the data for initial assessment and selection of clinical agencies. Further, teachers who work in a particular agency with students can provide ongoing input into the decision about whether that agency continues to provide the desired experiences for a specific group of students.

A tool outlining specific criteria for the selection and continued use of a particular agency is helpful for accomplishing the task of selection with the least amount of frustration and time. Several resources are available to help with this task (Hawkins, 1981; Murdock, 1978; National League for Nursing, 1973; Schweer, 1972). Examples of important areas in which to collect data for determining the potential for learning experiences of students are:

1. Agency philosophy and goals. Are they compatible with those of the educational institution?

2. Kind of agency and type of clients. Are the available clients appropriate to the type of experience needed?

3. Staffing patterns. Is staffing sufficient to provide an appropriate model of care? Is staffing adequate to allow staff involvement with students? Are staff members responsive in a positive way to the presence of students?

4. Geographic location. Is the agency accessible by public and private transportation? How far is it between the educational institution and the clinical setting (if students and faculty must travel between the two)?

5. Census statistics. Is the client population adequate to provide experiences for the anticipated number of students? To what extent is the agency being used by students from other nursing programs or health care fields?

6. Support services and human resources. Is the agency one that provides adequate exposure to a total health care team concept (residents, interns, pharmacists, occupational therapists, physical therapists, respiratory therapists, infection control personnel, dietitians, social workers, and other specialists)?

7. Available physical facilities. Do the physical facilities allow for desired practice? Are appropriate facilities available for conferences and consultation with students and for storage of educational materials and personal items? What facilities are available for student needs (library, cafeteria, parking)?

8. Special requirements of the agency. Does the agency require screening tests not already required by the educational institution (e.g., rubella and varicella titres)?

If these areas are carefully scrutinized, the agency selected for specific student experiences will more likely be appropriate. However, one must be aware that the health care delivery system is complex and everchanging. Health care programs and populations may change drastically from year to year. Thus, the tool that is developed for initial assessment of an agency should be used regularly (and revised if necessary) to decide if the agency is still appropriate to provide the experiences for which it was originally selected.

Competition for agencies among various types of educational programs for health care personnel has presented problems in recent years. Desired placements and times are not always possible. Overcrowding of clinical agencies with students may have a negative impact on both students' learning and the agency. Where such competition exists, the need for a close working relationship among the educational institutions involved and the available clinical agencies cannot be overemphasized. The situation also underscores the importance of using nonclinical settings, as mentioned previously, to prepare the student for the experience so that the emphasis in the clinical setting is on application and validation rather than on initial learning. The various programs needing clinical settings for student experiences also need to investigate possible alternatives. Greater flexibility is possible by using nontraditional agencies, when appropriate to learning objectives (possibilities include day-care centers, senior citizen centers, women's centers, self-help clinics, prisons, and other community settings), and by scheduling student experiences at other than traditional times (weekends, evenings, and nights).

Limitations on the degree of flexibility possible must be recognized, however. Certain types of clinical experiences, as in community health and some hospital areas, may not be available at nontraditional times. Some educational institutions restrict the scheduling of clinical classes to certain days and hours. Agencies accrediting educational programs place restrictions on the use of nonaccredited agencies. The situation requires discussion, negotiation, and creativity in order to deal with the limitations and obtain desired experiences for students.

Once the collection of data has been completed and it is decided that an agency is appropriate for the desired student experiences, a formal contract is signed by designated representatives of the clinical agency and the educational institution. The contract specifies the responsibilities of the agency and its personnel and those of the educational institution and its personnel.

PLANNING SPECIFIC CLINICAL EXPERIENCES

Once an agency has been selected and an agreement has been made between the agency and the educational institution, the specific planning to be done usually falls to the faculty member(s) working with students in that setting. There are a number of things that need to be done so that the chances for success of the relationship are increased.

Preliminary Planning with the Agency

One of the major areas of concern in preliminary planning with an agency is the dual orientation of faculty and staff. The faculty member needs to be oriented to the agency and the specific unit(s) to be used. Staff members need to be oriented to the goals and expectations of clinical experiences. Understandings need to be reached about individual responsibilities and expectations.

Faculty Orientation.   Orientation to the agency may be accomplished in a variety of ways. Some agencies require that faculty members attend the orientation for new staff members. At times, only selected parts of the orientation program will be required. In other instances, a person in the agency may be designated to provide a modified orientation program for those faculty members assigned to the agency. The faculty member can also complete independently much of the orientation to agency policies, procedures, and philosophy by observing, talking to selected people, and reading available manuals and publications.

Orientation to a specific unit within an agency is usually the personal responsibility of the faculty member, although unit personnel assist to varying degrees. It is helpful for the faculty member to spend time in the unit becoming familiar with staff members, clients, practices, and procedures. The amount of time required will vary, but it needs to be sufficient to allow the faculty member to function without unnecessary dependence on the staff for knowledge about everyday operations and standard nursing procedures. It must also be adequate to demonstrate that the faculty member is competent in the common nursing activities of the unit. Otherwise, a faculty member may be viewed as a highly educated person who is not competent in practice (Remember the old saying, "Those who can—do; those who can't—teach"?). This establishment of both collegiality and credibility is important to future successful working relationships between the faculty member and clinical staff. Other methods of instructor involvement with the staff that can help achieve collegiality and credibility include working with the staff on nursing care plans, presenting teaching conferences for staff, and sharing new and varied educational resources.

Staff Orientation and Involvement.   Agency personnel must be made aware of the goals and objectives for the specific clinical course. They need to know the level of the students, what the students can and cannot do, expectations for student performance, and what faculty and students expect of staff members. Ways to accomplish this include sharing course materials, individual and group conferences, informal conversations, and answering specific questions. After these have been done, it would also be helpful for the faculty member to write a formal letter to staff members summarizing the main points that have been discussed.

Teaching in the clinical area is seen as a major responsibility of nursing faculty members (McCabe, 1985). Staff members are involved in varying degrees, depending on the desired outcomes for the experience. Efforts to enhance student-staff relationships are desirable. Unfortunately, with the advent of nursing programs in educational settings rather than in service settings, clinical staff members have often been expected to practice a "hands-off" policy where students are concerned. Although the faculty member is seen as ultimately responsible for arranging and overseeing student experiences, students can gain much from a close working relationship with the staff. Certainly, the student becomes more acutely aware of the "real" world. Although this may not always be ideal, it allows a student to gain insight into what problems exist in daily practice. Further, the extent of learning experiences to which the student can be exposed will be greater since the base of supervision and guidance is more extensive.

Working with a student also provides the staff member with certain advantages. Greater insight into student needs and what part the available experiences and the staff member can play in meeting those needs can make the job of the staff member more satisfying. Depending on the level of the student, staff members also gain awareness of the capabilities and strengths of students and their potential for future employment in that setting. From the standpoint of recruitment, it is more likely that students who have positive experiences in a particular setting will return to that setting seeking employment after graduation (Joachim & Karampelas, 1982).

In many agencies classified as "teaching" institutions, working with students from various health fields is a prerequisite for a staff member's advancement in professional rank. Regardless of this requirement, there are staff members who will not want to work with students; some will feel threatened by the questions that students invariably ask. Others relish their involvement with students and the stimulation it provides in increasing their own knowledge base. The faculty member may have no control over which type of staff member a student will be working with. Those who feel threatened may be helped by a faculty member who reinforces observed strengths and offers guidance in how to increase positive feelings about working with students. Those who enjoy working with students need to have that behavior rewarded by positive feedback and by having contact with students who are well prepared and motivated.

There are many ways that staff involvement with students can be enhanced. As a result of working directly with students, staff members can provide valuable input to the faculty member about student needs and problems, as well as level of performance. They may be asked to participate in joint care-planning conferences with students. They may be invited as guest speakers/lecturers for clinical conferences or other classes. The various members of the health care team—nurses from specialty areas, such as a burn unit or an intensive care unit; nurses with special skills, such as working with abusive families; enterostomal therapists; respiratory therapists; dietitians; infection control nurses; and others— can inform students about their roles and responsibilities in relation to the care of clients in all settings and help acquaint students with a holistic health team concept.

Mutual Decisions.   Joint concerns, goals, and expectations between faculty and staff need to be established early in the relationship (Joachim & Karampelas, 1982). Faculty members and staff members need to be open about what these are. Certainly, client care is a major concern for both. In all types of settings, the staff member who would normally be responsible for a client retains that responsibility when a student is assigned. In fact, the staff member needs to maintain close contact with both the client and the student to insure that proper and safe care is provided.

Lines of Communication.   The lines of communication to be used are usually a concern of both faculty and staff. In the acute care setting, since staff members are still responsible for patient care, it is generally best if they give the report on a specific patient to the student assuming care. This direct contact permits the staff member to establish expectations for care and to inform the student about any special requirements for that patient. At the same time, the student can ask questions, share ideas about care, and let the staff member know if there is anything that the student will not be able to do or with which help will be required. During the time of care, it is also best for a student to go directly to the responsible staff member with questions, comments, and problems related to a patient. It is important for faculty members to inform students that it is useless to go to those not directly involved in the care of an assigned patient unless the responsible staff member is unavailable. Further, it is the staff member responsible who needs any information the student has related to that patient.

Staff members also need assurance that the faculty member has discussed with students the whole area of questions and comments about clients. Although questions and comments are certainly desirable and warranted, students need to develop an awareness of when and where they are appropriate. This is particularly true in a hospital setting. A student who asks a question or tries to give information about a patient when the staff member is involved in something that calls for full attention is likely to cause negative feelings on the part of the staff member. A student who asks a question or shares information in the presence of a patient, family members, or visitors when that is inappropriate is also likely to be perceived negatively.

Staff members also have certain responsibilities to students and faculty members in the area of communication. Reasonable expectations in a hospital setting include the availability of an up-to-date nursing care plan and medical plan, availability of the medical and nursing records, timely sharing of information about changes in patient status or care, prompt reporting of results of diagnostic tests, and assistance in those situations for which the student cannot yet assume responsibility. Such measures help to keep students and faculty members fully informed, decrease the need for questions from students, enhance the relationships of staff members with students and faculty members, and enhance the quality of care given.

Selection of clients.   Another area requiring discussion and joint-decision making is the procedure to be followed for client selection. The student is primarily a learner rather than a provider of service, thus the central aim is to provide the student with required learning experiences. The faculty member is the one who knows the objectives that must be achieved. However, staff members in all types of agencies must be involved in the selection of clients with whom students are to work. If staff members have been well informed about the objectives and the needs of students, they can provide valuable assistance to the teacher who may be in the clinical setting only 1 or 2 days a week. Staff members can provide vital input that can help a faculty member determine if assignment of a particular client will or will not be a good learning experience for a particular student. They are aware of clients or families who do not wish to have students assigned. They are aware of each client situation and the level of complexity. They are aware of specific client needs. They are aware of diagnostic tests or special procedures with which students may assist or which they can observe. Without such information from staff members, the task of client selection for student experience becomes much more difficult.

Policies and Procedures.   Specific policies and procedures to be followed within the agency by students and faculty members must be considered. For example, a faculty member needs to be well informed about policies of medication administration and any special guidelines and limitations. Possible questions include: What drugs require verification of dosage calculation by an R.N.? What drugs require supervision during administration? Are students restricted from giving medications by a particular route (e.g., IV push)? What is the procedure to be followed when errors are made? What are the procedures used for emergencies or fires?

Another important area is record keeping. The faculty member needs to know about any specific requirements or practices. Possible questions include: What type of charting is used in the setting? What are all the different places where a particular piece of information must be noted (bedside records, team leader's worksheet, client's chart, and so forth)?

Timing of Student Experiences.   Staff members need an opportunity to give input about timing of student experiences. In a hospital setting, for example, it may be viewed as disruptive to have students entering a unit midshift. At the same time, it may be next to impossible for a student just entering a unit to locate a patient's chart or care plan at the end of a shift. If any flexibility is possible, the faculty member may find it advantageous to adjust the time that students are entering a unit, leaving a unit, or both, so that disruption is kept to a minimum while assuring student access to necessary resources for learning and patient care. Generally, it is most helpful if students are present for an entire shift. This pattern follows the natural flow and normal operation of the unit. If students will not be in a unit for a whole shift, the faculty member needs to look carefully at what learning experiences are desired and when they can best be obtained. The major factor limiting the ability to practice such flexibility would be the presence of different student groups in the same unit.

IMPLEMENTATION OF STUDENT EXPERIENCES

Once all necessary preliminary arrangements and discussions have taken place, the faculty member is ready to initiate the actual experiences with students in the selected agency. Areas to consider are student orientation, assessment of students, and daily operations.

Student Orientation

Ample orientation of students to the agency and the unit will pay off in dividends of decreased student anxiety and improved student assimilation of orientation content. With less clinical time, an instructor may feel the need to limit orientation and provide more time for contact with clients. However, just as with faculty members, students must be adequately knowledgeable about basic policies and procedures in order to make the best use of the time and the facilities with as little interruption in the usual routines as possible. Students' presence will invariably alter the operation of the staff to some extent, but every effort must be made to make any changes that occur as constructive as possible.

Basic methods of student orientation include tours, games, conferences, and special assignments. Although students cannot be expected to remember everything they are told and shown during orientation, they should be able to get an overall picture of the agency and unit, types of clients served, policies, and daily routines. Important areas to include in general *agency* orientation are location and general function of various departments; titles and roles of selected personnel; location of areas that will be used throughout the experience (conference rooms, cafeteria, library, pharmacy, radiology department, medical records, and so forth); and information about parking and transportation. In a *hospital* setting, important areas for orientation to a specific unit where students are assigned include type of patients; physical setup of the unit and what can be found in each area (patient areas, kitchen, utility room, supply room, linen room, and so forth); regular personnel and staffing patterns; unit policies and daily routines; and standard forms and their use.

Tours are helpful for providing an overview of the agency and the unit. Tours are more informal and allow time for highlighting important points by the faculty member and asking questions as needed for clarification by the student. Following a tour, time may be allotted for students to work individually or in pairs to further their own orientation by completing a directed activity using a modification of the old treasure hunt game. It is designed according to specific goals and needs of a particular group and the characteristics of a particular setting. An example of an activity used in a pediatric, acute care setting with students in their first experience with sick clients is shown in Appendix 1. It directs students to relocate those items and areas seen during a tour of the unit which are especially pertinent to their experience. Further, students have an opportunity to spend some time analyzing and making notes about use of standard forms with which they will have to work. The game helps reinforce what has been covered during the general orientation and decreases the amount of stress a student feels by allowing time to reinvestigate and assimilate what has been included.

Another activity that may be useful for a more complete orientation to a unit is to give each student a short assignment with a specific goal and purpose. One example is to have students work with a patient alongside regular staff members for a designated period of time on the first or second day on the unit. Such an activity could focus on one or more areas of concern. Possibilities include initial assessment of a patient, unit routines, use of bedside records, and getting to know staff members. The experience provides low-stress contact with a patient, an introduction to staff members and routines, and an opportunity for self-assessment in relation to requirements and activities of the course. An additional benefit (through vicarious learning) can be achieved by having students share their impressions, experiences, and feelings with the whole class during either an informal discussion or formal conference, and the teacher can answer questions or explain further about future experiences and expectations. Other activities, such as review and discussion of nursing care plans or nurses' notes from the unit or role-played situations on areas of student concern, may also be a part of the orientation conference. The selection of specific activities depends on the objectives of the course, the level and needs of the students, and the type of hospital unit.

A group orientation conference is also necessary so that specific objectives, requirements, and expectations of the course can be discussed. Some of this may be done verbally, but it is also helpful to have handouts or written guides to which students can refer later when their anxiety level is lower and they are involved in doing the required activity. Included are instructions about required written work and special clinical activities. Selected materials may be given to students ahead of time so that they can read and jot down questions before the orientation period. Along the same line, specific readings or audiovisual media related to the client population with which the students will be working may be assigned before the orientation. Such advanced preparation saves orientation time and makes use of the time that is available more productive.

Although the focus of the preceding discussion has been on a traditional clinical setting in a hospital, it applies equally well to any other agency used for student experiences. Some adjustments are required with different settings, but major areas of concern and the basic process remain the same.

Assessment of Students

In any setting it is essential that the teacher obtain information about individual students so that appropriate learning experiences can be selected. While much of this information comes directly from the student, additional resources include the student's record and previous instructors. Ultimately, the current instructor needs to develop a picture of student strengths and limitations, barriers and positive influences, goals and aspirations, extent of motivation, and student perceptions of learning and the instructor (Little & Carnevali, 1972). Much of the data in these areas may be obtained by having the student answer several open-ended questions. Examples of useful questions are:

1. What nursing experiences have you had before entering this nursing program?
2. If you are currently working, describe briefly the type of work, number of hours worked per week, and what impact this is likely to have on your school work.
3. What degrees or educational experiences besides nursing do you have?
4. What other responsibilities do you have that may affect your school work?
5. What do you hope to accomplish during this clinical experience? Be as specific as possible about personal educational goals, interests, and needs.
6. What do you see as your major strengths?
7. What are the major areas in which you feel you need to improve?
8. What type of teaching behaviors work best in helping you learn?
9. Is there anything else that you would like your clinical instructor to know?

Options for getting the responses to these questions include interviewing, using a standard written format, or using a computer program into which student responses can be recorded and filed. The student may also be asked to provide other basic information needed by the teacher and the agency, such as the student's telephone number, status

of malpractice coverage, information about specific health requirements, and currency of CPR certification. Whatever method is used to
obtain this information, it is helpful if the instructor also has a follow-
up conference with each student in order to initiate the teacher-student
relationship and provide clarification as needed.

Daily Operations

Once the basic orientation has been completed and the teacher has obtained needed information about each student, planned student experiences with clients can begin. The first thing to consider is the selection
of clients with whom students are to work. By being aware of student
strengths and needs and by knowing the emphasis of concurrent nursing courses, the teacher will be able to guide the selection of clients who
will best help the students achieve course objectives.

Making the Assignments.   The teacher can make the assignment, have
the students select their own clients, or select a pool of clients from which
the students then make their own selection. If the students have the
option of personal selection, the teacher must participate by helping the
student know how different assignments can help achieve course objectives and by guiding the student in selecting according to degree of complexity, type of experience, and opportunities for growth. Throughout
the selection process, staff members need to be given an opportunity to
provide information that relates to the assignments made. Specific types
of useful information available from staff members have already been
discussed.

Once assignments are made, they must be posted in a predetermined
location for both students and staff. Further, depending on the standard
forms used in a particular setting, additional methods of communication
can be used. In a hospital setting, for example, it is helpful to attach a
note to the patient's nursing care plan, medical plan, and medication
record so that the responsible staff member knows immediately that a
student is assigned.

A teacher may choose to use different types of assignments in different situations, depending on the type of client, the learning level of the
student, and the objectives of the course. Several types to consider are
individual assignment, dual assignment, alternative assignment, and
preceptorship.

Individual Assignment.   Individual assignment is when one student is assigned to one or more clients. The student may be responsible for only certain aspects of care or for total care.

Dual Assignment.   Dual assignment is when a student is assigned to work with one or more clients along with another student or staff member. This type of assignment is particularly appropriate in a hospital setting when the level of complexity of care is beyond the capabilities of an individual student although certain elements of care can be performed. Benefits of dual assignment include decreased anxiety and the development of a mutually supportive relationship. When the dual assignment pairs a student with a staff member, further benefits include establishing a relationship between staff member and student, decreasing the extent of reality shock for the student, providing a role model for the student, and enhancing the socialization of the student into the practice role. It is vital that the instructor orient the staff member to what can be expected of the student and what the specific objectives are for the assignment. Otherwise, the experience may become fragmented and undirected, or the student may become nothing more than a "go-fer."

When two students are assigned to one or more clients, it is vital that they work closely together so that important aspects of care will not be overlooked. Dual assignments often help to lower students' stress level, thus increasing their ability to focus on desired learning. Also, particularly with beginning students in a hospital setting who require closer supervision and lots of support, dual assignments decrease the number of clients with which the teacher must become familiar and increase the ability of the teacher to be available when needed.

Another type of dual assignment may be used when the teacher wishes to give students more responsibility but the patient population does not permit assigning several patients to each student. In this case, it is possible to have two students work with three clients, sharing responsibilities. This not only increases the amount of responsibility for each student but requires that they communicate clearly and plan carefully what each will do.

Dual assignments may also be used in community settings with students making initial home visits. The student may make early home visits with a staff member as role model or with another student as peer and support person. In the latter situation, the students can help one another in collecting important data, determining needs of clients, doing necessary teaching, making referrals, and recording what has occurred. Although one of the students would have primary responsibility, the other serves as an observer and helper. The roles then would reverse for the next client. An important teacher role in using this type of assignment is the appropriate pairing of students and the use of methods to assure that both students are meeting desired objectives and that both students are fulfilling individual responsibilities. One suggestion is to have intermittent individual and paired conferences with the students.

Alternative Assignment.   Alternative types of assignments may be utilized when the individual needs of students call for different types of experience, when the available number of patients drops below that desired for the number of students, and when the alternative assignment helps to meet specific objectives of a course.

One example of an alternative assignment in a hospital setting is that of "helper." Basically, this assignment involves a student working in a support capacity with several other students in their individual assignments with patients. It is most useful for those students who are enrolled in beginning clinical courses but who have had some prior experience and need more of a challenge and expanded contact with a greater number of clients. It is also useful when the available patient group does not permit individual assignment with several patients. Major benefits for using this technique accrue from the broader experience and from the emphasis on time management, communication, expanded knowledge base about various aspects of care, involvement with a greater number of nursing care procedures, and more extensive exposure to clients and other members of the health care team. The helper is involved in all aspects of care—assessment, planning, implementation, and evaluation—and assists with various procedures, obtaining required materials, communicating with staff members and physicians, and documenting nursing observations and actions. Also, the helper gains increased awareness about how other students function and an increased understanding of the roles of both staff nurses and instructors.

Other types of alternative assignments are possible, depending on the particular clinical setting in which the student is located. For example, in a pediatric, acute care setting, students may be assigned for one experience to provide diversional and social activity for a group of selected children. By doing so, the students have an opportunity to gain in-depth knowledge about growth and development, how illness and hospitalization affect children of different ages, and how the nurse can intervene to decrease the negative impact of illness and hospitalization and enhance the opportunities for growth. A similar activity could also be used with adult patients.

Presently, faced with a declining client population in acute care settings, it is increasingly important that faculty members consider other settings besides hospitals where students can get experience in working with adults and children who are ill. One way to accomplish this is for the student to work through a home care agency in providing needed services to patients who are being discharged from the hospital setting at a higher level of acuity. Such an alternative assignment would only be appropriate when the individual student has the skills needed for a particular situation or when the student can be assigned with a more experienced practitioner.

Ideally, the greater the flexibility in a particular curriculum, the more varied the types of assignments that can be used. For example, in a modularized curriculum, the precise types of experiences desired in a clinical setting are identified. If this involves working with a diabetic client, the student would complete a theoretically based independent learning module covering concepts about diabetes mellitus. Once that module is mastered, the student would complete other modules on such topics as diabetic teaching and administration of insulin, skills needed for work with the diabetic client. As part of the skills modules, the student would have to schedule independent practice in a simulated environment and demonstrate proficiency at a prescribed level (as measured by stated competencies) before having contact with a client. Once both cognitive and psychomotor skills are mastered at the prescribed level, the student would contract with a teacher in different clinical settings for actual experience with a diabetic client. The clinical setting could be the home, a nursing home, a clinic, or a hospital, depending on which aspect of care is desired for the student. Another possible requirement might be that the student have contact with a diabetic client in at least two different settings. Thus, different students could be doing different things at the same time; a student could progress at a faster or slower rate; and there would be less need for a particular type of client, in a particular setting, at a particular time for an entire student group.

Preceptorship.   Although preceptorships may be viewed as a type of dual assignment, they are considered separately here since they usually involve a more formal relationship and some type of formal agreement. An in-depth discussion of preceptorships is beyond the scope of this chapter; however, it is mentioned as a type of assignment especially appropriate to use with undergraduate students nearing graduation and employment and with graduate students learning a clinical or functional specialty.

In a discussion of the historical development of use of clinical preceptors, Backenstose (1983, p. 9) reviews the changing relationships between nursing education and nursing service and their individual roles in teaching nursing students. It is her contention that the use of clinical preceptors is not new since, before the advent of nursing programs in college and university settings, practicing nurses were the ones who taught nursing students. Once nursing education began its movement into academic settings, nursing service and nursing education became more and more separated. Those teaching nursing students were educators who were often far removed from the practice setting. Nursing service personnel were less and less involved with teaching.

At present, nursing students assigned to clinical agencies invariably have contact with staff members in that agency who serve as role models and mentors. The extent of involvement of staff members with student teaching depends on the type and level of student, the staffing patterns in the agency, the willingness of the staff member to be involved, and the receptiveness of the faculty member to that involvement. The amount of direct teaching a staff member does can range from none to a great deal.

Although the term, preceptor, simply means "tutor" and *could* apply to any teaching activity between one person and another, it generally is used in nursing to refer to a more formal arrangement that pairs a novice with an experienced person for a specific educational purpose. As used in this chapter it refers to a formal relationship between a student (novice) and staff member (experienced nurse) in which the staff member serves as mentor, role model, consultant, supervisor, and facilitator for a designated period of time. Its specific purpose is socialization into a new role (Morrow, 1984, p. 4) while facilitating the student's development of clinical competence and decreasing the amount of reality shock experienced. The student will experience the full impact of the reality setting yet have the preceptor readily available for consultation and support.

This more formal type of preceptorship has existed in nursing education since the 1960s (Mahr, 1979). They were first introduced using physicians as preceptors in teaching physical assessment skills to nurses who were being prepared as primary health care practitioners. More recently, preceptorships have been used in both elective and required courses with graduate and undergraduate students (Adams, 1980; Archer & Fleshman, 1981; Chickerella & Lutz, 1981; Christman, 1979; Clark, M.D., 1981; Crancer, Fournier, & Maury-Hess, 1975; Dobbie & Kalinsky, 1982; Ferguson & Hauf, 1973a and b; Limon, 1984; Mahr, 1979; Maraldo, 1977; Stuart-Siddall & Haberlin, 1983; Walters, 1981).

Preceptorships are also widely used in other areas of nursing. Maraldo (1977) discusses their usefulness for improving health care in underserved areas and helping experienced nurses get instruction in a specialized role. Others describe the use of preceptorships for new graduate orientation (Dell & Griffith, 1977; McGrath & Koewing, 1978; May, 1980) and staff development (Morrow, 1984). The increasing use of preceptorships reflects a willingness by both education and service to share the responsibility for educating the novice (Limon, 1984) and helping students to "bridge the gap" between being a student and being a graduate. Also, preceptorships expand the available number of clinical placements, thus improving the quality and appropriateness of the type of experience that can be provided.

As with any other educational endeavor, a careful planning process is crucial to the success of the preceptorship experience. Two critical elements to consider in the planning phase are the characteristics of the preceptor and desired learning outcomes for the student. Preceptors are selected using criteria established by the educational institution in relation to the objectives. Some educational settings require that preceptors have a master's degree, although the most critical requirement is clinical expertise and experience. Amount of experience required may be regulated by state law. In California a "clinical teaching assistant" must have had at least 1 year's experience within the past 5 years in the practice of professional nursing in the clinical area to which assigned (California Board of Registered Nursing, 1985, section 1427[5]). Other areas to consider include interpersonal skills, teaching and leadership ability, and professional attitudes and commitment (Morrow, 1984, p. 52).

Selection of the preceptor is closely related to the student's learning objectives, since they will determine which preceptor in which setting would be most appropriate. Identification of specific objectives and determination of the time frame in which they are to be accomplished are usually arrived at jointly by the teacher and student. Objectives indicate to all participants what the student is to know and do by the end of the experience.

The various aspects of the student-preceptor relationship are negotiated, and the responsibilities of the preceptor, student, and faculty member are clearly delineated. The culmination of the negotiation process is a formal contract or letter of agreement between the educational institution and the agency/preceptor. An example of a preceptorship contract used in the Rural Clinical Nurse Placement Center—California State University, Chico, is shown in Appendix 2. A more in-depth discussion of the use of contracts and the process involved in their development may be found in Chapter 14.

The benefits of preceptorships to those involved are enumerated by Backenstose (1983, pp. 11–15), Limon (1984), and Morrow (1984, pp. 10–13). Benefits to the student include improved socialization into the professional practice role; involvement in learning activities that more closely parallel personal learning needs; ability to learn about the requirements of actual practice without assuming full responsibility; accumulation of practical knowledge; development of collaborative relationships with practicing nurses and practitioners from other disciplines; decrease in the impact of reality shock; increased awareness of problems, conflicts, and relationships in the clinical setting; and increased confidence and competence when performing clinical skills.

Benefits to the preceptors include professional stimulation and increased opportunities for learning; improved knowledge and skills, particularly in teaching and evaluating the performance of others; development of new professional relationships; satisfaction of having an impact on the teaching-learning process of the student; and increased status in the agency and among peers.

Benefits to the agency include improved recruitment and retention of recent graduates; development of a closer working relationship with the educational institution; increased availability of faculty members for consultation; and, ultimately, improved quality of care.

Benefits to faculty members include increased opportunities for collaboration and communication and the development of collegial relationships with those in clinical agencies; improved insight into the roles and responsibilities of the staff nurse; increased satisfaction from more successful student experiences; and availability of more time to focus on student objectives and provide guidance for the application of theory to practice.

Helping Students Learn in the Clinical Setting. A teacher is usually more directly and personally involved with students in the clinical setting than is possible in other types of courses. Through this involvement, the teacher is in the unique position of having a major influence on student learning, motivation, and overall progress toward development as a health care professional. Teacher activities include working with the student during preparation for the clinical experience, at the time of actual client care, during follow-up activities, and for evaluation of student learning and performance.

Preparation. Once an assignment is made, the student needs an opportunity to prepare for what will be involved in working with the client, whether in a hospital or community setting. In a hospital setting, total care is usually the desired goal; however, it is dependent on the level and abilities of the student. It may be necessary, for example, to ask staff members to carry out certain requirements of care when the student has not yet learned about a particular area needed for total care. Although the student may not be directly responsible, it is still important that preparation in that area be done so that care of a client is seen in its total context.

One format for preparation includes a combined use of the case study and the nursing care plan. The case study method requires that the student obtain information about the various aspects of a client situation including diagnosis and treatment regime, while the nursing care plan focuses on specific and individualized care in relation to identified nursing problems.

Preparation starts with obtaining information about current status of the client. Available resources include the medical care plan, the nursing care plan, the client's record, the medication record, bedside records (if they are used), members of the health care team, and the client and/or family. For the beginning student, a guide that helps to focus the collection of data on vital information is helpful. Suggested areas to include are client initials and age, diagnosis, surgical procedures, treatments, medications, and laboratory or other diagnostic tests.

After this basic information about the client is gathered the student will need to review theoretical content, which will clarify and explain the client situation as well as determine specific nursing implications associated with the medical regime. Resources needed to complete these tasks include textbooks, notes or other materials from related courses, agency manuals, and nonprint audiovisual materials. Depending on the type of resource, they may be owned by the student or available in the clinical unit, an agency library, or a learning resource center or library on campus. The shorter the amount of time allowed for preparation, the more lenient the teacher needs to be in the depth and breadth of what is expected.

Several possibilities exist for specific areas to include in student preparation. The following are suggested as elements of a basic framework through which students can gain insight into a client situation in which the person has been hospitalized:

1. Writing a definition of the diagnosis and describing the related pathophysiology
2. Describing past or planned surgical procedures
3. Stating why various treatments are required and identifying related nursing responsibilities
4. Describing each medication in relation to action, effects desired, dosage range, side effects, and major nursing implications
5. Describing each diagnostic test in relation to normals, what is

being tested, existing variations from normal in the client, and related nursing responsibilities

Study in these areas, along with the data obtained about the specific client situation, serves as the basis for identification of major nursing problems and the development of an individualized nursing care plan. Development of a nursing care plan is believed to help students become more effective decision makers when applying knowledge to the clinical situation. Jenkins (1985) stresses the importance of clinical decision making and states the belief that decision making is a skill that can be learned and that effective decision making is enhanced through education and opportunities for practice. One format to provide this practice may simply be a listing of identified nursing problems followed by an outline of major assessments, planned interventions, and measures to evaluate effectiveness of care in each problem area. The teacher can then review the student's work before and during client care and react to ideas presented, guide the student in new directions, make suggestions about care, and correct misconceptions. Other strategies to help students learn and practice clinical decision making are discussed elsewhere in this book. (See Chapter 3 for a discussion of simulations, Chapter 10 for a discussion of Guided Design, and Chapter 15 for a discussion of computer simulations.)

In addition to the development of a nursing care plan for major problem areas, the student needs to prepare an organizational plan for the designated time in the clinical area. Questions suggested by Predd (1982) to help in preparing such a plan are:

1. What must be done immediately?
2. What must be done on a schedule?
3. What must be done sometime during the shift?
4. What would be good to do if time permits?

One tool that can be used is a timed card on which a brief note can be made at specific times for checking such things as IVs and dressings, giving medications, and performing specific procedures. Notes can also be made about necessary observations. Students can then carry the organizational plan with them, refer to it throughout the time in the clinical area, check things off as they are completed, make additions as needed, and use the card as a guide for documenting care in the patient's record. As with the proposed nursing care plan, the teacher can review the organizational plan before and during patient care. The teacher will then be able to determine when students will need assistance, how well they have identified appropriate priorities, and make suggestions for change, if needed.

Depending on the particular focus of the clinical course, other areas of preparation may also be necessary. Possibilities include preparation about team leadership, primary nursing, time management, communication strategies, and clinical problem solving. Whatever the specific focus of the clinical experience, students are usually required to establish personal learning goals and objectives that reflect that focus. Often these will involve application of theoretical content or the performance of psychomotor skills. Upon the completion of each clinical experience, the student would then document what learning occurred and describe how that learning was applied to client care.

In all areas of preparation, students need specific guidelines to help them prepare in the way desired by the teacher. Guidelines may be provided both in written and verbal form. Each is helpful for reinforcement so that students clearly understand what is expected of them. One method of verbal input is preconferencing with students individually or as a group. In this way, the teacher can ask questions to stimulate student investigation, provide feedback on student work and plans, and make specific suggestions as required.

Client Care.   Valuable experience is gained from working with clients. It is only through the contact with actual clients that a student has the opportunity to use knowledge, processes, and skills and progressively develop the level of functioning desired for a beginning health care professional. The purpose, then, of clinical teaching is to assist students in making the necessary applications and developing the desired competencies.

The learning climate established by the teacher has a major impact on how well students are able to achieve this goal. The teacher needs to be able to provide support, yet allow the students freedom to test individual abilities and ideas. The teacher needs to be able to encourage students to do their best, yet keep stress at an optimal level so they *can* do their best. Neither of these is an easy task in a situation where the primary concern is client safety and welfare.

Thus, the clinical situation is one that provokes anxiety for both the teacher and the student. Stress experienced by nursing students is seen as a significant deterrent to success in nursing schools (Policinski & Davidhizar, 1985). These authors view stress as a special problem of beginning students who are insecure about new procedures and afraid of forgetting something important or hurting someone. Most students are motivated to do well in the clinical setting. When they appear disinterested and unmotivated it may be that they fear making a mistake or failing. Students do not intentionally harm anyone. They do not purposely make mistakes or overlook key observations.

The teacher is concerned about providing the best learning experiences while maintaining client safety. The problem is magnified, particularly in hospital settings, when student groups are large, the level of acuity is high, the available patient pool is too low for the number of students, staff members are minimally involved with students, or there are one or more students having difficulties with learning or performing in the clinical situation.

Policinski and Davidhizar (1985, p. 35) discuss the role of faculty members in working with the novice. They stress the importance of the teacher focusing less on supervision and more on guidance.

> The faculty-student relationship required by the novice is less that of supervisor to student and more that of clinical advisor to novice, the 'mentoring' relationship. In the mentoring relationship an older, wiser, and more experienced person guides and nurtures a younger individual. The mentor maximizes student accomplishments by providing warmth and empathy, decreases feelings of inadequacy, and assists the mentee through stressful experiences. The mentor focuses less on criticism, authority, and grades, and more on support, affirmation, and problem-solving skills.

Student motivation and learning are enhanced when the teacher is closely and purposefully involved with them. Providing supervision and support during student activities with clients is a major part of clinical teaching. At the same time, the teacher needs to use various strategies to help the student learn as much as possible. Strategies for preparation already discussed help to focus the student's attention and influence the quality of performance. A common teaching strategy during actual care that helps the student relate theory to practice is directed questioning and discussion. Kilty (1982) differentiates between learning "by" experience and learning "from" experience. To facilitate learning "by" experience while involved in a particular learning situation, the teacher can ask the student about thoughts and feelings or to identify what is noticed in a particular situation. Craig and Page (1981), Morrow (1984, pp. 162–163), and Wenk and Menges (1985) provide specific guidelines for the effective use of questions. An adaptation of their work pertinent to clinical teaching is presented here:

1. Questions should make students think and respond in relation to the current clinical situation.
2. Terminology used must be clear and familiar to the student.

3. Divergent questions (those for which there are several possible satisfactory answers) are most useful for clinical learning.

4. Open-ended questions elicit a greater amount of information.

5. Once a question is asked, the time allowed before an answer is demanded should be adequate to let the student think about and organize an answer. Increasing the amount of wait time is thought to create an atmosphere more conducive to higher-level thinking.

6. Techniques for reinforcement during questioning that are most likely to motivate and help students with clinical application are attentiveness, encouragement, patience, and positive comments about efforts.

Questions can also be a useful technique for directing student attention to important points. In some cases, it may even be useful to let the student know in advance what questions will be asked later. This technique is particularly useful with beginning students who need direction in identifying the most important areas for which to prepare. (See Chapter 5 for a more in-depth discussion of the use of questioning to facilitate learning.)

Transfer of knowledge and skills to the clinical area is not an automatic process. Students need help in recalling and applying theoretical concepts and principles to the present situation. They also need a lot of support and guidance while performing basic skills until they reach the same level of proficiency in the clinical laboratory as they had previously attained in a simulated setting. Often the achievement of true proficiency is unattainable, since a student may not have more than one opportunity to perform some skills in the clinical setting. These students need to be reassured that they will have similar experiences later and that greater competence and confidence will be attained with continuing experience.

Follow-up Activities.   Topics in this section include postcare conferences, logs and diaries, nursing care plans, and process recordings. Each can help students learn from their experiences and document the learning that has occurred. Learning "from" experience focuses on reviewing the experience to identify the learning that has occurred (Kilty, 1982) and to help give meaning to the experiences. As with transfer of learning, this does not happen automatically. Students must be helped to bring learning to a conscious level, to analyze adequacy of performance, and to identify areas and plans for change. These activities also provide the teacher with tools for evaluation of learning and performance to augment the observations made in the clinical setting.

Postcare conferences are one of the most common forms of retrospective review of clinical experiences. The most common site used is a classroom or conference room, although walking rounds in the clinical unit may be used as well. One format recommended is student presentations and discussions. A major emphasis should be placed on the conscious recall and application of knowledge to the clinical situation, particularly in relation to theories, processes, and skills being taught in concurrent and previous courses. The teacher's roles include listener, moderator, questioner, encourager, and facilitator. While the content of postcare conferences should be focused, an open format allows freedom of discussion and requires a teacher who is able to tolerate a low level of structure. Major advantages of conferences in which students participate with their peers include feedback to one another about learning, multiplication of the scope of learning, help from others in the group for solving clinical problems, increased self-confidence in participation in group discussions, and increased cooperation among students (Krawczyk, 1978).

A clinical log or diary includes a record of personal experiences, observations, and thoughts in relation to the clinical setting. Its purposes are to provide a method for student review and reaction to experiences and provide data to the teacher upon which to base decisions about the teaching-learning process (Crowley, 1965). It demonstrates how well the student is assimilating and applying content from other classes to clinical practice. As Cooper (1982) points out, content in diaries or logs should be more than a mere description of the learning experience. Thus, an analysis of what, why, where, and how forces the student to think about the experience, reinforces the learning that has occurred, and indicates areas that require further study.

At times, students may feel that logs or diaries and the documentation for learning are "busy work"; however, this is less likely to occur if the teacher shows evidence of thoughtful consideration of what has been included through comments, positive feedback, and suggestions for further study. In addition, the prompt review and return of these assignments will be more likely to have a positive influence on student perceptions of their value.

The nursing care plan is an extension of the work done by the student in preparation for client care. It involves a thorough analysis of each client situation in relation to major problem areas, goals, desired outcomes, interventions, and evaluation. It should also include theoretical support for problems identified and scientific rationale for actions taken. In contrast to the tentative plan completed in preparation for care, the nursing care plan completed as a follow-up to the clinical experience reflects what actually occurred, how well tentative plans were accomplished, and any changes needed in approach. Analysis of nursing care is used in an attempt to help students relate theory and practice, face new situations logically, and solve current problems using previously learned materials (Bell & Marcinek, 1985). The nursing care plan is a tool that stresses both process and content and helps students develop a pattern of problem solving that will be useful throughout their nursing careers. The use of the tool operates on the assumptions that decision making can be learned and that one can become a more effective decision maker through education and practice.

The process recording is another method used in some areas for clinical teaching (Morrow, 1984, p. 146; Schweer, 1972, pp. 167–170). It is an individual learning activity that supplements the nursing care plan for the analysis of nursing care. Process recordings contain verbatim notes of what was said during a student-client encounter. It provides an opportunity for retrospective analysis of interactions, thoughts, and feelings that occurred during contact with clients. Although process recordings can be used anywhere, the two areas in which they are most commonly used are psychiatric and public health settings.

EVALUATION OF STUDENT LEARNING AND PERFORMANCE

The purpose of this section is not to discuss the how and why of evaluation, but rather to comment on the dilemma facing teachers and students in the clinical setting when learning and evaluation are occurring simultaneously. As stated above, if learning opportunities are limited so that all students cannot have repeated contact with a particular situation in order to gain proficiency, evaluation becomes extremely difficult. It may even be unfair to evaluate the performance of a student who is doing something for the first time in a "real" setting. For example, although a student is able to give a polished performance of administering an IV medication via piggyback method in a simulated setting, that same student must be considered a new learner when it comes to performing the same skill in an acute care medical-surgical setting. So many new variables are present that were not factors in the simulated setting—doctors and other staff members may be present, the patient may be asking questions, family members may be at the bedside (also asking questions), the equipment may be different, plus others. The problem is magnified if there has been a lapse of time of more than a few days between practice in the simulated setting and performance in the clinical setting. At most the student can be evaluated on the ability to recall certain specifics from prior learning—what basic supplies are needed, how to do necessary calculations, how to reconstitute the drug, and key steps to take in giving the medication—but not on the finesse or speed of performance. In fact, even in the above areas, it is essential that the teacher focus the student's attention on pertinent points and ask specific goal-directed questions to assist the student with transferring knowledge from the simulated setting to the reality setting. Further, each clinical teacher must remember that the objectives of courses are designed to be accomplished by the *end* of the course and that students, along the way, need to be able to function and develop without always being evaluated.

Although the student must be given some freedom to make mistakes, the clinical setting deals with "real" people, and it is not possible to purposely allow mistakes when safety of the client may be jeopardized. Any situation in which a client is perceived at risk because of student action must be carefully analyzed and discussed with the student. For most students, making a mistake in the clinical setting is a powerful basis on which to base learning and improved performance. Rarely do students appear unconcerned that they have made mistakes and, if they do, it is very likely a defensive, protective mechanism against fear of failure.

Another factor placing limitations on teacher-student interaction for the purpose of learning in the clinical area is time. There are many occasions when a nursing procedure must be accomplished without delay. In this situation, the teacher needs to become more directive in helping the student perform the procedure rather than using time for discussion and questioning. Hopefully, the desired discussion and questioning can occur soon after the procedure is completed.

A fundamental responsibility of the teacher in a clinical setting is to give students feedback and suggestions about their learning and performance. Using multiple and varied sources of data increases the possibility that a truer and more complete picture of student learning and performance will emerge. Methods commonly used include teacher comments while observing or working with a student, teacher comments on performance after each clinical experience, client and staff remarks about performance, and teacher analysis of materials developed by the student in preparation for, during, and after the clinical assignment.

Teacher observations are made throughout the clinical experience in an effort to obtain a sampling of behaviors that will reflect quality of care provided and the extent of student learning. One method used by many teachers to record those observations is writing anecdotal notes. In these, the teacher records in objective terms the specific behaviors or incidents observed during the clinical experience. Behaviors may be either positive or negative and are used as the basis for feedback to the student. Feedback can be provided in various forms—audiotape, written notes, or orally. One suggestion is to give the student an exact copy of the anecdotal note written by the teacher. In this way, the student is aware of all impressions of the teacher. Whatever the form utilized, it is vital that feedback be given regularly throughout the experience as soon as possible after the experience so that students are fully aware of the teacher's perceptions about their performance and areas of desired change.

As discussed previously, student-developed products are another area for ongoing evaluation of student performance and learning. These materials developed in preparation for, during, or as a result of client care are helpful in illustrating the level of preparation and actual care provided. Examples of such materials are organizational plans, nursing care plans, case studies, drug cards, logs/diaries, diet plans, teaching plans, developmental studies, process recordings, and student entries on clinical records like nursing care plans and nurses' notes. One or more of these is usually required for each clinical experience and provides an additional perspective on student learning and performance besides direct observations. Ultimately, all data collected using the various sources mentioned will be used by the teacher to develop interim and end-of-course evaluations. It is helpful to students and to those who will teach the student later to provide summary statements about strengths and specific areas where improvement is needed. The student can then use the evaluation to continue purposeful development in areas of strength and to identify strategies for change in those areas where improvement is needed.

SUMMARY

Clinical teaching is an activity in which most nursing faculty are involved. Learning in the clinical area is viewed as vital to the overall development of the nursing student. Clinical teaching involves a number of important activities in assessing and selecting the clinical agency to be used, preliminary planning for the experience, implementation of actual clinical experience with students, and evaluation of learning and performance of the student.

APPENDIX 1
PEDIATRIC UNIT TREASURE HUNT

Department of Nursing

Pediatric Unit Treasure Hunt

** Locate the following key areas and items and check each off as you find it:

___ Kitchen
   ___ Patient refrigerator with popsicles, juices, special formulas
   ___ Staff refrigerator for lunches
   ___ Microwave oven
   ___ Ice/water machine
   ___ Infant formulas, glucose water, sterile water, Pedialyte
   ___ Calibrated infant feeder
   ___ Nipples
   ___ Baby food
___ Linen closets (2)
___ Linen cart with infant shirts & child PJs
___ Visitor restroom
___ Staff restroom
___ Wheelchairs
___ Utility room
   ___ IVACs and IMEDs
___ Treatment room
   ___ IV tray
   ___ Band-Aids
   ___ lb & kg scales
   ___ gm scales
   ___ BP cuffs
   ___ Emergency cart
   ___ Tape
   ___ 2 × 2 & 3 × 4 gauze pads
___ Tub room
   ___ Infant seats
   ___ Disposable diapers
   ___ High chairs

___ Medication room
   ___ Refrigerator for drugs
   ___ Narcotic locker
   ___ Narcotic record
   ___ Syringes & needles
   ___ Alcohol wipes
   ___ Sterile water and normal saline for injection
   ___ Flashlights
   ___ IV poles
   ___ Sp. gr. refractometer
   ___ Urine dipsticks
   ___ Hemocult test
   ___ cm tape measures
   ___ Monitor electrodes
___ Supply room
   ___ Urine collection bags, single specimen and 24-hr
   ___ Clinitest & Acetest
   ___ Sterile specimen cups
   ___ Soft restraints
   ___ Kerlix gauze roll
   ___ IV armboards and sandbags
   ___ IV solutions
   ___ IV volutrol & tubing
   ___ IV filters
   ___ IV extension tubing
   ___ Infant & child feeding tubes
   ___ Sm. tubs for bathing
   ___ Incontinent pads
   ___ DDST kit
___ Medication carts (3)
   ___ Medication rands

___ Individual medications	___ Patient charts
___ 1- & 3-oz med. cups	___ Nursing care plans
___ Sterile gauze pads	___ Medical care plans
___ Needles and syringes	___ Small conference room
___ Sterile water and normal	___ Patient worksheets
saline for injection	___ Reference books
___ Alcohol wipes	___ Playroom
___ Drug order form	___ Play cabinet with play supplies &
___ Desk area	references

** Go to a room where there are patients. Locate the following items and make notes about the type of information recorded:

1. Patient care worksheet
2. I&O worksheet
3. V/S record
4. Graphic sheet

** Go to one of the medication carts. Notice how the medications for each patient are stored. Practice unlocking and locking the cart. Look at the medication record and notice how the drugs are charted. Write down questions if there is anything you do not understand.

** Get one of the patient rands and review both the nursing care plan and the medical care plan for one patient. Make any notes that will help you remember the contents of the forms and how to use them.

** Get a patient's chart and review its contents. Notice the location of the doctor's orders and progress notes. Pay particular attention to the 24-hour I&O sheet and the nurses' notes. Make notes to help you remember how to use these forms. Write down questions for discussion later.

MAT/December 1985

APPENDIX 2
SAMPLE PRECEPTOR CONTRACT

LETTER OF AGREEMENT

The_____ , the Rural Clinical Nurse Placement Center,
     Educational Institution

Calfor[nia] State University, Chico, and _____
                                        Health   Agency/Individual

hereinafter referred to as the health agency, agree to the following responsibilities to students enrolled in _____ who are
                                               Educational Institution

participating in the Rural Clinical Nurse Placement Center and receiving field instruction in the above agency.

I. The Educational Institution shall:
  A. Select educationally prepared students for this rural clinical placement experience.
  B. Provide for a nursing faculty member to collaborate with the health agency clinical preceptor and Rural Clinical Nurse Placement nursing staff.
  C. Approve the student's learning objectives which will then be sent to the RCNPC and the Clinical Preceptor.
  D. Determine the units of academic credit to be granted to the student who successfully completes this clinical option.
  E. Provide an evaluation form for the student and clinical preceptor to complete at the conclusion of the student's experience.
  F. Submit an evaluation of the student's learning experience to the Rural Clinical Nurse Placement Center upon completion of that experience.

II. Rural Clinical Nurse Placement Center—California State University, Chico, shall:
  A. Have nursing staff available at all times for consultation to students, faculty, and clinical preceptors.
  B. Make regular and requested visits to clinical placement sites where students are assigned.
  C. Provide the health agency with information about the student prior to his/her arrival.
  D. Notify the educational institution of the placement site and preceptor the student will be assigned to.
  E. Orient clinical preceptors to the placement program and their role as clinical preceptors as needed.
  F. Orient students to the program, the community, and the agency to which assigned as well as their responsibilities as participants in this placement program.
  G. Obtain documentation demonstrating that each student is covered by professional liability insurance.
  H. Will not assume financial responsibility for student while he/she is participating in this placement program.

III. The Health Agency shall:
  A. Provide each student with clinical experiences necessary to meet his/her learning objectives.
  B. Designate an appropriate staff member to act as the clinical preceptor who will assume responsibility for student supervision.
  C. Provide the resources needed for a desirable learning climate.
  D. Assure that staff is adequate in number and quality to insure safe and continuous health care to individuals.

    E. Provide Rural Clinical Nurse Placement nursing staff and faculty access to the agency and agency staff.

    F. Orient Center staff or faculty and students to the agency purposes, policies, and procedures.

    G. Within its limited service capabilities provide emergency care for students in case of injury, with any financial liability assumed by the student for that service.

    H. Shall not financially compensate any student receiving academic credit according to this Agreement nor shall students be considered employees of the health agency.

    I. Have the right, after consultation with the Rural Clinical Nurse Placement Center and the educational institution to refuse to accept or continue any nursing student, who in the health agency's judgment, is not participating satisfactorily or safely in this placement.

    J. Any problem reflecting on the qualifications of a student shall be immediately called to the attention of the Rural Clinical Nurse Placement Center and the educational institution.

    K. Maintain standards accepted by appropriate accrediting bodies, as applicable.

    L. Participate in written evaluations of the student's performance and of the Rural Clinical Nurse Placement Center.

  IV. The parties of this Agreement shall not discriminate against any student because of age, sex, or national origin.

   V. Financial responsibility:
By this Agreement none of the parties incur any responsibility for financial exchange whether in monies or in kind.

  VI. Period of Agreement:
This Agreement shall be in effect beginning _____, 19 ____ and shall remain in effect for one year from the date of Agreement or until terminated by one of the parties who shall provide three (3) months written notice of their decision. This Agreement automatically terminates upon the termination of the Rural Clinical Nurse Placement Center.

  VII. This Agreement may at any time be altered, changed or amended by mutual agreement of the parties in writing.

IN WITNESS WHEREOF, this Agreement has been signed by and on behalf of the parties identified above.

For the Educational Institution:

By _____ Date _____
    Chairperson, Nursing Program

By _____ Date _____
    Representative of Educational Institution

    For the Rural Clinical Nurse Placement Center:

By _____ Date _____
    Director

    For the California State University, Chico:

By _____ Date _____
    Purchasing Officer

    For the Health Agency:

By _____ Date _____
    Nursing Service Administrator

By _____ Date _____
    Agency Administrator or Physician

Stuart-Siddall, S., & Haberlin, J. M. (1983). *Preceptorships in nursing education.* Reprinted with permission of Aspen Publishers, Inc.

MAT/December 1985

PART 3

STRATEGIES FOR TEACHING INDIVIDUAL STUDENTS

12

Individualizing Instruction

Individualization of instruction as a desirable goal has, in recent years, gained increasing acceptance among educators in various fields. Reports appearing in educational and nursing journals attest to the fact that there have been many attempts to achieve this goal. Traditional teaching methods have been and are being challenged for several reasons. Among them is the growing awareness of individual differences among learners. As individuals mature and are exposed to varied experiences, the differences become even greater.

Presently, the student population in nursing programs is widely diverse. Many students now entering nursing are older, both men and women, and from many cultures and ethnic minority groups. Some return to school after raising a family. Other choose nursing as a second career. Those who are already R.N.s are returning for associate and baccalaureate degrees. Others have had previous education and experience in health care in the military or by their involvement in vocational/ practical nursing or as a nursing assistant. Each of these makes the nursing student population of the 1980s quite different from that of the 1950s when most nursing students were female, white, and recent high school graduates.

Such diversity calls for varied approaches to teaching. Traditional lockstep methods, in which all students in a class are expected to study the same thing at the same time, are no longer adequate (and probably never were). The present and future challenge for nurse educators is to respond to the unique needs of individuals and provide equality of educational outcomes while still providing education that achieves the standards of the profession and is relevant to the needs of society.

There are many examples of efforts being made to individualize education in nursing programs throughout the country, but nursing education is still highly traditional. There is still regular use of large lecture groups that all students must attend, written and clinical assignments that are the same for all students, and, at times, limited formal recognition of previous education and experience. Rarely are students tested to determine their perceptual strengths and weaknesses and decide which teaching strategies would be best. Rarely are several options of media, assignments, and experiences offered from which the student can select. Seldom are students allowed to take a different route to meet the requirements of a course. Some methods, including independent study and learning modules, have become traditional in the sense that they are often required of all students at the same time and at the same rate. Such practices are not responsive to the special and individual needs of students.

This chapter will present three main topics: tools for determining individual learning styles, research about learning styles, and characteristics of individualized instruction. This chapter serves to introduce three other chapters, each of which will discuss one strategy that can help to individualize instruction.

TOOLS FOR DETERMINING LEARNING STYLE

Learning style refers to the unique ways in which a person perceives, interacts, and responds to the various elements in a learning situation. Identification of learning style classifies individuals according to the educational conditions that are most likely to result in learning. The dominant learning style indicates one's preferred way of receiving and processing input from the learning environment. Using methods reflective of the dominant learning style is usually considered the best way to produce the greatest learning achievement. Several examples of specific tools that may be useful for diagnosing one or more aspects of an individual's learning style follow:

1. The Learning Style Inventory developed by Renzulli and Smith (Ferrell, 1978) is an instrument for determining student attitudes about nine specific learning methods: projects, simulation, drill and recitation, peer teaching, discussion, teaching games, inde-

pendent study, programmed instruction, and lecture. Student attitudes about each are obtained by responses on a Likert scale, from "very enjoyable" to "very unpleasant."

2. The Autonomous Learner Index developed by Southern Illinois Collegiate Common Market (Ferrell, 1978) is an attitude scale designed to determine the level of an individual's self-direction in learning. Somewhat related to this is Rokeach's Dogmatism Scale, which reveals the extent of open-mindedness or closed-mindedness of an individual (Osborn & Thompson, 1977).

3. The Productivity Environmental Preference Survey (PEPS) (Dunn & Dunn, 1978, pp. 5–17; Price, Dunn, & Dunn, 1979) is an inventory for the identification of individual adult preferences for conditions in a working and/or learning environment. The individual responds on a Likert scale indicating strong agreement to strong disagreement with statements reflecting conditions in 21 areas of four stimulus categories: environmental, emotional, sociological, and physical. An individual score indicates student preferences in each of the 21 areas.

4. Kolb's Learning Style Inventory (LSI) (1978; 1981, pp. 237–238) is a self-description inventory that measures differences in learning styles along the two basic continuums, concrete-abstract and active-reflective. Four basic learning styles have been identified: converger (preference for abstract conceptualization and active experimentation), diverger (preference for concrete experience and reflective observation), assimilator (preference for reflective observation and abstract conceptualization), and accommodator (preference for concrete experience and active experimentation).

5. The "cognitive mapping" technique of Hill (Cranston & McCort, 1985; Cross, 1976, p. 126) includes a battery of tests to assess student preferences and yield a profile that reveals a student's cognitive style. Major components are theoretical symbols, qualitative symbols, cultural determinants, and modalities of inference. Data obtained are fed into a computer to produce a cognitive map that can then be used to prepare a "personalized educational prescription" (PEP).

6. The Grasha-Riechmann Student Learning Style Scales (Garity, 1985) are used to assess student attitudes toward teaching methods and peer relationships. Six styles are measured: independent, dependent, participant, avoidant, collaborative, and competitive.

7. The Group Embedded Figures Test (GEFT) (Hodson, 1985; Partridge, 1983; Witkin, Moore, Goodenough, & Cox, 1977) is used to determine the relative field-dependence–field-independence

of individuals. The results indicate how a person perceives surroundings. Field-dependent individuals experience their surroundings in a global fashion and see the whole rather than parts of a situation. On the other hand, field-independent people experience their environment with individual objects separate from their background. Witkin and coworkers (1977, p. 7) indicate that socialization plays a major role in the adoption of preferred styles, with women in Western cultures tending to be field-dependent. Field-dependent people are more likely to choose people-oriented professions like nursing (Witkin et al., 1977, pp. 40, 43).

RELATED RESEARCH

There is ample research to support the assertion that each student learns in ways that are different from others and that students learn best when they are taught using preferred methods. Witkin (1973, p.1) stressed the importance of cognitive style in relation to other life events by stating, "Cognitive style is a potent variable in students' academic choices and vocational preferences; in students' academic development through their school career; in how students learn and teachers teach; and in how students and teachers interact in the classroom." Although limited in number, a few studies are available that investigate the learning styles of nurses or nursing students. A few examples follow:

1. The research by Bradshaw (1978) has already been cited on page 31. Bradshaw concludes that most students in nursing programs are of "sensing-feeling" type who perceive the world more clearly through the use of the five senses, thus achieving the greatest learning benefit through involvement in concrete experiences.

2. A group of adult learners in an ADN program were found to have a slightly positive attitude toward all of nine teaching methods investigated, except simulation (Ferrell, 1978). They were also determined to have a tendency toward being self-directed learners. Posttest results, although not statistically significant, showed a slight increase in student preference for the traditional strategies of drill or recitation and lecture.

3. In an investigation with first-time employed graduate nurses, Garity (1985) found that their preference was for concrete and teacher-structured learning experiences. This study supported earlier research in which baccalaureate nursing students were

found to prefer traditional learning strategies that were teacher directed, highly organized, and denoted student passivity (Ostmoe, Van Hoozen, Scheffel, & Crowell, 1984). Students of allied health professions showed similar attitudes (Rezler & French, 1975).

4. Merritt (1983), when comparing generic and R.N. students on the basis of age and length of career employment, found that these factors did not account for differences in learning preferences. Conclusions from this research included (1) the preference by both groups for structured environments with clear definitions of course requirements and expectations and presentation of content in a logical, organized manner, (2) that neither group was particularly interested in setting their own goals or pursuing their own interests, and (3) that both groups tended not to prefer competitive and teacher-controlled learning environments. Further, R.N. learners were less positively oriented than were basic generic students toward formal teaching methods and environment and more positively inclined toward reading than generic students.

5. A study by Hodson (1985) revealed that field-dependent nursing students spent more time more often with the instructor, spent more time with patients when other persons were also directly involved, were more likely themselves to initiate activity units, and were more likely to engage in social contacts than the field-independent students. There was no indication whether the nursing students were primarily field-independent or field-dependent.

6. Physical therapy and nursing students in baccalaureate programs expressed significantly stronger needs for organization and direct experience than other groups studied (1974 study by Canfield and Lafferty cited by Payton, Hueter, & McDonald, 1979).

Research investigating a match between teaching methods and learning styles in nursing education is even more limited than that identifying learning styles. From what is available, it is apparent that matching teaching method with learning style results in cognitive and affective gains. Three available studies are summarized here:

1. In a 1972 study, Lange (reported in Garity, 1985) determined that the failure-withdrawal rate in specific nursing courses was lower when teachers and students were matched on learning style than when teachers and students were not matched.

2. Skipwith (cited by Garity, 1985) reported that students who had access to their learning styles were more successful in course work,

experienced more efficient learning, and exhibited more responsibility in manipulating learning activities according to their specific needs.

3. Open-minded students (as determined by Rokeach's Dogmatism Scale) achieved a significantly higher mean posttest score on learning modules than did their closed-minded peers (Osborn & Thompson, 1977). Thus, the closed-minded student benefited less from the use of this independent learning strategy.

The above evidence supports the theory that individuals have definite learning styles and preferences for certain teaching methodologies. In general, it indicates that nurses and nursing students prefer direct, concrete, teacher-structured experiences; have a positive attitude toward most teaching methods, both traditional and nontraditional; and prefer highly organized activities with clearly stated requirements and expectations. Certainly, there is a lack of support for the full-scale use of nontraditional strategies with all students. Perhaps we should ask instead, "Which method is most useful for an individual student at a particular stage of development?" and "Which method is best for the subject matter and desired outcomes?"

WHAT IS INDIVIDUALIZED INSTRUCTION?

Basically, individualized instruction (II) is the use of teaching approaches that focus on individual learning needs and styles and allow the highest level of achievement by each student. It is a goal that many nursing educators have been working toward for several years, although it is difficult to achieve without major changes in traditional philosophies and procedures. Those interested in moving in the direction of a more individualized approach may gain insight into the requirements of II by looking at its specific characteristics. The following list reflects a synthesis from several resources (Clark, 1981, pp. 584–596; Cross, 1976, pp. 52–55; Forman & Richardson, 1977; Weisgerber, 1973). The major characteristics of II are:

1. an II program requires active involvement of the learner and places the responsibility for learning on the student.
2. the teacher in an II program is a facilitator, manager, resource person, and consultant in the total learning process.
3. II requires specification of explicit objectives.

4. feedback and evaluation are integral parts of II.

5. II is flexible by providing the student considerable choice in selecting from alternative activities and multisensory resources, the sociological pattern to be used, and the pace at which learning will take place.

The Student's Role in Individualized Learning

The role of the student in individualized learning is one of an active, responsible participant. Active rather than passive involvement of the learner has long been recognized as desirable. Markle (1977, p. 13) stated: "It is not what is presented to the student but what the student is led to do that results in learning." If one believes that learning is a lifetime process and that nursing requires a practitioner who can think and make decisions independently, then active involvement is crucial in the educational preparation of the nurse. While traditional classroom situations encourage the participation of some but not others, individualized programs require the participation of every student.

Active involvement of a student can include either mental or physical processes. The student should be required to participate, recall information, think through problems, and use judgment and reasoning, that is, to be personally involved with the materials for learning. Many examples of active involvement of a learner are available. The list of ideas that follows is particularly pertinent to nursing education. It is given in the hope that it will help each reader generate other ideas that are applicable to individual settings. The student might:

Answer questions about a topic or a printed or medicated clinical situation

Compute problems in drug doses and intravenous rates

Prepare a nursing care plan, drug study, diet plan, or teaching plan

Manipulate equipment, materials, and models

Interview an individual or a family

Work with one or more peers on a particular learning task

Apply what has been learned to an actual situation in various clinical settings—hospital, home, clinic, community, and so forth

Role play

Research/investigate available community resources for health care, transportation, or shopping

Demonstrate a procedure

Diagram a process

Collect prepared resources for teaching peers or clients

Produce learning materials for teaching peers or clients

Write reports

Conduct experiments

Play games or complete puzzles

Participate in groups—brainstorming sessions, task groups, panel discussions, and so forth

These and other activities will involve the student directly in the learning process, which may help, in turn, to increase motivation, interest, and learning. Students who have become accustomed to traditional methods will require guidance and assistance in becoming more active, responsible participants in learning. Thus, some students will, at first, require more structure than others but can progress, if supported and encouraged, to become more actively involved in their own learning.

The Teacher's Role in Individualized Instruction

The teacher's roles in an II program have been discussed by various authors (Clark, 1981, pp. 596–598; Cross, 1976, pp. 205–208; Rogers, 1969, pp. 103–126). It is clear that II teacher roles are quite different from the roles of teachers using traditional methods. Central teacher activities with II deal with determining learning needs, organization of materials and methods to provide the means for learning, assisting students to use materials productively, and determining if desired learning has occurred. Four specific roles will be discussed: diagnosis and prescription, management and facilitation, evaluation and remediation, and motivation.

Diagnosis and Prescription.   In the area of diagnosis and prescription, the teacher is responsible, at times in conjunction with the student, for determining the variance between objectives and the present status of the student. This may be done in a conference or through pretesting and serves as the basis for deciding what is to be learned. The prescription then becomes that which must be done to achieve those objectives that have not already been met.

Management and Facilitation.   Once what is to be learned has been established, the teacher manages, facilitates, coordinates, and guides the student in the required learning process. Teacher responsibilities include designing, structuring, selecting, and arranging any activities, experiences, or resources that are expected to lead to the desired changes in behavior. This may involve developing instructional materials in a subject area, coordinating activities in the community, leading discussions, having conferences to monitor progress, providing real-life experiences, elaborating on and interpreting experiences, and, for some students, providing structure and direction.

Rogers (1969, p. 105) was among the first to express the belief that the aim of education is the facilitation of learning. He also identified the personal relationship between the facilitator and a learner as a critical element that is dependent on the facilitator's possession of three attitudinal qualities: (1) realness and genuineness, (2) nonpossessive caring, trust, and respect, and (3) empathic understanding and sensitive listening (Rogers, 1969, pp. 106–112).

Evaluation and Remediation.   During and after the various learning activities, it is the teacher's duty to assess progress and evaluate outcomes. This may be done in face-to-face conferences, observations in simulated or real settings, written testing, evaluation of products, and so forth. Feedback about progress is given so that students are aware of their standing and what has to be done to achieve learning if any gaps exist between objectives and performance. This function of the teacher is closely related to diagnosis and prescription, except that diagnosis and prescription imply initiation of a new learning sequence while evaluation and remediation occur during and after a learning episode. The reader is also referred to Chapter 1 for a discussion of reinforcement and to the section in this chapter on feedback and evaluation.

Motivation.   Closely related to the role of facilitator and evaluator is the role of motivator. There is general agreement among learning theorists that the learner who is motivated learns more readily than one who is not. Through the use of various motivational devices, the teacher sets a climate conducive to learning and stimulates the student to learn what is required. The teacher helps a student set goals, assume responsibility, and identify appropriate learning materials. The teacher provides support, encouragement, and praise and establishes a cooperative, friendly environment.

The importance of the personal relationship between the teacher and student has already been noted. Associated with the function of the teacher as motivator is that of serving as role model. Bandura (Knowles, 1978, pp. 87–89) established the label of "social learning" for the process of imitation and identification associated with role modeling. Through role modeling, the teacher demonstrates the actions and attitudes that a student should imitate. This is a particularly important mechanism for demonstrating appropriate interpersonal behaviors in nursing and for establishing learning as a lifetime process. By functioning in a "humanist" role along with the other roles in II, the teaching-learning experiences can become more creative, enjoyable, and productive for both the teacher and the student.

Explicit Learning Objectives

A learning sequence that is purported to be individualized requires a clear statement of what the student is to accomplish and how achievement will be measured. In this way, students know exactly what they are accountable for and can go about reaching stated objectives instead of having to guess what the learning requirements are. Only by specifying what is to be learned can the teacher verify when it has been taught. Moreover, active involvement is futile unless learners know what it is they are supposed to accomplish (Cross, 1976, p. 52).

An explicit objective leaves no doubt about its meaning. Vague terms, such as "appreciate" or "understand," should be avoided, and behavioral terms that are observable should be used instead. However, objectives should not be stated in such minute detail that they become overly lengthy and burdensome. A useful guideline is provided by Wilson and Tosti (1972, p. 18):

> The objective should be stated in only enough detail to enable several knowledgeable observers to agree that the observed student behavior represents an adequate accomplishment of the objective.

For example, consider the objective: Describe in 20 words or less what is meant by a physician's order that reads, "NG replacement, ml for ml." Knowledgeable observers would agree that each milliliter of nasogastric tube drainage is to be replaced with 1 milliliter of an ordered intravenous solution.

Just as an explicit learning objective is of benefit to the student so it is also to the teacher. It will help the teacher clarify instructional goals, select or design instructional materials, identify entering and terminal competencies of the student, and evaluate the instructional program itself.

The discussion in this section has focused only on the importance of making objectives explicit. Many other excellent references that discuss types and levels of objectives and provide guidelines for writing objectives are available. Further discussion of objectives in relation to mastery learning will be presented in the next section on feedback and evaluation.

Feedback and Evaluation

Any teaching method will be improved by prompting and feedback. Individualized instruction requires the establishment of a monitoring and evaluation system for ongoing assessment of individual performance. Objective evaluation based on clearly stated behaviors, helps the learner to develop expected competencies. Knowledge of results is important so that the student knows when objectives have been achieved or when something else must be done in órder to reach them.

The emphasis in individualizing instruction is on the mastery of *all* objectives by *all* students rather than on how well or how poorly objectives are met by students in comparison with one another. Evaluation of a student against stated objectives is called mastery learning, criterion-referenced evaluation, or competency-based evaluation in contrast to normative evaluation, in which students are compared with one another by the use of the "normal curve." In mastery learning, standards are often stated at a minimum performance level; however, a higher level is possible and desirable if educators encourage higher quality performance of all students and allow students to have more time, if needed, in which to achieve objectives. Objectives at varying levels may also be stated if it is necessary, within a particular setting, to designate desired student performance level for assigning letter grades.

Cross (1976, pp. 14–15) summarized research that indicates that the level of achievement in a more traditional curriculum has little to do with success later in life. It is her belief that learning to achieve and to develop one's best talents is more likely to lead to self-fulfillment and, perhaps, success. Learning theorists agree that reward is preferable to punishment for increase in learning. Changing the focus from differential grading to grading based on standards of performance provides students with greater reward and positive reinforcement for continued achievement rather than constant reminders of their relative standing in a group.

Bloom (1968) reports both cognitive and affective gains from the use of mastery learning. He claims that 95 percent of students can attain mastery of most learning tasks if given sufficient time and adequate human and educational resources. In fact, II is based on this premise. According to Cross (1976, p. 8) many people mistakenly equate the preservation of the normal curve with the preservation of academic standards. She advances the idea that standards are best served when students learn the material.

Affective gains include the belief that one can attain mastery and competence, a view of oneself as adequate, more positive feeling about the subject, increased cooperation among students, and an increased interest and motivation for learning, both in relation to the subject at hand and lifelong learning (Bloom, 1968). Thorman and Knutson (1977) provide similar results in the areas of attitude toward learning and degree of motivation. Ely and Minars (1973) further corroborate the positive affective outcomes by showing improved scores for students on a self-concept scale after using mastery learning.

As with any learning situation, evaluation is of two types: formative and summative. Formative evaluation is continuous and is used to provide feedback to the student and the teacher regarding the progress toward achievement of objectives. It tells what has been learned and what still needs to be learned. It may be carried out as part of a unit of study or as part of an entire course. It serves, in either case, to help a student move toward the desired competence. If there are areas not yet mastered, the use of formative evaluation provides feedback about those areas. Such a process implies that activities and resources that can help students correct any deficiencies must be readily available for use.

There are different methods for providing ongoing feedback. One involves the use of self-evaluation or peer evaluation of performance using videotaping or criteria check lists. Other forms include responding to a clinical situation, answering questions, filling in crossword puzzles, creating a product, applying past learning to a clinical situation, and responding to attitude scales. The related role of the teacher is to determine what needs to be done next. If the evaluation is part of a clinical experience, the teacher may also provide feedback in the form of written, verbal, or taped anecdotal notes. Regardless of the method used, the student should be aware of progress and/or problems at all times and have the opportunity to do what needs to be done to reach objectives. This is in contrast to the inadequate learning that may occur when a student is a member of a large group and does not receive individual feedback or assistance.

As with formative evaluation, summative evaluation provides evidence of learning success or lack of it. However, summative evaluation is carried out at the end of instruction, either in a unit or a course, and is used as final evidence of mastery of stated objectives. Typically, students in traditional courses do not have an opportunity to correct errors or be retested. In mastery learning, if objectives are not reached, the student continues to work until they are.

Summative evaluation shows how students have changed as a result of learning activities and tasks. It may involve the same tools used in formative evaluation or they may be different as long as the behaviors that are part of the learning objectives are reflected. Summative evaluation can include performance in a simulated or clinical setting, participation in group discussions or reports, responses to attitude scales, performance on various types of written exams, developing a product, or answering questions about a videotaped episode. One technique for helping a student know which objective has not been met is to key each test item to its related objective(s) and learning activities. In this way, the student is able to restudy the area needed and to retest at a later time. This does, of course, require the availability of alternate test forms so that the student actually demonstrates mastery of an objective rather than memorization of a test item.

Flexibility of Student Choice

Adult learning theory suggests that the maturational process amplifies the differences among individuals (Knowles, 1978, p.31). It further suggests that older learners prefer instructional situations that allow them (1) to be self-directing and actively involved, (2) to utilize past experiences in new learning situations, and (3) to deal with current life situations and problems more effectively (Knowles, 1978, pp. 55–59). Thus, providing choices is a response to the needs of adult learners.

Three areas in which the student in an individualized learning program should have considerable choice are (1) pacing of study, (2) selecting the sociological pattern to be used, and (3) choosing from among alternative activities and multisensory resources.

Self-Pacing. Pacing has already been mentioned in the previous section on feedback and evaluation by referring to Bloom's view that most students can learn a subject to a high competency level given sufficient time and appropriate help for doing so. Self-paced learning recognizes that students learn at different rates and encourages/allows the student to use the amount of time needed to reach stated objectives.

Just as self-pacing is closely aligned with mastery of stated competencies, it is also closely associated with placing the responsibility for learning on the student. One related problem is that a student may not be self-disciplined, motivated, or adept at managing time for learning so that the objectives can be met within a reasonable period of time. Depending on the limitations of time (such as a semester or a year), the teacher can assist a student in dealing with these problems and in making the involvement with self-pacing a positive, growing experience. The teacher provides encouragement, guidelines for the amount of work that should be done by a particular time, orientation about what is expected, and continued interpersonal contact. It is also crucial that the amount of work be realistic for the unit structure and the time period involved. Experience indicates that there are more lack-of-completion problems when the student in a self-paced course is also taking traditional courses that have definite deadlines and examinations. If this situation is unavoidable, it is even more crucial to provide the type of assistance already outlined.

It would be erroneous to conclude that a self-paced course or program is automatically individualized. Other characteristics, referred to in this chapter, must also be present. However, there are real advantages of self-pacing in and of itself. It allows some students to move more slowly and others to progress more rapidly; it responds to the needs that most students have at some time or other to be absent in the event of unavoidable occurrences, such as illness; it allows students to take time off for financial, physical, or emotional rejuvenation; and it permits scheduling of learning as an important, but not the only, event in one's life.

Although self-pacing in an unlimited period of time is theoretically possible, this presents significant management problems associated with credit for courses; registration and add-drop procedures; determination of student-teacher ratios and teaching loads; and the use of clinical agencies, classrooms, and other resources. It would be worthwhile for those in nursing education to continue to deal with these problems. In spite of them, however, there are many ways to increase the number of self-pacing opportunities in nursing programs. Techniques include the use of independent study, modules, contracts, and computer-assisted/managed instruction. Independent study will be discussed in the next section, and the specific strategies of learning modules, learning contracts, and computer-assisted instruction will be discussed in Chapters 13, 14, and 15.

Sociological Pattern.   Sociological pattern refers to the number and type of people present in a learning situation. The student who has full control over the selection of the sociological pattern to be used for learning can decide whether to work alone, with one or two peers, with a small group, with a large group, or with a combination of these. Although such a choice may not be fully realized, in many instances the student can select the pattern to be used. For example, a student who is learning facts about a particular clinical situation may be given a choice of which sociological pattern to use. At other times, when involvement in group or cooperative effort is deemed necessary, the teacher may require the student to work with others. Even then, however, the student may choose with whom to work. As the unit of study is being prepared by the teacher, an effort can be made to include various options so that the student can either select the favored pattern or understand why a teacher believes that a particular pattern is desirable for a certain objective or group of objectives.

The discussion of types of sociological patterns will take place under two main headings: independent study and learning with others.

Independent Study. Independent study (IS) literally means that a student carries out the activities for learning independently of the teacher. Other terms that may be used synonymously with IS are self-study, self-instruction, self-directed study, and autotutorial study. It is, perhaps, the use of these terms that has led some people to believe that the teacher is uninvolved in the learning process or that the student alone decides what, when, and where to learn. Neither is the case; however, both teacher and student roles change. Both are involved in a different way than in traditional education. The student has a greater responsibility in all aspects of learning and is more actively involved in deciding what, when, and where to learn and what activities will be completed. However, the teacher who designs or approves the study determines how much flexibility will be allowed. The unit of study may be highly structured, very flexible, or somewhere between the two extremes. Faculty members who have no more to do with the student's experiences after objectives are devised are abdicating their responsibility. Sommerfeld and Hughes (1980, p. 416) believe that student performance in independent experiences "must be carefully developed in much the same way as other well structured learning activities." They go on to say that allowing students complete freedom without holding them accountable is not educationally sound. On the other hand, any study unit that requires all students to use IS entirely or that is so heavily structured that there are no options cannot be called individualized.

Independent study in some form is probably the method most widely used by nursing educators in an attempt to individualize instruction. Early efforts involved students who had special interests and talents that teachers wished to address. Independent study permitted and/or encouraged enriching experiences for those students who wished to go beyond the minimum requirements of a course (Sorensen, 1968). It was generally reserved for the academically superior student who wished to investigate a topic or problem of personal interest.

Progressively, the design of the IS project was seen as a joint effort between the student and teacher. While viewed by Hanson (1974) as an opportunity to promote personal and professional growth, it was pointed out that both the teacher and student must agree on the goals of the study, how student progress will be monitored, how experiences will be recorded, and amount of supervision the instructor will provide.

The concept of self-directed, independent study is now widely accepted among nursing educators. However, as reported by Bartol (1984), there is a wide variation in faculty perceptions and practices in the use of IS in nursing education. IS, or self-study, is regularly mentioned as a central strategy for basic nursing education (Bartol, 1984; Blatchley, Herzog, & Russell, 1978; Cudney, 1976; Dick, 1983; Honey, 1975; Jones & Kerwin, 1978; Layton, 1975; Paduano, 1979; Rochin & Thompson, 1975; Swendsen, 1981). Other researchers discuss IS from the student's perspective (Hanson, 1974; Kilcullen, 1985) and in relation to in-service and continuing education (Huntsman & Thompson, 1977; Reinhart, 1977; Schmidt, 1977; Sherer & Thompson, 1978; Smith, 1980). In fact, IS is the basic sociological pattern required with learning modules, learning contracts, and computer-assisted instruction, discussed in the next three chapters.

From the reports it is clear that there are definite values to the use of IS. Besides increasing student responsibility and participation, IS increases motivation and allows for differences in student needs, interests, and learning rates. It permits students to study required content at a time that is most appropriate to a particular clinical setting and most convenient for them. IS units help to establish a minimal level of knowledge in a particular subject that is required of all students, provide enrichment experiences for some students, and allow some students to move more rapidly through learning experiences. IS materials are particularly helpful in providing background and preparation information to a student preparing for a specific clinical experience. In this way, teachers and students have more time for clinical practice, the quality of the clinical practice is improved, and discussions on the application of content to client needs can take place. Further, IS cultivates the skills and attitudes that are essential to lifelong learning and provides practice in analyzing, evaluating, and using information.

Learning with Others. Just as students should be given the option of learning independently at times, so should they be provided opportunities to learn with others. Nursing is a profession that requires the effective use of interpersonal skills and the ability to work cooperatively with others. The instructional sequence, then, should provide options in the type of social environment to be used in order, first, to provide more individualized learning and, second, to provide social interaction that will facilitate the development of skills for working effectively with others.

The involvement in a social situation may be an end in itself for those who need human warmth and support in order to function and learn effectively. Social situations offer highly effective learning experiences. Specific support for the value of learning with others is offered by Knowles (1978, p. 112) in his discussion of adult learners. He states that the maturing adult, by having participated in many previous experiences, is a rich resource for learning through the use of such experiential techniques as discussions, laboratory, simulation, field experience, team projects, and other action-oriented techniques. Consequently, nursing educators should provide such experiences and, in addition to rewarding independent thought and action, foster and reward the student's involvement in cooperative interaction with others.

There are many positive aspects of learning with others. The list that follows is not an exhaustive one but is given in an effort to enumerate some of the benefits of social interaction during learning. Learning with others:

1. fosters cooperative effort and democratic participation
2. prevents isolation of the learner
3. increases motivation and interest
4. enhances the development of analytical and problem-solving skills
5. provides practice in development of ideas
6. facilitates the development of interpersonal skills
7. increases sense of responsibility for shared learning
8. broadens exposure to others' ideas and ways of thinking
9. increases confidence of the individual
10. broadens knowledge base through collective participation
11. provides practice in integrating information from varied sources

The two main forms for individualized learning with others are pairs and small groups. Research evidence indicates that students who desire "close, friendly interpersonal relations develop problem-solving skills better when they are assigned to work on the problem in pairs . . ." and that "weak students are especially likely to profit from peer tutoring" (Cross, 1976, p. 125). Furthermore, those students who are uncomfortable in teacher- or authority-dominated situations profit from learning with their peers (Dunn & Dunn, 1978, p. 12).

Several arrangements of peers working together in learning situations can be found in the literature. Each of these seems to support the notion that mutual learning is more productive for some students and that teaching something to a peer is an excellent way to increase one's own understanding. McKay (1980) describes a peer group counseling model in which peers are used as support persons. In this method, students are trained to provide listening, support, and interaction with the primary goal of enhancing problem-solving skills of the person being counseled. DiMinno and Thompson (1980) report on the use of an interactional support group for graduate nursing students.

Several examples of the use of peer teaching or evaluation are also available. The proctor-managed system and the peer-proctor system are described by Wilson and Tosti (1972, pp. 61–72). In the proctor-managed system, a student who is more advanced than the proctored student provides a supporting role and gives feedback and evaluation of learning at specified points in the learning sequence. Their scope of responsibility is well defined, with the authority to evaluate student performance (rather than teach) and to indicate to the student what the next assignment should be. On the other hand, the peer-proctor system uses either an advanced student or one who is presently enrolled in the course to work with an assigned group of students or to be "on duty" at certain times to serve all students who need help. Another variation of the same system is to select proctors on a rotating basis in relation to which students are able to complete a particular unit of study most quickly. In the peer-proctor system described, student proctors work for either credit, bonus points, or pay.

Rochin and Thompson (1975) reported on a variation of the peer-proctor system in a nursing education setting. They described the use of student "facilitators" who work for either credit or pay and dispense learning materials for student use in a learning center, grade module posttests, and provide assistance with learning in relation to assigned learning modules.

Several authors discuss the value of peer teaching for the development of skills needed in the future practice of nursing. Burnside (1971) believed that assigning a student to supervise another student in the clinical setting increased autonomous functioning and helped the student develop teaching behaviors, expand resources for learning, and obtain feedback about behaviors. Clark (1978) believed that student interaction with one another as student, teacher, and peer helped to prepare them for future experiences with peer review. Boguslawski and Judkins (1971) stated that the opportunity for peer observation and counseling was an important factor in the development of independence and creativity.

There are other, less formal, ways to pair students for learning. In a particular unit of study the student may be given the option or may be directed to work with a peer. This method is particularly useful in a basic skills course so that each student will have a partner with whom to work, try out ideas and techniques, and provide mutual feedback and encouragement about performance of the skills. A student can also be encouraged to work with another student in answering a specific set of questions, generating ideas about dealing with a certain clinical situation, or doing research on a particular topic. Ways to encourage peer interaction and learning in the clinical arena include dual assignments, having one student serve as "helper" on a rotating basis to three or four other students, or assigning a student at least one time during a clinical rotation to work as a "free agent" and become involved in a variety of activities that may not be possible with a regular assignment. Each of these is useful at different times to increase peer interaction, enhance the use of limited clinical facilities, and allow the student to function in different roles.

In addition to learning in pairs, small-group techniques are helpful for achieving the positive results of learning with others already listed on page 197. It is crucial that nursing students learn to work effectively as members and leaders of groups in situations that are reality oriented (Clark, 1978). Only by having such experiences can the students, upon graduation, be expected to assume those roles in their work and community lives. The use of small groups has been one of the most pronounced trends in educational practice during the last 2 decades (Knowles, 1978, p. 94). Small-group involvement provides interpersonal benefits through interaction with peers and helps students grasp complex ideas and relate more effectively to subject matter (Phillips, 1973, p. 52).

A small group is usually made up of five to nine people and may work in either a formal classroom setting or in other, less structured settings. When a specific learning assignment is involved, it may be one that has been designed by the teacher alone, the teacher and students together, or students alone. Learning activities often include individual or collective reading or viewing; the use of case studies, critical incidents, or clinical situations; consideration of a particular problem; answering questions; or development of a care or teaching plan.

Three types of small-group techniques that seem particularly helpful to learning in nursing will be summarized. They are supportive, teaching, and task groups (Clark, 1978). The supportive group is usually an informal one in which students select one another when they have mutual needs. However, the peer-counseling model by McKay (1980) also had support as one function with upperclass students trained as peer counselors. Both formal and informal groups can be helpful in decreasing the level of stress of nursing students so that energies can be used more productively for learning. In addition, the peer-counseling model can be used as the training ground for students who are learning to lead groups and developing counseling skills; thus, for the student in the group it is a supportive group and for the student serving as counselor it is a teaching group.

The task group and teaching group are the major types with which formal education is concerned. In general, all group work used in education has some elements of both teaching and task since students are involved in completing some type of task assignment in order to achieve certain knowledge and skills. Therefore, there will be no attempt to differentiate between the two types of groups except to make a few comments specific to task groups that are not true of the usual teaching groups.

The primary purpose of small-group or team learning is to involve the members of the group in a cooperative effort to learn about a particular topic that is of interest to all members of the group. The group members often serve as catalysts to each others' ideas so that combined learning is increased. As an added benefit, the students gain knowledge about group dynamics. Although any small-group work may be thought to be involved in the completion of a task, there are some unique characteristics of "task groups." Participants are organized around a particular task only for the duration of the specific job to be done; leadership evolves and changes depending on the strengths of individual members at different times; and members participate equally in some portion of the task (Bevis, 1982, pp. 237–239). In addition, much of the work of the task group can be carried out individually or in pairs and then brought back to the total group for presentation, consolidation, and agreement. Thus, each member has a particular job that is important to the work of the total group. Any member who does not complete a subtask interferes with the accomplishment of the primary task for which the group is responsible.

There are a number of ways in which task groups can be used in the educational process. A few possibilities are listed below:

1. Demographic study of a community
2. Research on various aspects of a selected topic, such as child abuse
3. Preparation of an annotated bibliography on a specific topic
4. Investigation of problems of particular groups, such as housing, transportation, medical care, and recreation for the elderly

Regardless of the procedure for small-group work that is used, it is important for the teacher to meet certain responsibilities in order to increase the chance for group effectiveness. A clear goal or task must be established; real and meaningful problems that stimulate interest must be selected; guidelines for group operation must be provided; expectations of group participation and activity must be clarified; required resources for group work must be accessible; and constructive feedback during the task must be given. Furthermore, the teacher should remember to give options for independent and paired learning in addition to group learning when a specific sociological pattern is not a requirement of the activity or necessary for the educational goals.

Alternative Activities and Multisensory Resources

The term "media" includes all resources used in a learning sequence to help the student achieve stated objectives. When there is a combination of several communication media, the term, multimedia, is used.

Diversity of learning style in relation to type of media is well recognized (Ward & Williams, 1976, p. 69). Some people learn best through the written word and reading; others through spoken instruction and hearing; others through visual presentation and seeing; and some by handling concrete forms. For many, learning is enhanced with a combination of two or more media forms. Table 12-1 includes examples of media appropriate to nursing education in relation to the four main learning modes: reading, seeing, listening, and manipulating.

Learning activities must include a variety of media so that people who learn best in a particular way can use their preferred method. Individualized instruction presumes the availability of alternate routes to reaching the objectives (Dirr, 1976). Whether or not the use of media improves instruction and increases individualization depends on how media forms are used in the instructional sequence. To be effective, media should not be merely attached to traditional instructional procedures simply for the sake of using media. Rather, each learning resource should be selected because it is believed to be the most useful for achieve-

Table 12-1
Learning Modes, Formats, and Representative Examples of Media

Learning Mode	Medium Format	Representative Examples of Media
Reading	Print materials	Textbooks, reference books, charts, pamphlets, outlines, workbooks and studyguides, handouts, crossword puzzles, printed programmed instruction, journals, newspapers, scripts
Seeing	Pictorial materials, visual representations	Filmstrips, filmloops, videotapes, television, 8-mm and 16-mm films, displays, exhibits, posters, photographs, slides, overhead transparencies, diagrams, cartoons, simulated activities, demonstrations, flow charts, graphs, sketches
Listening	Auditory	Lectures, seminars, paired and small-group discussions, skits, audio and videotapes, one-to-one interaction with teacher, peer, or client, oral presentations, panel discussions, debates, simulations
Manipulating	Tactile, kinesthetic	Practicing with real or simulated items, lab activities, manipulating or constructing models, playing games, drawing, filling in worksheets or workbooks, preparing bulletin boards, charts, graphs, or displays

ment of instructional goals. At times, several different types of learning resources may be equally appropriate.

An important function of the teacher is the use of a variety of methods so that each student is able to choose one that is personally most productive for reaching objectives. The degree of individualization increases when the student is provided with options about learning activities to be completed and type of resources to be used. Secondarily, student attitude toward learning will be improved since there is a greater degree of control over the learning situation (Ward & Williams, 1976, p. 22). At the same time, learning productivity is increased since perceptual strengths are supported.

If there are several ways to present the same subject matter, and exposure to each would result in extensive repetition, it is undesirable to require that a student use all media forms. Rather, the teacher should determine what alternatives are possible and allow each student some choice among the different media. The choice might be between a reading activity in a textbook or journal and a viewing/listening activity using a filmstrip and audiocassette. Too often students have no choice—a list of learning resources is given and students are instructed to study everything. This may occur because the teacher feels that, otherwise, "something will be missed." It may be because objectives are not yet well enough defined in relation to the topic for a particular level of student. Thus, it is easier to require students to complete all related activities than to specify objectives to reflect exactly what is expected of the student.

There are valid reasons why the degree of flexibility of student choice is restricted at times. Desired experiences and available resources may be limited due to overcrowding of clinical facilities, lack of fiscal resources to purchase or develop media, or lack of quality or availability of commercial media. In such situations, it may still be possible to allow individual choice through the creative use of those resources that are available. A few examples follow: (1) reporting on a topic in written, verbal, visual, or auditory form or a combination of these; (2) writing personal learning objectives for an experience; (3) attending a lecture or completing a guided, independent learning activity (such as a module or audiotutorial lesson); (4) selection of a client with whom to complete an interview, carry out some type of physical or developmental assessment, or apply prior learning; (5) selection of one or more peers with whom to work on an activity or project; (6) selection of one topic from a list of several on which to report to a group; (7) deciding level of mastery in relation to desired grade (contracting to do a specific amount and quality of work for a specific grade); and (8) choosing from among two or three optional plans for how to complete a learning experience or project.

When it is not possible to provide choices, every effort should be made to use activities and resources that are multisensory. In this way, the perceptual strengths of the student can, at least, be accommodated for a portion of the learning experience, and each medium helps to reinforce another. For example, if there is a filmstrip/audiocassette and a chapter in a text that discusses different aspects of a topic, the student might be required to study both but would achieve greater gains using the medium that is preferred. Learning can be increased in the nonpreferred medium if it can be supplemented with teacher-developed materials that focus or direct student learning. One example of the latter would be the preparation of a study guide or an audiotape to be used by a student in combination with the required media.

Another example, in a motor skill area, is when the student is learning to thread intravenous tubing through an infusion pump and put the pump into operation. The best learning result would probably occur through a combination of several activities—reading the procedure, seeing a demonstration, seeing a diagram of proper threading, and, finally, manipulating the tubing and the pump. Further, typical problems may be simulated in a controlled setting so that the student has an opportunity, in a safe environment, to learn to deal with them. It is easy to visualize the difference in level of clinical performance between a student who has participated in all of these and a student who has had an opportunity only to read the procedure and see a demonstration.

There has been no attempt made to discuss which medium is best in different situations. The reader is referred to some excellent references that do so (Kemp, 1985, pp. 136–140; Price, 1971; Diamond, 1977).

FUTURE IMPLICATIONS

It seems clear, from the evidence presented early in this chapter, that students do benefit from a matching of teaching methods with learning styles. It is also important to consider the possibility that a preference for passive learning experiences and teacher-structured activities is a result of many years of educational conditioning. It may be more important to concentrate on broadening the learning styles of our students so that they will be able to benefit under more varied conditions, rather than always trying for a precise match of teaching method and learning style. Partridge (1983, p. 247) agrees by stating, "if a student habitually utilizes only one learning style, he may be at a serious disadvantage when confronted with the necessity to utilize a different mode."

If this is to occur, not only do we need more research on the relationships of learning styles and teaching methods but also on specific techniques for helping students learn to use different styles under different circumstances. This also requires the inclusion of more content on learning styles in graduate programs and the expanded evaluation of *all* learning methods in relation to whether desired outcomes are actually achieved. In the future, we may decide that truly individualized learning occurs when the students achieve what is desired in a way that will be most beneficial to them over the long term rather than what they prefer at the moment.

SUMMARY

Individualized instruction is a valuable approach for meeting the unique needs of diverse student populations. There is considerable evidence to suggest that increased learning gains occur as a result of matching teaching styles with learning styles. Various tools are available to ascertain individual learning styles. In order for instruction to be labeled "individualized," it must meet basic criteria for student involvement and responsibility; teacher roles; specification of learning objectives; feedback and evaluation; and degree of flexibility in selection of media and activities, sociological pattern, and pacing. Questions have been raised about the need to help students expand the methods by which they learn, the importance of further study about learning styles and teaching methods, the inclusion of material on learning styles in graduate programs, and the purposeful evaluation of all learning methods.

13

Developing and Using Modules for Instruction

One strategy by which mastery learning and individualization can be achieved is the learning module. In the past 2 decades, the use of modules for teaching a variety of subjects at all educational levels has been described in educational literature. In fact, Cross (1976, p. 75) credited the learning module with being at the heart of an "instructional revolution" in which the accent is on learning. Previously, Novak (1973, p. 4) had observed: "The use of some form of modular instruction is probably the fastest-growing trend in the history of Western education." Three surveys support these conclusions in relation to community colleges in general and to associate and baccalaureate degree nurse education programs. In a survey of community colleges (Cross, 1976, p. 75), almost three-fourths of the respondents reported some use of learning modules. A survey of associate and baccalaureate degree nursing programs (Thompson, 1980) revealed that almost two-thirds of the respondents were using modules or learning packages in their programs. And in a later survey of baccalaureate nursing programs (Knippers, 1981), 76 percent of the respondents indicated that modules and packages were used in some courses. There are many reports in the literature that describe the use of modules or other closely related strategies for nursing education at the undergraduate, graduate, and postgraduate levels. Many of these will be cited in this chapter.

A problem that confronts anyone who wants to gain a historical perspective of utilization of learning modules is that a variety of terms are used to describe essentially the same approach. One of the earliest educational uses of the term module was in 1971 by Craeger and Murray. Others who have used the term since include Russell (1974), Rochin and Thompson (1975), Cross (1976, pp. 75–110), Shute (1976), Magidson (1976), Swendsen, Meleis, and Hourigan (1977), Bell and Miller (1977), Hinthorne (1980), Zebelman, Davis, and Larson (1983), Armstrong, Toebe, and Watson (1985), and Reilly and Oermann(1985, pp. 133–136). Other terms were used during the same period to describe approaches that had varying degrees of similarity to learning modules. Representative of these are Minicourse (Postlethwait & Russell, 1971), Audio-Tutorial Package (McDonald & Dodge, 1971), Learning Packet (Ray & Clark, 1977; Ubben, 1971; Ward & Williams, 1976), Learning Activity Package (Brock, 1978; Cardarelli, 1972; Layton, 1975), Interactive Learning Package (O'Connor & Jones, 1975), Individualized Instruction Package (Duane, 1973), and Self-learning/Self-instructional Package (Gentine, 1980; Rufo, 1985). Blatchley, Herzog, and Russell (1978) used the terms module and minicourse synonymously. The term module will be used throughout this chapter as a more descriptive and inclusive term.

WHAT IS A LEARNING MODULE?

The learning module, a strategy for individualizing instruction, is a self-contained instructional unit that focuses on a single concept or topic and has a few well-defined objectives. Although other instructional formats may be (and should be) incorporated, independent study is central to the use of learning modules. Through independent study, the student has increased control over when and where learning will take place. At the same time, a learning module should reflect other characteristics typical of individualized instruction (II) as given in Chapter 12.

The design of a learning module determines the degree to which the learning situation is individualized. Design depends on the philosophy and expertise of the developer, specific concept or topic of the module, and availability of learning resources for use with the module. The finished product should demonstrate a close integration of the individual components of instruction—objectives, strategies, and evaluation. This is most likely to occur when one uses a systematic approach while developing a learning module. One such approach is described by Thompson (1978), the steps of which are paraphrased below:

1. Select a topic and describe its general purpose or intent.
2. Outline the pertinent characteristics of the student group that will use the module.
3. List learning objectives and complete a task analysis to determine what tasks a student must perform to reach objectives.
4. Identify content pertinent to each behavioral objective.
5. Develop learning activities for each objective.
6. Select or develop media (all materials) to present the content and allow variations in learning style.
7. Validate instructional media and techniques with content and/or instructional experts.
8. Develop tools for testing and evaluation to reflect each objective.
9. List any required prerequisites.
10. Identify and arrange for any necessary support services.
11. Develop the guide that the student will use for completion of the module.
12. Develop a tool for feedback from the student about the module.
13. Use the module in a trial run with a student group.
14. Make necessary revisions.

Elements of a Learning Module

What does a module look like? An outline of typical components is given below:

1. Table of contents
2. Introduction, including purpose, terminal objective, and general directions
3. List of prerequisites and suggested resources
4. Instructional objectives
5. Pretest
6. Resources
7. Activities
8. Self-checks of progress
9. Posttest
10. Feedback on module

Each of these components will be discussed briefly. The reader is also referred to the sample module included at the end of this chapter for an illustration of each of the elements (Appendix 1).

Table of Contents.   If the printed packet of the module is more than a few pages long it is helpful to have a table of contents to identify each section and its page location. This allows the student to find a section quickly and easily with minimal confusion and frustration. A table of contents is especially helpful for the student who has already had an introduction to the subject covered by the module and who wants to locate the objectives and the pretest to decide if the module or parts of the module have been previously mastered. A table of contents is also useful for the student who wants to review the list of resources to be used so that resources and where they are located can be determined ahead of time. In this way, time for study of the module can be planned and organized more productively. Furthermore, a table of contents aids the student in locating a particular activity or section when self-check or posttest results indicate the need for further study in order to achieve mastery.

Introduction.   The introductory section of the module lets the student know the purpose of the module, the significance of study of the material covered, the terminal objective, and how best to advance through the module. The language should be directed to the student and written at a level that the student can understand. In this section, as in others, every effort should be made to avoid typographical and grammatical errors that distract or hamper progress of the student.

Prerequisites and Suggested Resources.   A list of the prerequisite knowledge and skills is given so that students are able to determine if they have the background necessary for success with the module. Prerequisites are best stated in specific behavioral terms so that the student can understand more clearly the required entry behavior for module study. A list of suggested resources is useful for the student who needs to make up deficiencies before beginning study of the module. Notice in the sample module that alternative resources are given. This allows the student more flexibility in selecting which resource to use.

A prerequisite test and key can be included to help the student make a quick self-assessment of desired knowledge and skills and indicate the direction that review should take, if needed. Bloom (1980) suggests that teachers should pay greater attention to entry characteristics of the student. He believes that what a student brings to a course may have more to do with achievement than the course itself. Thus, greater gains can be assured in a particular learning situation if the student is first brought to the desired level of achievement on prerequisites for that learning task.

Instructional Objectives.   Well-defined learning objectives specific to the module are stated so that expectations are clear to the student. As stated in the definition of learning module, only a *few* objectives should be included. Although the actual number depends on specific content, it is preferable if the number is limited to 15 or less per module. If more than 15 objectives are necessary for a particular topic, the developer of the module should consider narrowing the topic further so that fewer objectives will be covered in the module. For example, this may require that modules be developed on two subtopics rather than one module on one major topic.

Ideally, objectives should require more than simple recall and involve the student in using the content in a practical learning situation. The objectives should be relevant to the experiences of the student and the goals of the course in which the module is used. They must be matched precisely with module content, resources, activities, and items for evaluation and testing. In some cases, each objective is listed separately with directions and a list of resources and activities specific to that objective given immediately after the objective. In other cases, all objectives for the module are given and resources and activities keyed to each objective. The latter is the format used for the objectives in the sample module.

Pretest.   A pretest representing all learning objectives is a vital part of every module. Length of the pretest will vary depending on the level of complexity of the objectives and the type of activity required to demonstrate mastery. However, if the objectives are few and well defined as specified in the definition, a pretest representative of all objectives would not be lengthy. A maximum time period of 15 to 30 minutes is recommended. This does not seem unreasonable when one considers that traditional testing usually involves the use of a 1-hour examination to cover lectures, readings, and so forth for one-third to one-half of a semester or quarter. The difference is that the objectives for a module are more delineated so that the student knows exactly what is required and can, thus, be expected to reach each objective.

The pretest is primarily a mechanism for assessing prior knowledge and skills to determine if a student must complete all, part, or none of the activities of the module. For the student with previous exposure to

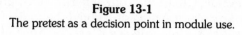

Figure 13-1
The pretest as a decision point in module use.

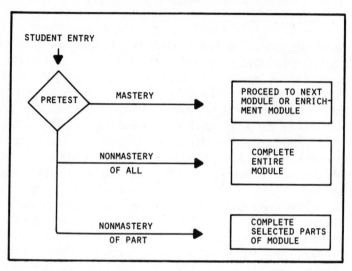

the module subject area, success on part or all of the pretest serves as positive reinforcement and recognition of that learning. It is possible, then, to give credit for previous learning and allow the student to progress more rapidly through required learning experiences. The pretest thus represents a point at which decisions about prior mastery or nonmastery are made. For the student who demonstrates nonmastery of all or part of the module, either the total module or selected parts of a module can be completed based on exact pretest results. Figure 13-1 depicts the pretest as a decision point and shows the possible routes indicated by pretest results.

The pretest also serves other functions that are useful to the learning process. By providing a preview of what is in the module, it "sets the scene" so that the student knows what to expect. In addition, since it tests the same objectives, the pretest gives an indication of what the posttest will look like. Because of this, the pretest may be used, if desired, as an alternate form of the posttest or as a self-evaluation tool by the student to determine readiness to take the posttest.

The key for the pretest can be included in the module for the student to use independently for self-assessment or self-evaluation. However, if the student is to be given formal credit for prior learning, it is probably necessary for the teacher or an assistant to retain the test key and review pretest results personally. If performance of a skill is involved, the student may demonstrate competence in different ways. A skill may be performed in front of an observer who is using a criteria checklist, or the performance of the skill can be videotaped by the student for review later by an evaluator. The latter provides greater flexibility for both the student and the teacher and can decrease the amount of stress felt by the student during a testing situation.

Notice that the format of the pretest in the sample module includes a notation with each question telling which objective is being tested. In this way a student with prior learning is able to determine more easily which activities can be skipped and which ones must be completed. A key provides immediate feedback about level of knowledge if the pretest is being used independently by the student. The key can be placed immediately after the pretest in the module or at the end of the module with other keys to self-checks and the posttest. The key can also be provided in other than written forms, such as on an audiocassette tape, for the student who prefers to listen or who gains more from listening and reading at the same time.

Resources.   A list of alternative or required resources must be given so that the student will be directed to materials to be used in the achievement of objectives. Alternate resources from which the student may choose increase student options to select preferred materials. When such alternatives are given, it is important that each provides equal access to achievement of objectives. One alternative may be a visual and auditory experience using either a filmstrip and audiocassette or a videotape. Another may be a reading activity using either a textbook or journal. Another may have the student handling and manipulating real objects or models. One important advantage to giving a choice of resources is that limited resources or those housed in a learning center are used more efficiently when a number of students need the resources at the same time. If alternatives cannot be given, it is important to use a variety of multisensory resources so that, at least, different perceptual strengths are addressed during a learning experience. Such variety also helps to increase motivation and maintain interest.

A listing of resources also indicates if there are limitations in their availability. For example, a module that requires the use of a videotape would require the presence of the student in a learning center or viewing area. On the other hand, a module that requires the use of a textbook owned by the student can be completed wherever and whenever the student chooses. A module that directs the student to discuss a particular topic in a small group cannot be completed without the availability of a group. In all of these instances if the student is aware, in advance, of such limitations or special requirements, time for study of the module can be planned more effectively. Student frustration will thus be decreased since the student will not begin study of a module only to discover that an important resource is not readily available.

Self-Containment. A module is self-contained since it is made up of everything that is required to reach the objectives and to measure their achievement. Self-containment can take two forms: (1) all module components are under one cover or in one package that is portable, and (2) the module is made up partially of peripheral components that are not easily transportable. When all module components are in one package, access and convenience to the student are increased. For example, in a module on the topic of Clinitest urine testing, everything required can be contained in a small carton. Such a module is usable either in a learning center or skills laboratory or, if sufficient kits are available, may be transported to any location selected by the student. Often, as in this case, portability is easily accomplished by the use of kits to be checked out by the student. When such kits are involved, it is important that someone be available and responsible to check them out to the student and to check and replenish the contents when returned.

Portability can also be achieved by synthesizing material from various resources and putting the information under one cover—the all print module. This type of module, however, has some distinct disadvantages. First, it is in print and may not be the best type of learning experience for many students. Second, it requires greater time for development and is more difficult to revise and update than one using peripheral resources that can be readily deleted or added.

In some cases, portability is increased by using easily transported equipment and materials for checkout. For example, a compact filmstrip-viewing and audiocassette playback unit and a copy of a filmstrip and audiocassette program available for checkout broaden accessibility and add to the convenience of the student. An arrangement of this type requires ample equipment and materials as well as personnel for their dispensing and servicing. It is also crucial that some understanding be reached and communicated about responsibility for replacement or repair of lost or damaged items.

Portability is difficult or impossible to achieve in many instances: when heavy or expensive equipment is involved; when format or cost limits availability of media resources; or when location of required resources is specialized, as in a clinical setting or the community. In such cases, self-containment at a specific location is the only alternative. For example, a module that requires the use of a computer, specialized medical equipment, or media of which there are limited copies would necessarily require completion where those resources are located. This is restricting to the student in one sense because the student must go where the resources are—often in a learning center or skills laboratory with limited hours of operation. If this is required, it is imperative that adequate hours be scheduled so that learning requirements can be achieved within a reasonable period especially if time for completion is limited. Although operating hours may be limited, the student still has some important options: selecting a personally convenient time within specified hours, deciding which resources to use if alternatives are stated, and choosing whether to work alone or with a friend.

Activities.   Learning activities that direct the student's use of the resources focus the student's efforts on the objectives to be mastered and give the student practice in reaching objectives. Directions provided with each activity must be clear so that the student is able to use time productively and avoid unnecessary confusion. Activities must reflect the type of action specified in the objectives and involve the learner in active participation with the content. Participation can take the form of mental, written, interactive, or manipulative exercises and can involve the use of study questions, guided reading, worksheets, projects, charts, diagrams, puzzles, simulated or actual clinical experiences, practice with models or actual items, interaction with others, and so forth. As stated previously, activities may be listed with each objective in turn or each activity can be keyed, as in the sample module, to indicate which objective it is addressing.

Some activities are required of all students. This is particularly true when resources are limited or different resources are not comparable. Even when students are completing the same activity, they may be given an option of which medium to use when the content among the various media is similar. It is desirable, when possible, to use alternative activities to allow some choice by the student. The choice could be either to complete a short paper on a particular topic or to give a 5-minute speech on that topic to a group or on an audiocassette. Another choice could be to select a drug or clinical situation to be used for more in-depth research. The possibilities are limited only by the availability of resources and the creativity of the person designing the learning experience.

Some activities are completed by only a few students for the purpose of enrichment when a student is able and interested in studying a topic to a greater depth. They may be designed by the student, by the teacher,

Figure 13-2
The progress self-check as a decision point and alternative routes indicated by self-check results. Adapted from Wilson & Tosti, 1972, pp. 138–139. Used with permission of Individual Learning Systems, Inc., P.O. Box 225447, Dallas, Texas 75265.

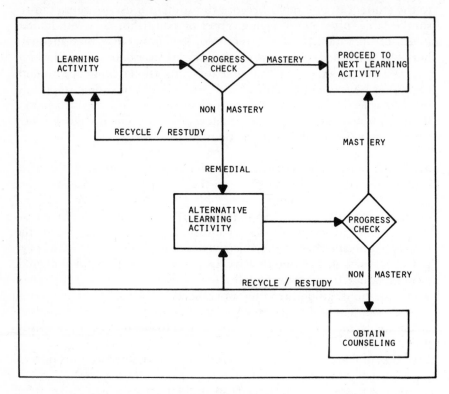

or by both. When modules are used in conventional grading situations, enrichment activities are often used to differentiate among the various grade levels.

Self-Checks of Progress. Self-evaluation checkpoints are included to provide immediate feedback to the student about progress toward meeting each learning objective. They let the student know if an objective has been reached; if not, the student is directed to repeat an activity, do an alternate activity, or seek counseling from the teacher. Figure 13-2 illustrates the use of the self-check as a decision point in the learning module and shows different routes that the student can take depending on self-evaluation results.

The self-check also serves secondary purposes by indicating readiness for the posttest and giving the student clues about what the posttest will be like. Self-checks may be similar in form to pretest and posttest items or may have a different form as long as learning objectives are clearly reflected.

Posttest.   A posttest is used to determine whether or not the student has achieved mastery of the learning objectives stated in the module. As with the pretest, the posttest covers all objectives and should take no longer than 15 minutes to complete. It is helpful when each posttest item has a notation to indicate which objective is being tested so that a student is readily aware of which sections to study further when a question is answered incorrectly. If posttest results indicate that objectives have been met, the student can proceed to another module or learning experience. If objectives are not met, the student must repeat activities or do alternate activities in order to achieve what is required. Figure 13-3 shows the posttest as a decision point in the module and indicates the different routes by which mastery can be achieved.

The posttest is used by the student, the teacher, a teacher's assistant, or a computer to provide data that indicate what the next learning experience should be or the need for restudy of material. If used by the student alone, the posttest is often a part of the printed module packet. If it is to be graded by someone other than the student, the posttest is usually retained by the teacher or an assistant or generated by a computer.

Posttest items, like the pretest and self-check items, can take various forms—multiple-choice, fill-in, short answer, true-false, essay, performance—depending on the content and level of objective. It is desirable, when possible, to use test forms other than written. For example, diagrams, slides, videotaped situations, and exhibits offer testing variations that increase interest, capitalize on different perceptual strengths, and add realism.

The pretest and the posttest can be the same, especially if the teacher wishes to determine exact gains from module study. Broader evaluation might be accomplished, however, if the two tests are different. Alternate forms of the posttest are needed when retesting on a module is required. The pretest, if different, serves as one form, or a computer can be used to generate alternate test forms. In addition, the teacher who maintains a file of questions related to each objective will be able to construct an alternate posttest, if necessary.

Posttest results, in addition to indicating mastery or nonmastery of objectives, provide feedback about effectiveness of module design. If a number of students study a module and the posttest confirms that they

Figure 13-3

The posttest as a decision point, with alternative routes indicated by posttest results. Adapted from Wilson & Tosti, 1972, p. 140. Used with permission of Individual Learning Systems, Inc., P.O. Box 225447, Dallas, Texas 75265.

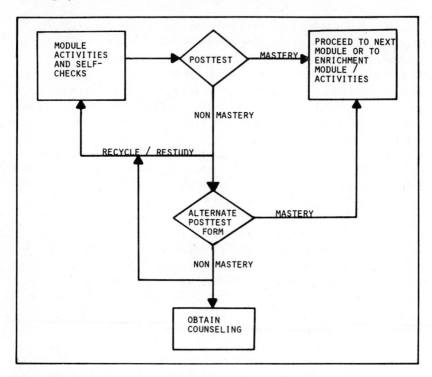

have met the objectives, posttest items are validated and the design of the module is supported. If, on the other hand, nonmastery is evident, it is necessary to analyze the posttest and module design to determine what revisions are needed. The objectives may need to be rewritten. Resources and activities may be inappropriate. Posttest items may not adequately reflect the objectives. Whatever the case, analyzing posttest results provides data that help a teacher to make alterations that will increase the effectiveness of the module as a learning tool.

Feedback on the Learning Module. Students may be requested, usually on a voluntary basis, to give their impressions about each module used. They may be asked to write out general impressions or be given a tool that will direct their attention to certain important aspects for evaluation. This feedback provides information from the student's perspective that is helpful for making revisions in the learning module. The sample module includes one example of a feedback form for use by students (see p. 251).

RESEARCH ON EFFECTIVENESS OF LEARNING MODULES

More research into the effectiveness of modules for learning nursing content is needed. Although there are many reports in the nursing literature that describe experiences with the use of modules and other self-instructional packages, it is rare to find studies that investigate the effectiveness of the module as a teaching/learning method. Those that are available support the use of modules for learning content in various educational and practice settings. The results of three studies will be summarized here.

Osborn and Thompson (1977) studied several noncognitive factors affecting student mastery of learning modules in several baccalaureate programs. They found that students achieved significantly higher post-tests scores when the modules were used in traditionally graded theory courses instead of in credit/no credit clinical courses, when the posttest was not self-graded, and when the student was classified as more open-minded as determined by Rokeach's Dogmatism Scale.

One study investigating effectiveness of modules with graduate nursing students is by Huckabay (1981). She compared the amount of learning using objective cognitive tests with three groups: lecture discussion, module, and combined module/lecture discussion. Learning was found to be significantly greater with the combined module/lecture discussion group than with the lecture discussion group but not any greater than with the module group. Further, the module group showed significantly greater learning than did the lecture discussion group.

In one study in a hospital setting the effectiveness of self-instructional packages was compared with that of lecture/demonstration for orientation of staff nurses (Rufo, 1985). Five of the 10 self-instructional packages included were found to be significantly more effective. Three of the remaining five demonstrated a tendency toward greater effectiveness although the results were not significant. Only two content areas were found to be less effective in the self-instructional format.

Additional research is warranted in this area. A few questions suggested for further investigation are:

Figure 13-4
A modular system (Russell, 1974; Wilson & Tosti, 1972).

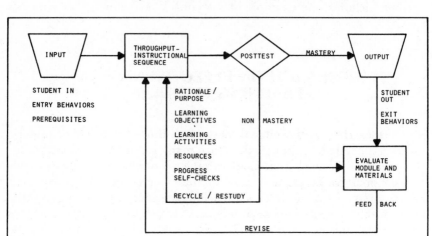

What type of content is appropriate to the modular method of instruction? Are certain types of content inappropriate for this method?

What are the learner benefits from this approach? What are the specific learning styles addressed by the use of learning modules?

How does module design relate to effectiveness?

Utilization of Learning Modules

The learning module represents an instructional *system,* since it involves an integrated assembly of components (resources, activities, equipment, people) that operate in organized interaction to transmit instructional messages designed for achievement of predetermined objectives and provide feedback about effectiveness of the system. Figure 13-4 depicts an operational diagram of the modular instructional system. Such systems can be used on a small scale to provide independent study options and enrichment or on a large scale to teach an entire course or all courses in a curriculum.

Common Uses. Learning modules can be used to teach any subject in any setting, including schools, places of employment, and the home.

They can be designed for formal credit, continuing education, self-improvement, hobbies, or other uses. In education, they are a mechanism for individualizing instruction and serve to extend the influence of a teacher over a great number of students and to take advantage of the contributions of experts on a particular topic. Russell (1974, p. 96) identifies the more common uses of modules as "regular instruction, enrichment, remedial instruction, establishing entry behavior, absentee instruction and correspondence courses." Russell's list will be modified somewhat and applied to situations in nursing education.

Regular Instruction and Absentee Instruction. Modules can be used to provide regular instruction in part of a course, an entire course, or all courses in a curriculum. Most of the reports in the literature in the last 10 years describing the use of modules (or other self-instructional learning packages) indicate that they have been used for regular instruction in different settings and for a variety of purposes. In nursing curricula, common areas of use include nursing theory courses (Blatchley et al., 1978; Rochin & Thompson, 1975), as an option for independent study in regular nursing courses (Layton, 1975), and for total curricula (Cowart & Burge, 1979; Ferrell, 1978; Rose & Riegert, 1976). However, the most common application of modules in regular coursework has been for teaching basic technical and physical assessment skills (Ray & Clark, 1977; Rochin & Thompson, 1975; Swendsen et al., 1977; Sullivan et al., 1977). In one of these settings (Rochin & Thompson, 1975), modules were used (to some degree) in more than half the courses in the nursing major to provide regular instruction. The independent learning module is the predominant teaching strategy in three sequential skills courses. Although each course is limited by the semester time frame and the student is required to complete designated modules each week, there are opportunities for selection of preferred media, pacing of study within each week, and choice of whether to study and practice alone or with one or more peers.

Each week's modules involve independent study; independent, paired, or small-group practice; and large-group lecture discussion. Independent module activities are to be completed by the student before the large-group lecture discussion and the scheduled practice lab. Some activities involve the use of audiovisual media, textbooks, journal articles, or other references located in the Nursing Learning Resource Center (NLRC), which is open Monday through Friday from 8:00 a.m. to 5 p.m. and two evenings a week until 9:00 p.m. Other activities require the use of textbooks, handouts, and equipment that each student owns. Some modules have alternative resources from which the student selects according to personal preference or access. Each module has a pretest, self-checks, and a posttest for which keys are included to help the student with self-evaluation of learning.

The large-group lecture discussion (1 hour) is attended by all students enrolled in the course. It is led by a faculty member and focuses on discussion of major concepts related to the skills being studied that week. There are opportunities for questions, clarification, and practice in applying the content to clinical situations. The lecture discussion is recorded, and the tape placed in the NLRC for those students who were unable to attend class or who wish to review the content discussed.

Following the lecture discussion, each student attends one of several scheduled practice sessions (3 hours) in a Skills Laboratory staffed by a faculty member. The lab period provides an opportunity for students to practice designated skills, ask questions, seek clarification, and obtain feedback about personal performance. A major technique used for self-check or peer evaluation and for testing is the "criteria sheet" outlining key points in the performance of each skill. The observer uses the criteria sheet to check each item as performed by the student.

Students are informed at the beginning of the semester how many points are needed for each grade. The total points possible in the course are distributed between "theoretical" and "practical" content. Theory examinations take place during the lecture discussion period and are composed of multiple-choice, objective questions. Item analysis and scoring of these tests are done by computer. The practical examinations take place during a lab period and are made up of exhibits about which the student must answer questions, make decisions, calculate mathematical problems, and so forth. Responses consist of item selection or short answer and are made on an answer sheet identifying each exhibit by number. Additional points are available through performance on written and practical quizzes given at intervals during the semester. Students do not know ahead of time which skill they will be asked to demonstrate. That is determined by teacher selection or by student blind selection from among five or six cards, each naming a specific skill. A teacher observing the performance uses a criteria sheet to evaluate and assign points.

Application of modules to regular instruction in practice settings has also been reported. When used for in-service/staff development, modules provide increased access to educational materials, broaden learning opportunities, decrease scheduling and management problems for groups who need the same instruction, and decrease per employee costs of instruction. For example, all new employees can be oriented to an agency through the use of modules that have been developed to incorporate the special characteristics and needs of the agency. Nurses in a clinical unit can be provided with specialized instruction unique to that unit.

Several reports are available describing the application of modules to regular instruction in staff development and orientation. Rufo (1985), cited previously, focuses on the use of self-instructional packages for orientation of newly employed nurses. Zebelman, Davis, and Larson (1983) describe their use of learning modules for orientation and staff development. They view staff nurses as adult learners who "are self-directed and who can identify and meet their own learning needs when given the necessary information, resources, and support" (p. 198). Huntsman and Thompson (1977) and Sherer and Thompson (1978) report on the use of modules for staff development in one setting. They contend that the program achieves not only the advantages cited above but also frees the staff development instructor to develop quality materials and spend time in the clinical units assessing and validating skills rather than planning, conducting, and repeating formal classes. Basic to this plan is the identification of learning needs by the head nurse and staff member involved and the subsequent independent use of the learning materials related to identified performance expectations.

According to another report (Schmidt, 1977), a modular curriculum was designed to teach 15 subject areas common to seven different intensive care units. Benefits identified were increased accessibility to learning materials, reduced costs, improved learning efficiency through immediate application in the clinical area, and more direct involvement of the clinical specialist in patient care and supervision of staff members' clinical performance.

Enrichment.   Modules can be used to provide an expanded, in-depth learning experience beyond the basic essential requirements for all students. Such experiences are enrichment opportunities for the student who is motivated or interested in pursuing a topic further or wishes to gain points or credit toward a higher grade. Russell (1974, p. 116) and Duane (1973, p. 172) refer to these as "quests" while Ward and Williams (1976, p. 32) use the label "DO-ITS" (acronym for Depth Opportunities-Individual Tasks).

Regardless of what they are called, enrichment activities or modules provide an opportunity for individual investigation and learning beyond the basic requirements. Enrichment can be achieved by providing optional activities as part of a module, by having separate, optional modules from which the student selects, or by allowing a student to design a learning experience related to a particular topic. When the optional activities are attached to the module, they are usually directly related to module content but provide an opportunity to gain greater knowledge about the topic or apply the knowledge or skills gained from the basic module in new and different ways. Optional activities should be meaningful to student experiences and appropriate to the level of the student so that interest is maintained and student time is used productively. Optional activities that are incorporated into a module for enrichment purposes can include:

Write a paper related to some aspect of the topic. (Length and number and type of references might be specified.)

Construct two learning aids to be used for client/peer teaching.

Prepare a short speech to deliver to peer group.

Prepare a demonstration of a skill.

Create a game or puzzle for teaching clients/peers.

If separate, optional modules are used, they are usually at least indirectly related to the basic learning experiences. Optional modules are often on specialized topics or issues that go beyond what can be included in the basic curriculum. The types of activities included should encourage projects or creative productions that require in-depth investigation and application of knowledge. Optional modules can include:

Complete research on a particular topic or on people and places associated with the topic.

Complete a survey of newspaper articles, magazine articles, and television reports relevant to a particular topic.

Prepare slides, tapes, posters, or bulletin boards that can be displayed or used by other people.

Interview a public official, members of a profession, or a client.

Locate and abstract three or four journal articles per week related to topics of weekly discussion.

Write a reaction paper to television specials, movies, or books associated with the topic being studied.

When the student is allowed to select a topic and design an enrichment activity, the teacher requires that the student prepare in advance and obtain approval for the plan of action, questions to be answered, type and number of resources to be used, and method of reporting. Teacher supervision is needed to provide necessary guidance and assure that the finished product is of the desired quality. (See Chapter 14 for discussion of learning contracts.)

Ideas for enrichment activities may be generated by the teacher or the student by thinking about experiences that are interesting and rewarding to them. The teacher may also consider the various aspects of topics for which there is not enough time in the basic curriculum and talk to other professionals about topics and issues or students about their interests and personal goals. Specialized topics or issues are particularly appropriate. A few examples are:

Moral or ethical issues, such as abortion, genetic engineering, right-to-die, and pollution of air, water, food

Professional issues, such as entry into practice, credentialing, standards of practice, and compulsory membership in professional associations

Social issues, such as crime prevention, segregation, welfare, overpopulation, rent control, child or spousal abuse, health care and living conditions of migrant workers, and rape

Special topics, such as genetic counseling, use of play with the hospitalized child, reactions of parents to the hospitalization of a child, compliance with immunization requirements or prescribed drugs, and client knowledge about side effects of drugs

Remedial Instruction and Establishing Entry Behavior.   These two uses are closely related in process. Modules can be used for remedial instruction when a student needs to review content covered previously for application to some current situation. For example, the student in a clinical course who is having some problem with dose calculation, remembering pertinent growth and development characteristics, or recalling certain physiological concepts can either repeat modules used before or use modules designed specifically for remedial purposes. Although remedial in nature, such modules help establish the desired entry behaviors for a particular learning experience and enhance the success of the student. Other modules designed for either or both purposes include a basic math computation module to determine if the student has the math skills necessary to master dose calculation skills, a module on basic research terminology or statistics to determine readiness for a graduate level applied research class, or a module on the physiology of glucose metabolism in preparation for study of diabetes mellitus. When modules of this nature are available, students can use them to develop necessary entry behaviors so that it is not necessary to devote limited class time to deal with material associated with course or topic prerequisites. Those who have fulfilled the necessary prerequisites are not required to use the modules; others can use them for review, if desired; and others can make up deficiencies resulting from a lack of earlier education or insufficient recall of content.

One example of the use of modules for establishing desired entry characteristics is given by Chinn and Hunt (1975) for graduate level child nursing instruction. Module pretests were used in that setting to determine a student's entry level of knowledge and skills and the results used to direct the learning experiences of the student. If the student lacked basic cognitive and performance skills in ambulatory child nursing, self-directed learning modules were used to provide a mechanism whereby these skills could be achieved before attempting advanced work in the clinical specialty.

Assessing Prior Knowledge for Advanced Placement.   Although related to the use of modules for establishing desired entry behaviors, assessing prior knowledge for advanced placement implies that the student has had previous course work or experience that may allow skipping of part or all of a course. Module pretests and posttests, or a sampling of test items, are used to assess individual ability and recognize previous learning. As a result, credit is given and the student placed at the proper level in the curriculum. This is particularly appropriate to determine if any part of a planned program can be eliminated for students with acknowledged previous experience—military hospital corps personnel, nursing assistants, licensed practical/vocational nurses, or registered nurses who have either a diploma or associate degree and are enrolled in a baccalaureate degree program.

Providing Nontraditional Options for Continuing Education and Degrees. There are several areas of need for educational opportunities beyond the basic nursing program. Among them are (1) many states now require or plan to require continuing education for relicensure of registered nurses; (2) large numbers of nurses desire courses for self-development or increase in professional status through upward mobility; and (3) there is a continuing information explosion.

In nursing, traditional forms of education have not been effective in meeting the needs of the nurse who is employed full time, has family responsibilities, and lives at a distance from educational institutions. Learning methods, such as the learning module and home study courses, help to provide independent and/or part-time study and flexible scheduling in a setting that is more readily accessible to the home or work setting of an employed nurse. Home study courses using modules are advertised in professional journals and newspapers. Study materials in modular form are now commercially available.* Such materials are useful for independent study at various levels of nursing education.

The large number of R.N.s returning to school in search of baccalaureate level education is documented by Smullen (1982) and Parlocha and Hiraki (1982). Currently, there are also many nurses seeking master's level education. In the past, R.N.s tried to achieve these goals through enrollment in traditional programs; however, they sometimes faced multiple barriers and found that prior learning and unique needs were not recognized. Typical of efforts to provide more flexible advanced educational opportunity for R.N.s are the "second-step" programs, which accept R.N.s only. Although these programs have met the needs of some, the increasing use of nontraditional methods must continue if higher educational opportunities are to be provided for greater numbers of nurses than in the past.

Two formalized nontraditional programs for obtaining advanced degrees are the "extended" or "outreach" program and the "external degree" program. They are specifically designed to meet the needs of adult learners. With extended or outreach programs, courses toward the completion of a degree are provided by an established educational institution in satellite locations convenient to learners' homes and work settings. At times the satellite center is in a work setting if there is sufficient demand to warrant it. Course offerings are of the same educational quality as those on campus, lead to the same credit, and are under the direction of faculty with regular appointments. Examples of the extended or outreach program include satellite programs for baccalaureate and master's education (White & Lee, 1977), an outreach baccalaureate program for registered nurses (Schoffstall & Marriner, 1982), and an extended master's program sponsored by a sister institution in a university with a baccalaureate degree only (Leveck, 1975). Although only one of the authors (Leveck, 1975) cited the use of modules, this teaching/learning strategy provides a viable way of expanding educational opportunities for advanced degrees and can be incorporated easily into either extended/outreach or external degree programs.

In comparison to the extended or outreach program, the external degree program emphasizes work and life experiences and credit by examination while deemphasizing time for completion. One well known program of this type is the Regents External Degrees Program, University of the State of New York, which offers associate and baccalaureate

---

*Learning materials in modular form are advertised by Addison-Wesley Publishing Company, Inc., Menlo Park, California; John Wiley and Sons, Inc., New York; AVC Nursing Series, Novato, California; and Mark-Maris Publishers, Buffalo, New York.

degrees in nursing (Lenburg, 1984). Degree requirements are similar to those in traditional educational settings. The hallmark of the Regents program is the competency-based examinations provided after students have availed themselves of a variety of personally selected learning opportunities. Candidates for the baccalaureate degree must complete five written nursing theory examinations and four performance examinations. Written tests are provided by the American College Testing Program (ACT), a service established to serve students who desire college credit for learning and experience accomplished outside the conventional classroom atmosphere. There is a national network of regional assessment centers where performance tests are conducted.

The Statewide Nursing Program (SNP) is another external degree program established by the Consortium of the California State University to expand educational opportunities for nurses who want a baccalaureate or master's degree (Consortium of the CSU, 1984). The program is designed for registered nurses who want to earn a degree but are unable to attend a regular campus program. Although similar to the New York Regents program in some ways, the SNP differs in several respects. In addition to focusing on assessment and credit for prior learning, the SNP offers specific instructional options, including self-directed learning modules and evening and weekend courses. The program is administered and taught by the regular faculty, and experts from the community are utilized.

Courses are offered in many locations throughout the state. The student has the option of earning academic credit through nontraditional course work (using learning modules) or assessment or a combination of both. Credit for prior experience may be obtained in several ways, including the New York Regents standardized tests provided by ACT. Student-designed learning contracts offer additional opportunities for individualized learning activities. Both the New York Regents program and the SNP baccalaureate program are accredited by NLN.

Similar educational opportunities, although not directed toward completion of a degree, are provided through outreach type continuing education programs. Outreach centers have been used to provide continuing education to nurses in underserved areas (McGill & Molinaro, 1978; Shockley, 1981). Independent study modules using cable and satellite television have been included in courses designed to provide continuing education to nurses in remote locations (Armstrong, Toebe, & Watson, 1985). The increasing availability of and access to computers and other technology further the expansion of educational opportunities for both continuing education and advanced degrees through the use of various independent learning methods, including modules.

Patterns of Module Use

The patterns of module use in a course or curriculum depend on several factors, including specific material, complexity of subject matter, and level of student. The patterns that will be discussed are time scheduling, subject matter sequencing, sociological format, and grading.

Time Scheduling. Time scheduling for module use falls into two general types, self-paced and specific scheduling. If fully self-paced, the student is given a list showing any required and alternative modules related to the course or the experience and allowed to complete them, including the necessary tests for competency, at a personally determined rate. The grade assigned is either one of mastery or a specific letter grade, depending on the type of course in which the modules are used. The amount of credit can be units per module, units for a certain number of modules within a course, or units for the course in which modules are used. For example, the faculty may decide that a particular module is worth a given amount of credit, such as ¼ unit, ½ unit, or 1 unit, depending on the amount of work and complexity of the module. Two or more modules could be combined and given a specified amount of credit upon completion. Or all the modules used in a course can be collectively assigned a certain amount of credit, such as 3, 4, or 5 units. At the present time, the most common pattern is one in which designated modules are used in a particular course, and the student receives credit upon successful completion of *all* the modules.

The same general pattern applies as well to specific scheduling, except that modules must be completed within a certain period of time. Modules can be assigned on a weekly basis or, when more flexibility is possible, a series of modules can be assigned to be completed within a certain period of time. That period of time might be 2 weeks, a month, or a quarter or semester. Specific deadlines are necessary when open time patterns are not possible within traditional settings and when testing must be done for all students in a course on a fixed schedule (e.g., midterm and final exams). At times, a fixed schedule is also necessary to help those students who are unaccustomed or unable to set their own timetables for completion. In a course with specific scheduling, the student who does not complete the designated work can receive an "incomplete" with the commitment to finish the required work within a designated time period in order to receive a grade for the course. Usually, the student is required to have completed a majority of the course at a satisfactory level in order for an "incomplete" to be assigned.

Subject Matter. The other pattern of module use relates to the sequencing of the modules themselves. The exact pattern depends on the determination of levels of complexity, structure of the curriculum or individual course, and interrelationships among subject areas. Usually the sequencing is established within a particular course or area of study. Basic patterns of module sequencing include single, serial, satellite, and stratified (Figure 13-5). Arrows indicate the sequence for study of the modules within each pattern.

Single modules are those that stand entirely alone. They are totally independent of other modules to be studied since they are not prerequisites to other modules nor do they require other modules as prerequisites. Modules in this pattern can be used in any order by students, thus allowing the student to select according to individual needs or preferences. Modules of this type can be used in a clinical course in which available experiences determine which modules need to be studied. Single modules within a course are usually of a similar level of complexity. Increased complexity is attained with other single modules in succeeding levels of the curriculum. A modification of this pattern, in order to achieve increased complexity using single modules within a course, is accomplished by two clusters of single modules with one cluster prerequisite to the other (Figure 13-6). Modules within each cluster are completed in any order; however, all modules in cluster 1 must be completed before beginning any of the modules in cluster 2.

Modules used in a serial pattern include those that are joined together in a row and that must be completed consecutively. Serial modules are content related, with each one serving as a prerequisite to the next one in the series. It is usually expected that the farther along a module is placed in a series, the more complex it is in comparison to earlier modules.

Modules in a satellite pattern are those that are joined by commonalities of content, perhaps an introductory or core module followed by several related, single modules that are completed in any order. Satellite modules vary in number, depending on the needs of the specific subject area. Shock is one example of a topic that lends itself to being taught in a collection of modules in the satellite pattern. The core module would include content on the concept, shock syndrome, common physiological mechanisms and results, basic nursing assessment and interventions re-

Figure 13-5
Basic patterns of module sequencing. Adapted from Bevis, E. O.: Curriculum Building in Nursing, ed. 3, St. Louis, 1982, The C. V. Mosby Co. Used by permission.

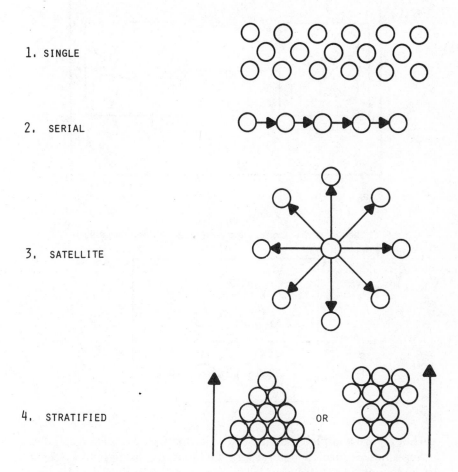

1. SINGLE

2. SERIAL

3. SATELLITE

4. STRATIFIED   OR

gardless of type of shock, and a brief introduction to the various shock types. Then, there would be individual modules discussing each shock category in more detail. The core module would have to be completed first, and then the individual modules could be studied in any order.

Stratified modules are those arranged in layers with all modules in each layer prerequisites to the modules in the next layer. Each layer represents a higher level of complexity than the previous layer. Modules at

Figure 13-6

Clusters of related single modules, with cluster 1 as prerequisite to cluster 2.

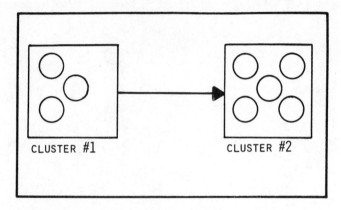

Figure 13-7

Stratified pattern incorporating both single and serial modules.

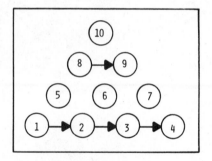

each level are completed in any order, at times, or completed serially, at other times. Figure 13-7 shows stratified modules using both single and serial sequencing at different levels. Modules 1–4 are serial and must be completed in numerical order. Modules 5–7 are single and can be studied in any order. Modules 8 and 9 are serial with 8 preceding 9. Module 10 is single but must be done after all the rest.

Courses may utilize a combination of these patterns of sequencing. For example, modules may be patterned as shown in Figure 13-8. There are 21 modules in the course. The modules are arranged in four clusters that are themselves in a serial order indicating that modules in each cluster must be completed before beginning any of the modules in the

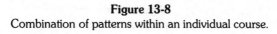

Figure 13-8
Combination of patterns within an individual course.

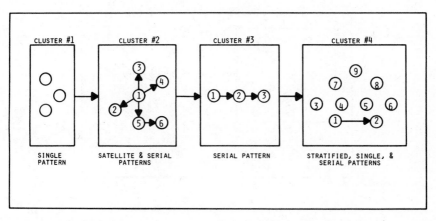

next cluster. Cluster 1 is made up of three single modules to be completed in any order. Cluster 2 has six modules in two patterns: satellite and serial. Module 1 must be done first; modules 2–5 may be completed in any order; and module 6 must be done after module 5. Modules 5 and 6 could be completed before modules 2–4, if desired. Cluster 3 has three modules in a serial pattern to be completed in numerical order. Cluster 4 is made up of nine modules in a stratified pattern, basically, but also incorporates single and serial patterns. This combination of patterns has already been seen in Figure 13-7. Many other variations are possible depending on specific material being taught.

The modules in the various patterns can have their own enrichment activities as part of each module or additional enrichment modules may be designated. For example, single enrichment modules to be done at any time, depending on needs and interests of the student, can be available or they can be attached to a cluster of related modules as shown in Figure 13-9. The modules in the cluster are required of all students, while the modules outside the cluster can be completed as desired by individual students. One student may decide to do neither of the enrichment modules; another may complete one only—in this case module 1 since it is prerequisite to module 2; and another may decide to do both.

Sociological Format. As stated previously, the primary sociological pattern used with learning modules is independent study (IS). This provides several advantages. IS allows the student to make some of the decisions about where and when to study. It also provides flexibility for

Figure 13-9
Enrichment modules attached to a cluster of required modules.

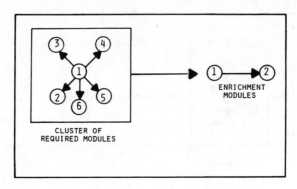

a student who wants to repeat difficult activities or move more rapidly through a module. Efforts should be made, however, to include activities that increase motivation and enjoyment for the student who learns best when involved with other people. Students should be encouraged to work with others when a complex learning task or situation is involved. If the goal of a module is to stimulate cooperative effort and problem solving, the student can be directed to participate with peers in companion or small-group activities such as data collection, brainstorming, or role playing.

The "people" component of the modular system (besides the student and peers) is also very important. Planned student–teacher interaction is crucial. The teacher must be available to answer questions, evaluate progress, diagnose learning needs, and prescribe learning requirements as well as to counsel, encourage, and motivate. This can be done on either a one-to-one or group basis and involve free discussion, questioning, testing, or observation of performance. It is possible to use auxiliary personnel to assist the teacher in these functions. For example, a baccalaureate prepared nurse, an undergraduate student, or a graduate student can observe student practice, grade quizzes, provide feedback about progress, keep records, or refer the student to the teacher when needed. People serving in this capacity are often referred to as "facilitators" (Rochin & Thompson, 1975) or "proctors" (Wilson & Tosti, 1972, pp. 69–72) and are expected to have mastered the material covered in each module so that they are able to help the students more effectively.

The extent and special needs of each modular program determine the requirements for support personnel. Clerks may be used to dispense and return learning materials to their proper locations, restock disposable materials as needed, assist students with minor problems with equipment or media, keep records of frequency of use of print and nonprint learning resources, and keep records of the number of students using specialized areas such as learning centers or skills laboratories. The record keeping role is particularly helpful for obtaining data needed to calculate costs per student and provide support for budgetary requests for personnel, facilities, equipment, audiovisual materials, and so forth.

When activities require the use of audiovisual or other specialized equipment, it is important that someone, such as a media technician or teaching assistant, be available to orient the students to its use and assist with special problems that occur with media or equipment. A media technician should be available to service audiovisual equipment and materials promptly, in order to decrease down time that affects the learning process. A media technician can also assist faculty with development and production of audiovisual learning resources.

The ready availability and organization of learning materials depends on having a person who is responsible for typing modules, cataloging various learning resources, ordering commercial materials, and having printed materials duplicated. When the use of modules or the number of support personnel is limited, it may be necessary to train one person to fill several positions in the basic operation of a learning center. If the one person is a secretary or clerk, it is vital to maintain a close working relationship with those personnel who provide services for equipment maintenance and repair, production of learning resources, and other specialized services.

Grading.   The normal curve has been used for grading for such a long time that current practices are still heavily influenced by it (Russell, 1974, p. 133). Some educators believe that there must always be a certain percentage of students who fail and that only a few students will be able to learn at a high level.

Bloom, Hastings, and Madaus (1971, p. 45), in their discussion of mastery learning, made the following statement about the normal curve:

> There is nothing sacred about the normal curve. It is the distribution most appropriate to chance and random activity. Education is a purposeful activity, and we seek to have the students learn what we have to teach. If we are effective in our instruction, the distribution of achievement should be very different from the normal curve. In fact, we may even insist that our educational efforts have been *unsuccessful* to the extent that the distribution of achievement approximates the normal distribution.

If one follows Bloom's philosophy, the majority of students, given enough time and adequate resources and assistance, would be able to achieve a high level of learning. Thus, if performance objectives and criteria of evaluation are clearly established for each module, and they are stated at a high level of learning, each student is able to work toward mastery of what is specified. Ideally, then, the grade is simply one of mastery with successful completion or nonmastery when additional work is needed. The formal grade recorded in this situation might be M for mastery, P for pass, or Cr for credit.

In actual practice, because of the influence of the normal curve, various grading patterns are seen. Several grading practices that illustrate a compromise between individualized and traditional approaches are outlined below. In general, they represent an attempt to provide some degree of individualization within the established educational structure. No attempt will be made to judge the quality or limitations of a particular grading system.

1. Objectives for modules are stated at a minimal, or C, level. The formal grade recorded upon successful completion of required modules might be C, representing achievement of the minimal objectives, M for mastery, P for pass, or Cr for credit. If provisions are made for higher grades, the student who desires a higher grade than C is required to complete enrichment activities, special projects, or additional modules for extra credit. One example of the use of modules for grade differentiation is when one series of modules must be completed for a grade of C, plus another series for a grade of B, and a third series for a grade of A.

2. Objectives for individual modules are stated so that those to be completed for each grade are specified. There may also be modules treating the same content area that are developed at different levels—one module with C objectives, one with B objectives, and one with A objectives—from which the student selects depending on the grade desired.

3. A certain number of modules to be completed at a satisfactory level are specified for each grade level. For example, in a course with 10 modules, the grading pattern might be as follows: (a) six or fewer modules completed satisfactorily, a grade of D, F, or *Incomplete;* (b) with seven, a grade of C; (c) with eight, a grade of B; and (d) with nine or 10, a grade of A.

4. Module posttests are used for self-evaluation only with other tests covering module content given at specified intervals. Students are

required to take all tests and to have a grade assigned based on the number of points received from those possible. For example, using total possible points the range for each letter grade is established, and a student knows ahead of time how many points must be attained for a certain grade.

5. A variation of item 4 is that tests over module content are given at specified intervals and the student is required to take a certain number of the tests as well as achieve a certain number of points for each grade level. A student who takes fewer than the minimum number of tests or makes fewer than the minimum points required receives an *Incomplete, D,* or *F,* depending on whether or not opportunities for further work exist.

6. Modules are used as one teaching strategy among others, such as lectures. The module is used for preparation for the lecture and the posttest of the module is used for self-evaluation only. The grade for the course is determined by performance on traditional course exams at specified intervals. The grade for an individual student represents the student's relative position in a normative grouping.

Problems Associated With Modular Learning

There are certain problems about which one should be aware when considering or beginning the use of modules in an instructional program. Some of these have been mentioned throughout the chapter. The intent here is to list potential problem areas and to identify possible interventions for dealing with them. Table 13-1 outlines three potential problems in relation to student role, whereas Table 13-2 identifies three potential problems in relation to teacher role and learning resources. Problems and interventions are examples only and are not presented as an exhaustive list.

SUMMARY

The learning module as a self-contained instructional unit offers one method for providing individualized learning. Available research in nursing supports the use of modules for learning content in various educational and practice settings. Development of modules requires a

Table 13-1

Potential Problems Associated With Student Role and Possible Interventions for Dealing With Problems

Problems	Possible Interventions
Student procrastination related to inability to manage self-paced study. Lack of prior experience Taking modular course along with traditional course with rigid schedules, requirements, grading	1. Provide thorough orientation to IS 2. Set up a suggested schedule for pacing of completion of modules 3. Begin with modules that are short and relatively easy to complete 4. Make modules as interesting as possible 5. Maintain contact with student for support, encouragement, assessment of progress, and assistance, when needed 6. Use modules in a more structured format at first 7. Provide positive evidence of success 8. Schedule quizzes and tests on module content at intervals
Insufficient learning related to failure of student to assume responsibility for own learning and to choose resources that increase learning effectiveness. Access to materials Prior experience in traditional courses that convinces the student that high level of learning is not attainable Using modules in a traditional course with a definite schedule regardless of level of mastery	1. Maintain contact with student for assessment of progress and assistance when needed 2. Set up evaluation/testing sessions so that student is made aware of problem areas/need for further practice 3. State objectives at a high level (traditional B or A level) and increase flexibility of time for practice and repetition 4. Devise ways to demonstrate increased learning quality that is possible with mastery learning 5. Include reality application experience as part of module so that importance of learning is demonstrated 6. Increase portability of learning materials and maintain as extensive hours as possible in practice labs and learning centers
Feeling of depersonalization by student related to the change in student and teacher roles.	1. Maintain face-to-face contact with student through conferences, seminars, personal appointments 2. Incorporate peer, small-group, and large-group interaction into modules 3. Provide personal attention as indicated by student need/progress

Table 13-2

Potential Problems Associated With Teacher Role and Learning Resources and Possible Interventions for Dealing With Problems

Problems	Possible Interventions
Poor teacher acceptance related to change in teacher role, lack of recognition of value of mastery learning, and lack of rewards	1. Have small group of faculty using modules at first to demonstrate educational benefits 2. Schedule workshops to aid in change of role perception and to assist with learning about module development and use 3. Establish incentives for use of nontraditional approaches that increase learning effectiveness 4. Set up research projects that will demonstrate the value of individualized instruction 5. Establish mechanisms that maintain teacher contact with the student 6. Provide recognition for involvement in efforts to increase teaching effectiveness, such as that found with involvement in research, community service, and committee work 7. Provide release time for faculty to develop learning materials and evaluate their effectiveness
Difficulty in keeping modules updated and revised related to rapid proliferation of knowledge	1. Provide faculty release time for revision work 2. Structure modules so that resources used can be readily changed without altering the total package 3. Utilize available instructional design/evaluation personnel to help with process 4. Develop modules around major concepts rather than specific content, which changes rapidly
Lack of appropriate learning resources (software) related to cost and failure of commercial media to meet local needs	1. Provide time and budget for in-house development of learning materials 2. Write instructional grant proposals that will provide additional funding 3. Let media publishers know what is needed and work with them to develop materials 4. Collect data to establish need for support of budget requests 5. Adjust commercial media (within copyright limitations) to meet local needs (adding slides, printed materials, or audiotape)

systematic process and an integration of objectives, strategies, and evaluation. They can be used in a variety of nursing settings to provide all types of instruction. As with any teaching strategy, an instructor needs to consider both strengths and limitations before embarking on the extensive use of modules in specific situations.

APPENDIX 1: SAMPLE MODULE
FETAL CIRCULATION AND CHANGES AT BIRTH

Table of Contents

Introduction

An understanding of the anatomy and physiology of fetal circulation provides a basis for the study of congenital heart abnormalities and increases the ease with which one can learn about the specific abnormalities. If the content of this module is mastered, you will be well prepared to study those congenital heart abnormalities referred to as cardiac shunts.

Terminal Goal

Upon completion of this module, you will have a knowledge and understanding of the anatomy and physiology of fetal circulation and those changes that normally occur at the time of birth.

Directions

Proceed through the module as follows:

1. Read the section on prerequisites below and review as necessary.
2. Read the objectives for the module on page 243.
3. Take the pretest if you feel you have prior background or experience that prepares you to meet the objectives. Grade the pretest using the key provided at the end of the module.
4. If you score less than 100% on the pretest, use the resources listed on page 242 to complete those activities and self-checks that have to do with the objectives you did not reach. If you scored 100% on the pretest, you do not need to do further work on the module.
5. Complete the posttest. Repeat activities if necessary in order to reach the objectives. If the pretest has not been completed previously, you may also wish to use it to further validate your learning.

Prerequisites

It is essential that you have certain background knowledge about normal circulation before you can expect to complete this module successfully. Be sure you are able to complete the following before beginning to work on the module. If you need help to meet the prerequisites, a list of suggested resources is given.

1. Name the four chambers of the heart.
2. Name the two veins that return blood from the body to the right atrium.
3. Name the artery that takes blood from the right ventricle to the lungs.
4. Name the artery that takes blood from the left ventricle to the body.
5. Define the terms: oxygenated blood, deoxygenated blood, systemic circulation, pulmonary circulation, artery, vein, arterial blood, and venous blood.
6. State whether the blood found in each heart chamber and each major artery leaving the heart contains oxygenated or deoxygenated blood.
7. Trace the route of blood flow from the time it enters the right atrium until the time it leaves the heart via the aorta.

Sources for satisfying the prerequisites:

1. Any college or university level anatomy and physiology test.
2. Guyton, A.C. *Textbook of medical physiology* (6th ed.). Philadelphia: Saunders, 1981.
3. Ross Laboratories. The normal heart. (Chart available in NLRC.)

Learning Resources for Module

Use any of the resources listed below as directed in each of the activities. The choice is yours and depends on which you have available or prefer to use.

1. Ross Laboratories. Fetal circulation (chart available in NLRC), or a labeled diagram of fetal circulation from any other reference.
2. Any recent medical, nursing, or anatomy and physiology text that includes content about fetal circulation. Suggested references:
   Jensen, M.D. and Bobak, I.M. *Maternity and gynecologic care—the nurse and the family.* St. Louis: Mosby, 1985, pp. 583–586.
   Guyton, A.C. *Textbook of medical physiology* (6th ed.). Philadelphia: Saunders, 1981, pp. 1040–1041.
   Ross Laboratories. Fetal circulation. (Discussion sheet available in NLRC.)

Pretest

100% mastery required. Each question is keyed to the objective(s) that it relates to. Complete the activities and self-checks for any objective that you cannot meet.

1. Place the letter of the item in column B in the blank next to the item it best matches or explains in column A. All items in the second column will not be needed. (Objectives 1, 2, and 3)

A	B
____1. Umbilical vein	A. carries deoxygenated blood from the fetus to the placenta
____2. Umbilical arteries	B. an opening between the right and left atria
____3. Foramen ovale	C. an increased RBC count
____4. Ductus arteriosus	D. carries oxygenated blood from the placenta to the fetus
____5. Polycythemia	E. an increased WBC count
	F. an opening between the right and left ventricles
	G. a connection between the aorta and the pulmonary artery

2. State the normal number of each of the blood vessel types found in the umbilical cord. (Objective 1)
3. What is the purpose of the foramen ovale and the ductus arteriosus in fetal circulation? (Objective 2)

4. In fetal circulation, the systolic pressure is greatest on the _____ side of the heart; therefore, the direction of blood flow through the foramen ovale is toward the _____ atrium. (Objective 2)

5. The blood found in the aorta of the fetus is _____ (oxygenated, deoxygenated, or a mixture of the two). (Objective 4)

6. What is the purpose of polycythemia in fetal circulation? (Objective 3)

7. Describe the alteration in relation to the route of blood flow through the heart, the pulmonary artery, and the aorta that should occur at birth or shortly after birth. Include the closure of fetal structures, changes in direction of blood flow, and changes in pressure and oxygenation levels, if any, in the chambers and major vessels of the heart (Use a separate sheet of paper.) (Objective 5)

8. Look at the two unlabeled charts depicting fetal circulation and normal circulation after birth. Identify which is which. (Charts are available in the NLRC.) (Objective 6)

Learning Objectives

Upon completion of the activities, you will be able to:

1. Name the two blood vessel types found in the umbilical cord, state the number of each, identify whether the blood found in each is oxygenated or deoxygenated, and state the direction of blood flow in each in relation to the fetus and the placenta.

2. Name and locate the two shunts that are normal in fetal circulation and state the purpose of each.

3. Define the term polycythemia, and state its purpose in fetal circulation.

4. Label a diagram of fetal circulation indicating differences in systolic pressure between the left and right side of the heart and between the aorta and pulmonary artery, the direction of blood flow through the foramen ovale and ductus arteriosus, and the level of oxygenation of blood in the four chambers of the heart and its four major vessels.

5. Describe the changes in circulation that should occur at birth or shortly after birth, including the closure of fetal structures, changes in direction of blood flow, and changes in pressure and oxygenation levels in the chambers and major vessels of the heart. Label a diagram indicating these changes.

6. Distinguish between two unlabeled diagrams or slides depicting fetal circulation and normal circulation after birth within the heart, pulmonary artery, and aorta.

Learning Activity 1 (Objectives 1, 2, and 3)

Refer to a labeled diagram of fetal circulation and a reference source that describes fetal circulation and answer the following questions:

1. What are the names of the blood vessels found in the umbilical cord?
2. How many of each of these vessels are there?
3. What is the direction of blood flow in each vessel in relation to the fetus?
4. Describe each vessel regarding content of oxygenated or deoxygenated blood.
5. What is the name of the fetal opening between the left atrium and the right atrium?
6. What is the name of the fetal structure connecting the pulmonary artery with the aorta?
7. What is the primary purpose of the two structures identified in questions 5 and 6?
8. Define the term polycythemia, and state its purpose in fetal circulation.

Activity 1 Self-Check

1. Name the vascular structures in the umbilical cord and state the number of each.
2. Place the letter of the item in column B in the blank next to the item it best matches or explains in Column A. All items in the second column will not be needed.

A	B
_____1. Umbilical vein	A. carries deoxygenated blood from the fetus to the placenta
_____2. Umbilical arteries	
_____3. Foramen ovale	B. an opening between the right and left atria
_____4. Ductus arteriosus	C. an increased RBC count
_____5. Polycythemia	D. carries oxygenated blood from the placenta to the fetus
	E. an increased WBC count
	F. an opening between the right and left ventricles
	G. a connection between the aorta and the pulmonary artery

3. On this diagram locate and name the two fetal structures that cause a normal shunting of blood before birth.

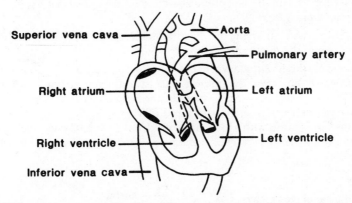

4. Write a sentence stating the primary purpose of the two structures identified in 3.

5. What function does polycythemia serve in fetal circulation?

Check your answers with those provided at the end of the module. If you did not answer all questions correctly, return to Activity 1, review the content, and repeat the Self-Check.

Learning Activity 2 (Objective 4)

Refer to any of the resources on fetal circulation and answer the following questions:

1. Where is the systolic pressure greater in fetal circulation? Right or left side of heart? Aorta or pulmonary artery?

2. What is the direction of the blood flow through the foramen ovale and the ductus arteriosus?

3. Determine the level of oxygenation of the blood in each of the following structures. Write "high" if highly oxygenated, "low" if deoxygenated, and "mix" if a mixture of oxygenated and deoxygenated blood.

　　　　　　　　　　_____superior vena cava
　　　　　　　　　　_____umbilical vein
　　　　　　　　　　_____inferior vena cava
　　　　　　　　　　_____left atrium and left ventricle
　　　　　　　　　　_____right atrium
　　　　　　　　　　_____right ventricle
　　　　　　　　　　_____pulmonary artery
　　　　　　　　　　_____aorta

Activity 2 Self-Check

Label the following diagram of the fetal heart according to the directions below.

1. Place an "X" on the side of the heart and on the artery that has the highest systolic pressure.

2. Indicate with an arrow the direction of blood flow through the foramen ovale and the ductus arteriosus.

3. Indicate the level of oxygenation of blood in each of the following: the superior vena cava, the inferior vena cava, the left atrium and ventricle, the right atrium, the right ventricle, the pulmonary artery, and the aorta. Write "high" or color in with a red marker if highly oxygenated. Write "low" or color in with a blue marker if deoxygenated. Write "mix" or color in with a green marker if a mixture of oxygenated and deoxygenated blood.

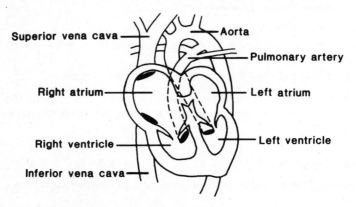

Check your completed diagram with the answers provided at the end of the module. If any answers were incorrect, return to activity 2 for further study and then repeat the Self-Check.

Learning Activity 3 (Objective 5)

There are many physiological adjustments that the newborn baby must make. These adjustments are great in the first moments of life and the first few hours after birth. Their magnitude is illustrated by the fact that there is a high rate of mortality during the first 24 hours after birth, with 30 percent of all infants who die in the first year of life dying during the first 24 hours.

Significant changes occur in the circulatory system at or shortly after birth. These changes involve both structural and functional aspects. Use any of the resources to write a description of the changes in the following areas:

1. Closure or obliteration of fetal structures. What are the structures, and why does each close?

2. With the closure of the structures, describe the change in the route of blood flow through the heart, the pulmonary artery, and the aorta.

3. With the closure of the heart and pulmonary artery (pulmonary circulation), and the left side of the heart and the aorta (systemic circulation).

Activity 3 Self-Check

Label the following diagram of the fetal heart according to the directions below.

1. Place an "X" on the side of the heart and in the artery that have the highest systolic pressure after birth.
2. Draw a line to show which structures close at birth or shortly after birth.
3. Indicate level of oxygenation of blood in each of the following structures after birth: the superior vena cava, the inferior vena cava, the right atrium and ventricle, the pulmonary artery, the left atrium and ventricle, and the aorta. Write "high" or color in with a red marker if highly oxygenated. Write "low" or color in with a blue marker if deoxygenated. Write "mix" or color in with a green marker if a mixture of oxygenated and deoxygenated blood.

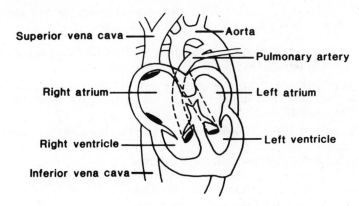

Check your completed diagram with the answers provided at the end of the module. If you missed any question, restudy Activity 3 and, then, repeat the Self-Check,

You have completed the learning activities for this module and may now proceed to the posttest, which begins below.

Posttest

100% mastery is required. If you miss any question or part of any question, review that section of the module until you can achieve 100 percent mastery. You may also wish to complete the pretest to further validate your learning.

1. What is the purpose of polycythemia in fetal circulation? (Objective 3)
2. What is the purpose of the ductus arteriosus? (Objective 2)
3. Place the letter of the item in column B in the blank next to the item it best matches or explains in column A. All items in the second column will not be used. (Objectives 1, 2, and 3)

<table>
<tr><td align="center">A</td><td align="center">B</td></tr>
<tr><td>
____1. Umbilical vein
____2. Umbilical arteries
____3. Foramen ovale
____4. Ductus arteriosus
____5. Polycythemia
</td><td>
A. carries deoxygenated blood from the fetus to the placenta
B. an opening between the right and left atria
C. an increased RBC count
D. carries oxygenated blood from the placenta to the fetus
E. an increased WBC count
F. an opening between the right and left ventricles
G. a connection between the aorta and the pulmonary artery
</td></tr>
</table>

4. Which two fetal blood vessels contain blood that is the most highly oxygenated? (Objectives 1 and 4)

5. In fetal circulation, systolic pressure is greater on the _____side of the heart and in the _____(pulmonary artery or aorta). (Objective 4)

6. In fetal circulation, the direction of blood flow through the ductus arteriosus is (Objectives 2 and 4)
   A. from the pulmonary artery to the aorta
   B. from the aorta to the pulmonary artery
   C. from the right atrium to the left atrium
   D. from the left atrium to the right atrium

7. In fetal circulation, there is a mixture of oxygenated and deoxygenated blood in the (Objective 4)
   A. right atrium
   B. pulmonary artery
   C. left ventricle
   D. descending aorta
   E. inferior vena cava

8. Indicate with an "X" in the blank if that situation normally exists in the newborn infant: (Objective 5)
   ____ A. a shunting of blood between the right and left atria
   ____ B. highly oxygenated blood in the aorta
   ____ C. an open ductus arteriosus
   ____ D. deoxygenated blood in the right atrium

9. After birth, systolic pressure is greater on the ⎯⎯⎯⎯⎯ side of the heart and in the ⎯⎯⎯⎯⎯ (pulmonary artery or aorta). (Objective 5)

10. What occurs at birth to alter the direction of blood flow and the level of oxygenation of blood in the aorta? (Objective 5)

11. After birth, the structure that contains the most highly oxygenated blood is the (Objective 5)
    A. right atrium
    B. pulmonary artery
    C. aorta
    D. inferior vena cava
    E. umbilical vein

12. Project the two slides of fetal circulation and normal circulation after birth on the screen. Distinguish between the two by identifying which is which. (Obtain slides in the NLRC.)

Keys to Pretest, Activity Self-Checks, and Posttest

PRETEST KEY

1. D, A, B, G, C.
2. One umbilical vein and two umbilical arteries.
3. To bypass the nonfunctioning fetal lungs in order to send blood, which is relatively high in oxygen, to body cells.
4. Right, left.
5. A mixture. Although a mixture, the blood in the aorta proximal to the ductus arteriosus is more highly oxygenated than that distal to this structure.
6. The body attempts to compensate for the resulting mixture of oxygenated and deoxygenated blood going into the systemic circulation by increasing RBC count and, thus, oxygen-carrying capacity.
7. The foramen ovale and ductus arteriosus should close, causing a cessation of shunting of blood from the right atrium to the left atrium and from the pulmonary artery to the aorta. A normal adult circulation pattern is begun. Pressure and oxygenation in systemic circulation are greater than that in pulmonary circulation.
8. Chart A is circulation after birth. Chart B is fetal circulation.

KEYS TO ACTIVITY SELF-CHECKS
Activity 1

1. Two umbilical arteries and one umbilical vein.
2. D, A, B, G, C.
3. Foramen ovale identified as opening between right and left atria; ductus arteriosus identified as connection between pulmonary artery and aorta.

4. These structures allow part of the more highly oxygenated blood to bypass the nonfunctioning fetal lungs and to send blood, which is relatively high in oxygen, to body cells.

5. The body attempts to compensate for the resulting mixture of oxygenated and deoxygenated blood going into the systemic circulation by increasing RBC count and, thus, oxygen-carrying capacity.

Activity 2

1. "X" should be placed on the right side of heart and pulmonary artery.

2. Blood flows through foramen ovale from the right atrium into the left atrium and through the ductus arteriosus from the pulmonary artery into the aorta.

3. *Low* superior vena cava; *mix* inferior vena cava; *mix* right atrium (note: although both are passing through the right atrium, most of the deoxygenated blood from the superior vena cava is directed downward into the right ventricle, and most of the more highly oxygenated blood from the inferior vena cava is directed straight across through the foramen ovale into the left atrium); *mix* left atrium and left ventricle; *mix* pulmonary artery; *mix* aorta (note: although there is a mix, the blood in the aorta which goes to the head and upper body is more highly oxygenated than that in the aorta distal to the ductus arteriosus since additional deoxygenated blood is shunted into the aorta at that point.)

Activity 3

1. "X" should be placed on the left side of the heart and on the aorta.

2. Lines should be drawn to close foramen ovale and ductus arteriosus.

3. *Low* superior vena cava, inferior vena cava, right atrium and ventricle, and pulmonary artery. *High* left atrium and ventricle, aorta. Should no longer be any mixture of the two in any structure.

POSTTEST KEY

1. To assure adequate oxygenation of body cells by increasing oxygen-carrying capacity by increasing number of RBCs.

2. To allow blood to be diverted from the pulmonary artery into the aorta in order to bypass the nonfunctioning fetal lungs.

3. D, A, B, G, C.

4. The umbilical vein and the inferior vena cava.

5. *Right* side and in the *pulmonary artery.*

6. A.

7. A, B, C, D, and E. Although there is a mixture in all of these, there is a relatively high oxygenation of blood in the right atrium and, thus, in the left side of heart and aorta proximal to the ductus arteriosus.

8. "X" should be placed next to B and D.

9. *Left* side and in the *aorta.*

10. Fetal lungs begin to function, which decreases resistance to blood flow and, thus, reduces pressure on right side of heart and in the pulmonary artery. Loss of placental blood flow increases systemic pressure on the left side of the heart and in the aorta. These changes in pressure cause the foramen ovale to close. The flow of oxygenated blood through the ductus arteriosus causes it to become nonfunctional; it is later occluded by growth of fibrous tissue.

11. C.

12. Slide A is normal circulation after birth. Slide B is fetal circulation.

MODULE FEEDBACK FORM

Title of module: _____

1. Make a check and comment in each of following areas:

Area	Relevance		Clarity		Organization		Comments
	Yes	No	Yes	No	Yes	No	
a. Content							
b. Objectives							
c. Activities							
d. Media (including articles and AV)							
e. Pre- and posttests and check-points							

2. Directions to the student were (circle one)

   very clear   very unclear
     1   2   3   4   5
   comments:

3. List those things about the module that you liked.

4. List those things about the module that you did not like.

5. What was your overall impression of the module? (circle one)

   excellent   poor
     1   2   3   4   5
   comments:

6. Please make specific suggestion(s) for revision of the module. (Use back of form, if necessary.)

14

Using Learning Contracts

The contract as a formal legal agreement is well known in American society. It is usually written but can be verbal. It binds two or more people or agencies in an agreement to carry out specific behaviors, usually within a certain period of time. It is essential before signing the contract that all parties are in agreement about goals and have a clear understanding of responsibilities of each participant. Legal contracts are often renegotiated when the situation of either party alters the ability to meet commitments.

In traditional learning situations, the contract between the teacher and a student is usually implied rather than explicit. Both teacher and student have certain expectations of themselves and each other. The student expects the teacher to provide appropriate learning opportunities so that the student can learn what the teacher requires. At the same time, the teacher expects that students will be motivated to carry out assigned activities and work to their highest level of potential to try to achieve the desired learning outcomes. Each participant may have greater expectations of the other person than of self, have unrealistic expectations, or feel betrayed when the other party does not behave as anticipated. The common results of such a situation are unclear expectations, unmet goals, anxiety, and frustration.

The type of contract referred to in this chapter is one in which there is an explicit agreement between the teacher and a student or group of students. It identifies exactly what each will do. It denotes a mutuality in establishing learning objectives, selecting resources and activities, and evaluating learning outcomes. It emphasizes learning rather than grading.

The use of learning contracts can be traced to 1919, with Parkhurst's development of "laboratory plans"—projects or units of study to be completed within a specified period of time (Dewey, 1922). Since then there has been ongoing discussion about the differences in learning styles among individuals, the needs of adult learners, the needs of students from diverse backgrounds, the importance of active involvement of learners, and the need for increased accountability of the learner.

The learning contract is one method that has been used in an effort to design a learning situation that is more individualized in these respects. In some higher education settings, the learning contract has been the only method used for an entire educational experience (Craig, 1975; Feeney & Riley, 1975; Worby, 1979), although traditional methods (lectures, seminars, and so forth) were also used as part of the contract.

In nursing, there is no evidence that an entire curriculum has been put on a contractual basis, although external and extended/outreach programs utilize this approach to varying degrees. Early descriptions of the use of contract learning for nursing education were by Layton (1972) and Rauen and Waring (1972). Since that time, a number of individual applications have been described in the nursing literature. Learning contracts have been used for undergraduate education in different subject areas, types of courses, and student levels (Aavedal, Coombe, Fisher, Jones, & Standeven, 1975; Beare, 1985; Bouchard & Steels, 1980; Dobbie & Karlinsky, 1982; Crancer, Maury-Hess, & Dunn, 1977; Kruse & Barger, 1982; Lord & Palmer, 1982; Martens, 1981; McFarland, 1983; Paduano, 1979; Price, Swartz, & Thurn, 1983; Sasmor, 1984; Schoolcraft & Delaney, 1982; Valadez & Heusinkveld, 1977). Learning contracts have also been used successfully for in-service or continuing education (Dougan, 1980; Reinhart, 1977; Smith, 1980) and for nurse-patient collaboration in community and hospital settings (Brykczynski, 1982; Herje, 1980; Zangari & Duffy, 1980).

DEFINITIONS

Definitions of terms associated with contract learning as used in this chapter are as follows:

LEARNING CONTRACT: An individualized learning plan that has been negotiated between a teacher (or committee) and a student (or group of students).* Al-

---

*Although the terms teacher and student are used throughout this chapter, they apply equally to any situation in which mentor/learner relationships are established, such as that of the staff development instructor-staff nurse.

though not a legally binding document, it is a written, signed agreement that specifies learning objectives to be accomplished; activities, materials, and procedures to be used; responsibilities of involved parties; criteria and methods for evaluation; and the reward that will be forthcoming to the student once commitments have been met.

CONTRACTING: The process of teacher-student negotiation and interaction in designing the learning plan (the learning contract).

CONTRACT LEARNING: Applies to either the process of using contracts for learning or the specific learning gains associated with their use.

VALUES

Fundamental principles underlying the use of learning contracts* include (1) the individuality of students based on unique learning styles, diverse backgrounds, and specific needs; (2) the need of adults to be self-directing and involved in learning choices; (3) the recognition that students should be held responsible and accountable for their own learning; and (4) the recognition that learning is a lifelong process.

There is widespread agreement among the nursing authors cited in the introduction to this chapter about the capacity of contracts to individualize instruction without compromising educational goals and objectives. Contracts respond to differences in learning needs, styles, and interests. They provide opportunities for independent learning and for variations in amount and rate of work. The use of varied resources and activities provides choices and addresses individual styles and interests. The extent to which contracts accomplish each of these depends, of course, on their specific design.

Contracts offer fulfillment of the adult's need to be self-directing. Tough (1981) and Knowles (1978) clearly demonstrated the ability of adult learners to design and complete their own learning projects. Knowles has credited the learning contract with being the single most effective tool for adult education. He says, "It solves the problem of the wide range of backgrounds, education, experience, interests, motivations, and abilities that characterize most adult groups by providing a way for individuals (and subgroups) to tailor-make their own learning plans" (Knowles, 1978, p. 127). The contract allows adult learners to build on broad human experiences and develop learning situations that

---

*Whenever the term "contract" is used in this chapter, it is referring to a learning contract, as defined previously.

will help them deal with problems they are facing in the work world. The choices made can reflect personal interests, unique ways of learning, or greater relevance to personal experiences and goals. By being more closely involved with planning and decision making, the learner is likely to be more strongly committed to the outcomes of the contract.

Some students may not be able to handle a self-directed learning experience. Traditional educational practices condition students to be dependent in the learning situation (Knowles, 1978, p. 176). For them, involvement in the process of negotiating and carrying out the activities of a contract fosters the development of independence and self-direction. Since students are heavily involved in discussions about objectives, resources and activities, and ways of evaluating, they are forced to think about personal educational goals and assume greater responsibility for their own learning.

Increased independence and responsibility for learning also help to teach students that learning is a lifelong process over which they have control. Chickering (1975, p. 63) stated the belief that the use of contracts gives students an opportunity to learn how to learn, a skill that is vital for continued learning throughout life. Students who learn to solve problems, manage their own learning situations, and develop independent, creative ways of thinking are better prepared to deal with the knowledge explosion and rapid changes associated with a field like nursing.

ELEMENTS

Many authors have identified the necessary elements of a learning contract. Some of these are Clark (1981, p. 588), Moran (1980, p. 82), and Reilly and Oermann (1985, p. 132). Although the organization and relationship among the elements vary with individual and institutional practices, the core of any learning contract is made up of objectives, activities to be completed, materials and methods to be used, and evaluation of outcomes. By focusing on these in the developmental process and then adding specific structural elements, the total contract evolves. The following list is provided as one framework for the development of a contract to use in a teaching/learning situation.

1. A general statement of the student's long-range goals, purposes, and objectives.

2. Clear statements of the specific objectives/learning outcomes to be accomplished upon completion of the contract.

3. A description of the learning activities to be completed by the student and the learning resources to be used, including identification of responsibilities of the teacher or other mentor and anyone else who may be supervising the work of the student.

4. Identification of what is to be used as evidence that objectives have been met and the criteria by which the evidence will be evaluated. Any responsibilities of the teacher or other personnel are also identified.

5. An indication of what reward the student is to receive upon satisfactory completion of the contract.

6. Time frame to be used.

7. Signatures of the teacher (or other mentor) and student.

Each of these elements will be discussed briefly. A sample contract is given in Appendix 1 to illustrate each element.

General Statement

The general statement of the student's long-range goals, purposes, and objectives is helpful in setting the parameters of the contract in relation to the specific objectives. For example, a student who wants to complete a contract in some area of pediatrics might have the general statement shown in the sample learning contract.

Specific Objectives

Specific objectives are required so that the student, the teacher, and anyone else involved will know exactly what must be accomplished by the student. The responsibility for identifying the objectives lies with different individuals, depending on the amount of structure in the situation in which the contract is being used. The amount of student independence in determining personal learning objectives decreases as the extent of faculty involvement increases. In one situation a student may have considerable freedom in deciding what the objectives will be. In another situation the student and teacher may work together to identify the objectives. And finally, in other situations the teacher alone may specify the learning objectives. If the contract is part of an independent study project (as shown in the sample contract), the objectives will be largely identified by the student with the teacher's guidance and approval. In a more structured situation, the objectives may be delineated by the teacher alone but with the student deciding, based on individual needs and preferences, which of several contracts to complete. If the contract is part of a course, broader course objectives are predetermined; however, a student may still have varying degrees of freedom to develop subobjectives that address personal interests, strengths, and needs. Even in more structured situations, students may be given options regarding desired level of accomplishment, types of activities to be completed, and resources to be used.

The ability to develop their own learning objectives depends on the level and experience of students. Many will need a great deal of guidance and assistance in developing realistic and measureable objectives for learning. In any case, objectives will either be negotiated or refined in consultation with the teacher. The teacher must ensure that the objectives are relevant to curricular or course goals, appropriate to the general goals of the student, and of satisfactory depth and breadth to warrant the reward established by the contract.

Learning Activities and Resources

The learning resources used in a contract should be available, up-to-date, and directly relevant to the desired learning outcomes. Depending on the subject matter and the availability of resources, various types should be used—reading, listening, viewing, and manipulating. Resources can include regular, correspondence, or noncredit courses, workshops, textbooks and articles, audiovisual programs, models, travel, and people. Some resources may not be identified ahead of time but, rather, have the student locate additional learning resources as part of the contract.

In utilization of the resources, attention should be given to providing choices to the student. Certain activities can be required while the student selects another from a list of two or more. Activities can include such varied things as reading a textbook or article; viewing/listening to an audiovisual program; completing a module; attending conferences, workshops, or scheduled classes; participating in field/practicum experiences; participating in study groups, committees, or task groups; visiting people or community agencies; doing an interview; completing research projects or surveys; conducting a library or computerized search; and others. The extent of possibilities is only limited by one's imagination and creativity.

See the sample contract for examples of learning activities and resources. Note that responsibilities of the teacher and others are identified. The teacher may need to meet with the student at intervals for conferences to determine progress or provide help if needed. Appointments for the conferences can be scheduled or left to the responsibility of the student. The frequency varies with the type of contract, level of student, and extent of a student's self-direction and discipline. The highly motivated and self-disciplined student may require little help after the contract has been negotiated and knowledge of how to demonstrate accomplishment of the objectives is clear. The student who is less motivated or has difficulty in maintaining self-discipline will likely need more frequent conferences to verify understanding, check progress, and provide encouragement and praise.

Evidence of Accomplishment and Criteria of Evaluation

The teacher and student work together to decide what evidence will demonstrate achievement of learning objectives. Since the student participates in the development of the contract and agrees to the standards for achievement, there is likely to be less anxiety over grades and less competition with other students. Two types of evaluation must be considered: ongoing, formative evaluation to determine progress and provide a basis for counseling the student and final, summative evaluation to indicate the achievements of the student in relation to the objectives in the contract. Consequently, as with other individualized methods, a student will be evaluated only on the basis of stated, desired competencies rather than in relation to the accomplishments of peers. In both forms of evaluation, the contract should state what, when, by whom, and how evaluation will be done.

When specifying desired results, tangible evidence of the activities and use of the resources must be identified. Evidence presented can include written reports, bibliography cards, logs, or journals; taped reports, logs, or journals; production of models or displays; critique of a chapter or article; development of mediated projects; development of care or teaching plans; conducting a class; oral reports to peers; preparation of an article for publication or filing in a resource center; and performance on attitudinal scales or standard tests. Again, the possibilities are limited only by the objectives of the contract and the imagination and creativity of the participants.

A major problem confronting teachers and students when contracts are used for grade level differentiation is that of quality versus quantity of evidence required. Every effort must be made to include evidence that demonstrates quality of learning rather than simply having a student do more work for a higher grade. Qualitative criteria for evaluation are vital in establishing credibility of the program and maintaining curriculum standards. The criteria for evaluation of each item must be shared with the student and/or mutually arrived at by the teacher and student. Either way, the student must be aware at the outset how the evaluation will be done. For example, if a care plan is used, a description of what must be included is identified. If an oral report is to be given, the student must know the length and how it will be evaluated. Often a rating scale is used for this purpose; if so, the student should have a copy to guide preparation of the report. The student's work may be evaluated by experts in the field, such as staff nurses working with a student in a clinical setting.

The student should also participate in the evaluation process, since self-evaluation provides an opportunity for growth. Students are encouraged to assess their learning in relation to objectives and criteria. However, teachers retain their responsibility to ensure that requirements of the specific contract have been met. See the sample contract for examples of evaluation measures and criteria. Note that different types of evaluation measures have been used and that the student is asked to complete an evaluation of the contracting process and teacher, in addition to the self-evaluation.

Rewards

Satisfactory completion of the requirements of the contract leads to the student's receipt of some type of reward (besides the learning that has occurred). It may simply be credit for completion of an activity or project or it may involve the more formal granting of credit or a letter grade. In either case, the student must know what the options are should the evidence presented be judged as unsatisfactory. Will the student have an opportunity to do further work or to complete an alternate activity? Will the student who does not meet the contract receive a failing mark, an incomplete, a lower grade, or will additional time be allotted? See Appendix 1 for an example of the reward associated with the sample contract.

Time Frame

A contract is usually designed for a set time period, such as a semester or quarter, although the amount of time can be open ended. Whatever time frame is established must be stated in the contract. The projected completion date must take into account the time needed to evaluate the work that has been done and the possibility that further work will be required. One way to decrease the need for additional work at the last minute is to set up a schedule of interim progress checks for presentation of portions of the evidence of accomplishment of objectives. Deadlines throughout the time of the contract can help to decrease procrastination. If deadlines are found to be unrealistic or other problems arise, such as illness and unforeseen commitments, the contract can be renegotiated as long as the final completion date is met or the completion date is renegotiated. The contract can also be renegotiated if the student wishes to increase or decrease the amount or quality of work so long as there is sufficient time remaining to accomplish the requirements of the contract. Renegotiation, when necessary, is the responsibility of the student.

The time frame for the sample contract shown in Appendix 1 was 1 semester; however, it required 3 weeks to negotiate and finalize the contract and the completion date for presentation of evidence was 3 weeks before the end of the semester. What remained was approximately 10 weeks for the student to do the required work. An initial progress check was established and the student was given the option of presenting other evidence at any time. For example, the care plan could be completed immediately after the clinical days and the exhibits could be done as part of either clinical day.

Signatures

The signatures required on all contracts are those of the teacher and the student. In addition, other signatures that may be required include those of people who are involved in some aspect of the contract. For example, a person who has agreed to supervise field work or evaluate the student's performance in some activity should formalize that agreement in some way. It may be by signing that section of the contract or it may be through a letter of agreement. Whatever the method used, the responsibilities and expectations of each person involved must be clearly spelled out and understood. Finally, all parties should receive a copy of the signed contract.

THE CONTRACTING PROCESS

The contract can be used with individuals or groups for one activity, a unit, part of a course, or an entire course. It can be used for independent study, establishing expectations for certain grades, providing flexible programs for those with prior experience, or continuing education and professional growth.

The process for use of contracts in nursing situations has been discussed by various authors, as cited on page 254. Further, others have discussed both general and specific aspects of use of contracts in educational situations (Knowles, 1978, pp. 198–203; Clark, 1981; Cooper, 1980). Important areas of the process to be discussed here include orientation of the student, diagnosis of student needs, development of the plan, completion of required activities, and evaluation.

Orientation

Since many students will not have used contracts before, orientation is vital. Significant areas to consider include the concepts and principles of self-directed learning and its components, purposes, and values. A handout summarizing major points and providing guidelines for contract development is useful. The orientation can take place in a group or individually, depending on the situation in which contracts are being used. A portion of the orientation process could include the completion of a mediated, independent learning module or some other independent study activity on the use of contracts as preparation for the initial group or individual orientation. Thus, those students who have not had previous experience with independent study or are completely unfamiliar with contracts will be introduced to the concept and process before the initial orientation meeting with the teacher.

Students who have never had any real control over the learning situation may be suspicious at first. Those who have always been dependent in a learning situation may have difficulty in dealing with the increased responsibility and need for self-direction. Either will require ongoing assistance in order to alter previous notions about learning and develop the skills required in becoming a more active, independent learner.

Diagnosis of Needs

An important part of developing a contract is the assessment of individual needs and goals. Areas can include levels of competence, future professional goals, personal interests, and analysis of qualities, strengths, and limitations. The key questions to be answered are "What does the student need (or want) to learn and why?" and "What prior learning in the area has the student had?" Diagnosis of learning needs and awareness of prior learning become the basis for the learning objectives of the contract. The assessment can be completed during a one-to-one conference between the teacher and student or the student can be asked to complete a self-assessment paper as part of the orientation process. In a well-developed contract program, the use of formal learning style inventories (as discussed in Chapter 12) will help students and teachers become aware of ways in which the students learn best and the variety of activities and resources that are needed. If used, the learning style inventory can be done during orientation so that the information gained is available to student and teacher at the time of an initial conference.

Development of the Plan

Once the actual plan is to be developed, energy is focused on how to go about achieving and evaluating learning objectives. As a basis for the initial teacher-student conference, in addition to the self-assessment, the student can be asked to complete a rough draft of ideas using a contract form. During the initial conference, such material is used to mutually establish roles and responsibilities, identify appropriate resources and activities, decide on evaluation procedures, agree on the amount of credit or other reward, and set time constraints, deadlines, and interim conferences. In most instances, the contract at this time is tentative; however, the student gains ideas and guidance about how to proceed. The student is then encouraged to continue the analysis of goals and objectives, find out what is available, and refine ideas for a later, scheduled meeting with the teacher for the final drafting of the contract. For students who have had no prior experience with contracts, it may be helpful to allow access to samples of completed contracts to help them gain ideas and increase understanding of the process. A sample contract could be included in an independent learning module as part of student preparation for the initial orientation meeting.

An area that the teacher must personally consider is whether or not one has the necessary skills and expertise to guide the student. If not, the teacher needs to help the student locate others who can provide the necessary service or refer the student to someone who is known to have the skills and expertise needed. In this way, the contracting process is one of learning for the teacher as well as the student. To have the student become aware of this adds to the knowledge that learning is a lifelong process.

Completing Required Activities

Once the contract has been established, the student proceeds to carry out activities that have been agreed upon by the teacher and student. The student should be encouraged to begin work immediately and develop, in areas where flexibility exists, a time frame in which to operate. Contact between the teacher and student should be maintained in some way so that the teacher is aware of progress and the student receives feedback and encouragement. It is desirable, especially for students who have never used a contract before or who have not developed self-discipline, to establish a schedule of conferences, either group or individual, during which there is assessment of progress, feedback and suggestions, and determination of any unexpected events and necessary changes.

Renegotiation is a key concept in the use of contracts. Students may not have a realistic view of capabilities or may become less (or more) motivated once involved in the contract activities. Thus, some students may overextend themselves beyond what is realistic, refocus their energies, or decide they can accomplish more (or less) than the contract states. In addition, unexpected events, including financial problems, family responsibilities, and illness, may interfere with the completion of the contract as planned. Renegotiation can include an extension of time, a change of activities and resources, or a decrease or increase in the requirements with accompanying alteration in the amount of reward. If contracts are being used for letter grades, sharing the specific criteria for all grade levels with students allows a student to "retreat" to a lower level or move up to a higher level, if desired.

Evaluation

Evaluation becomes an explicit part of the learning process when using contracts. It is clear to both teacher and student what the student must do to gain the rewards identified in the contract. Specific techniques of evaluation depend on the unique design of the contract but can involve self-evaluation; teacher evaluation of performance, projects, or papers; evaluation by supervisors or preceptors; ratings by peers; and performance on tests. It is also helpful to have the student evaluate the contracting process and the work of the teacher or other people involved in any part of the contract. Important areas for evaluation include clarity, fairness, ease of use, appropriateness and quality of feedback received, realism of scheduled time frames, flexibility, and quality versus quantity of work required.

Faculty Roles

The faculty-student relationship implied in the contracting process is one of mutual trust, responsibility, and decision making. The use of contracts requires the development of new faculty roles and skills from those of traditional transmitter of information. In discussions of faculty roles associated with the use of contracts (Boyd, 1979; Clark, 1981, pp. 596–598; Dougan, 1980; Lord & Palmer, 1982), a number of possible teacher roles emerge. Four key roles have been selected for discussion: counselor/adviser, negotiator, facilitator/mentor, and evaluator.

Counselor/Adviser. As a counselor/adviser, the faculty member helps the student to clarify professional and personal goals, understand general educational requirements, understand procedures and requirements, and establish a learning plan that is compatible with other areas of the student's life. Once the contract is established, the teacher helps the student set priorities, contact other people who will be involved, and arrange the necessary experiences to achieve learning objectives.

Negotiator. As negotiator, the faculty member works with the student to establish the specific requirements of the contract. This requires a cooperative rather than adversary relationship and the ability to listen and question in a way that will move the student toward identification of personal learning goals and methods. The teacher can help the student become aware of reasonable requirements for the reward desired and establish evaluation methods and criteria. Should contract disputes arise, either in initial or renegotiation processes, a mechanism for dealing with them should be available. If faculty and students know that there is a special committee or group who will be available to review objectively any disagreements, both will experience a greater sense of security.

Facilitator/Mentor. As facilitator/mentor, the faculty member is involved in the intellectual development of the student. The primary responsibility is to help students learn how to learn on their own. In this capacity, the teacher needs a knowledge of the variety of resources available or the ability to direct the student to places where desired information can be obtained. Teachers should be aware of, and readily admit, any personal limitations and be ready to refer the student to others who are experts in particular areas. As facilitator/mentor, the teacher assists in arranging placements in community/clinical settings and is the liaison with them for receipt of reports about student performance or evaluations of the contract experience.

Evaluator. The faculty member has a primary responsibility for assuring that contract activities are completed and that required standards are met. Evaluation is formative and summative in relation to both the student and the learning process. The teacher needs to provide the student with honest, regular, constructive criticism in a way that will motivate the student toward achievement of learning objectives. Once the contract is completed, the teacher either provides or obtains final evaluation of the products of achievement established by the contract.

RELATED APPLICATIONS

Although the discussion in this chapter centers on the use of contracts with individuals, they can also be used with groups of students (Bouchard & Steels, 1980; Clark, 1981, pp. 593–596). Group contracts are beneficial in bringing together diverse perspectives, values, and experiences and providing psychological support, criticism, and evaluation of one another's work (Clark, 1981, p. 593). With group contracts, each member of the group must be held accountable for providing individual evidence of performance, particularly if each member is to receive an individual grade. If a group grade is to be given, it becomes the responsibility of the members of the group to see that all individuals contribute equally to the achievement of the contract.

Most reports in the nursing literature dealing with educational uses of contracts describe their use in clinical courses, for increased flexibility of experiences for R.N.s returning for their baccalaureate degrees, and for in-service and continuing education. A few of these will be cited.

Several reports on the use of contracts in the clinical area with undergraduate generic and R.N. students are available. Beare (1985) used the contract approach to implement competency-based education. The clinical contract used was for grade differentiation with emphasis on evaluating clinical competency of students. Kruse and Barger (1982) described their use of a contract grading system. Their intentions were to provide increased flexibility and individuality while decreasing the anxiety related to grades. Schoolcraft and Delaney (1982) also reported on contract grading for clinical evaluation. They described their efforts in trying to confront the problem of quantity versus quality of work required. They conclude that contracts have improved the consistency of grading among faculty members and that there has been increased opportunity for individualized attention to student learning needs.

In respect to the use of contracts with R.N. students returning for a degree, Dobbie and Karlinsky (1982), Price and associates (1983), and Sasmor (1984) shared their experiences with using contracts in practicum courses. Their common aim was to utilize the principles of adult education by providing increased flexibility, self-direction, active involvement, and increased personal responsibility.

Although not strictly classified as a learning contract, the same philosophical base can be applied to nurse-patient collaborative relationships. Brykczynski (1982) described the use of contracts as a method of clarifying and making explicit the expectations and responsibilities of nurses and clients, increasing client participation in decisions, and increasing accountability of both parties. Zangari and Duffy (1980) discussed a similar contracting process in the hospital setting. Among positive outcomes cited for the inpatient setting were increased independence of patients, decreased patient and staff frustration and conflict, enhanced communication between patient and nurse, and increased accountability and responsibility of both patient and nurse.

Other related uses include student-family contracts (Sheridan & Smith, 1975) and student-agency contracts to increase student commitment and accountability (Rose, Koorland, & Reid, 1978).

POTENTIAL FACULTY PROBLEMS

Several problems that faculty may encounter with students at each phase of the contracting process have been discussed earlier in this chapter. Three that are specific to faculty themselves are mentioned here: teacher work load, faculty roles, and returns on efforts.

Teacher Work Load

Faculty work load, particularly in the early phase of contract use, is potentially greater than with traditional methods (Clark, 1981, p. 598; McKeachie, 1978, p. 118). Without question, teachers using contracts need a broad range of competencies to provide the necessary individualized guidance. New programs require significant planning and organizational efforts, although less time is required once students begin to work independently. The one-to-one contacts with students are frequent, especially in the early stages of contract negotiation. Some students who have had no prior experience with contracts or have difficulty with becoming self-directive may require continuing frequent contacts with the teacher. The investigation and development of outside resources is time-consuming. The amount of paperwork and the precise number of evaluative measures exceed most traditional courses. Even when the actual time spent overall is not greater, it may seem that way since it is more continually demanding of the energies and attention of the teacher.

In dealing with the problem of possible faculty overload, McKeachie (1978, p. 118) suggests that close attention be paid to the faculty side of the contract so that an excessive amount of one-to-one teaching time is avoided. Clark (1981, p. 598) points out the importance of training programs to help faculty develop necessary skills and the desirability of decreasing other faculty commitments when a new course using contracts is initiated. Faculty overload can also be prevented by the provision of adequate secretarial, administrative, and instructional development support staff so that the teacher can concentrate on the actual teaching-learning process.

Faculty Roles

Faculty members who have had training and experience in traditional roles only and are comfortable in them may find it difficult to adopt new roles or become anxious when placed in situations requiring different ways of behaving. Some will continue to "lecture" in spite of the situation. Some resist relinquishing control over students in order to keep them in dependent roles. Many will feel threatened by the need to admit to students that their knowledge is limited in some areas.

It is vital, if individualized programs are to be successful, that faculty roles be redefined and special training programs used to help those already in teaching develop the awareness and skills associated with the use of contracts. New programs have a greater chance for success if the faculty members associated with them are interested in providing instruction that is more individualized. Groups of faculty should be selected who are able to work well together and provide mutual support and education. Further, it is important for graduate nursing programs preparing teachers to expose their students to a variety of individualized teaching methods. New teachers are more likely to use a method with which they have had successful experiences as students.

Returns on Efforts

As with other individualized strategies, the teacher who uses contracts may receive little, if any, positive feedback from some peers and administrators. This is more likely to occur when the precise statements of expectations in contracts are viewed as "spoonfeeding," when materials are used at the local level only, or when grades of students using contracts are higher than those learning by traditional methods.

In dealing with this problem, the teacher using contracts will often have to educate peers and administrators about the reasonableness of increased grades when students are more aware of exactly what is expected. On the other hand, the teacher should make sure that the quality of work is adequate to merit the grade for which contracted. In line with this, grade level differentiation should be based on quality as well as quantity of work. Higher education settings also need to develop reward systems that recognize innovative teaching efforts at the same level as other professional accomplishments. Ways in which teachers might help to hasten that occurrence include combining their use of innovative strategies with some type of research or sharing their experiences through publications and conferences.

SUMMARY

The learning contract provides a mechanism for individualizing instruction with individuals and groups and establishing a pattern of self-direction and lifelong learning. It can be used in a variety of situations for individual activities and units or entire courses. Certain elements must be included to provide clear direction to both teacher and student about expectations and how the learning will be evaluated. The contracting process involves orientation, assessment, planning, implementation, and evaluation. Negotiation and renegotiation can occur throughout the process. Certain faculty roles are required when contracts are used, several of them different from those in traditional education.

APPENDIX 1
SAMPLE LEARNING CONTRACT

Student Name:	Mentor Name:
Address:	Address:
Telephone:	Telephone:

Long-Range Goals, Purposes, and Objectives

My goal is to complete the requirements of a baccalaureate degree in nursing and to obtain employment in an acute care pediatric setting.

Specific Objectives

Upon completion of the learning contract, the student will:

1. describe and analyze the general effects of illness and separation on young children of each age group.
2. describe and analyze the positive effects of the use of play with sick children in each age group.
3. apply theoretical content to the psychological/emotional care of children

in the acute setting with each of the following age groups: infant, toddler, preschooler, and school age child.

4. defend with the theoretical rationale the choices of specific play interventions with each age group.

Learning Activities and Resources

1. Select any text (less than 5 years old) on the nursing care of infants and children and (a) review the content related to growth and development of each age group and (b) read the material about the reactions of children of each age group to illness and separation. Prepare notes for each of the two areas in relation to each age group.

2. Contact the campus audiovisual center and arrange to view the film, "Let's Play Hospital." Take notes and write a brief reaction to the film in relation to each of the four objectives.

3. Contact the recreational therapist at the University Hospital and make arrangements to observe in that setting for at least one 8-hour period and to interview the therapist for approximately 30 minutes. The teacher will make a phone call to initiate the contact.

4. Schedule 2 clinical days of 8 hours each in the pediatric unit at Valley Hospital when an instructor is present. Arrange the time desired at least 2 weeks in advance with M. Thompson. Focus of the clinical experience will be on providing psychological/emotional care to children of different age groups. Patients will be selected jointly by student and teacher.

5. Read at least four journal articles or chapters specifically dealing with the use of play with hospitalized children and write a one-page reaction paper to each. Chapters must be in addition to those read for #1 above. Articles and chapters may be personally chosen, selected from a list obtained from M. Thompson, or a combination of the two.

6. Meet with M. Thompson on 2/23/85 at 10 a.m. to discuss progress and any problems. Present a plan for completing activities not finished before that date.

Evaluation

1. Prepare a written paper of not more than 10 double-spaced pages in which an integration of the theoretical study of the use of play with hospitalized children from the various resources is demonstrated. (Specific criteria are available from M. Thompson.)

2. Prepare a one-page care plan focusing on the use of play with one child in each age group. Each care plan must include an identification of a specific problem, a theoretical explanation of the problem, identification of at least two nursing approaches for dealing with the problem, an explanation of the rationale for selection of the approach, and the identification

of at least two objective criteria for the evaluation of success of each approach.

3. Develop some type of model or game for use with each of the four different age groups. These will be demonstrated to the nurses working in the pediatric unit at Valley Hospital, and a brief theoretical explanation will be given for each. The demonstrations can take place during either of the two clinical days. The nurses will evaluate each demonstration in relation to its creativity, ease of use, and appropriateness to the age for which developed.

4. Upon completion of the contract, write an evaluation of the project in relation to achievement of objectives and complete a teacher and self-evaluation using the rating forms provided.

Beginning date: 2/17/85   Ending date: 4/27/85

Credit: 1 unit of independent study under N180 to be used as an elective toward the degree

---

Student signature _____ Date _____

Mentor signature _____ Date _____

15

Using Computers
to Aid Learning

There is no doubt that computer technology is having a significant influence on all areas of our lives. Most readers are no doubt familiar with the everyday role of computers in automated banking, supermarket checkout, airline reservations, screening of income tax returns, and production of bank statements, billings, and junk mail. Applications that are common, although less apparent, include those in telephone and defense systems, medical diagnosis, air traffic control, assembly lines, weather forecasting, and predictions of business and political trends. Other applications, such as home management, financial planning, health record maintenance, and electronic mailing and newspapers, are now possible and may be commonplace in the near future.

Colleges and universities are already receiving students who are products of such technological trends. They will have been exposed to computers in every aspect of their lives—entertainment, daily living, work, and education. They will need computer skills for success in many professions. If students enter higher education in a field in which computers are not used for instruction, it may interfere with the student's ability to deal with massive amounts of information and technological changes, contribute to the culture shock of the computer illiterate, and impede success in work. In fact, Pipes (1980) predicted that those who are computer illiterate will, in the future, be as helpless as those who are now unable to read and write. Because of the pervasive influence of computers, it is vital that each individual learn about the nature and applications of this powerful tool in order to gain full benefit from its potential and deal effectively with its power.

Computers have been used for several years on college and university campuses—for some things. Common uses include scheduling of class-rooms and students, figuring payrolls, grading examinations, and pro-viding statistical analyses of examination results and research data. In a few areas, computers have been used for instruction; however, this has centered primarily around learning *about* the computer rather than learning *with* the computer. It is clear that higher education has not made full use of the technology that is available. Whether or not com-puters become a common part of the educational scene in colleges and universities is dependent on a number of factors. (A few of the barriers will be discussed later in the chapter.) The Carnegie Commission Report on Higher Education (1972, p. 1) predicted that by the year 2000, "a significant portion of instruction in higher education on campus may be carried on through informational technology. . . ." In light of current technological capabilities, that prediction could become a reality sooner than 2000 and be broadened to include all arenas in which education can occur.

Many changes have occurred since 1980 regarding the availability of and interest in the use of technology that relates to nurses and nursing. Without a doubt, nursing has been greatly affected by technology. Many hospitals now make extensive use of computerized information systems and patient-monitoring systems. Many nurses and nurse educators have home computers. Electronic bulletin boards and data bases provide ac-cess to tremendous amounts of information on a variety of subjects. Sev-eral interest groups for computer use in nursing have been established. Newsletters and journals focusing on computers in nursing are now being published. Several books and multiple chapters on computer use in nursing have been published. Descriptions of computer-assisted in-struction (CAI) use or research on CAI use are common topics of articles in professional journals and of presentations at conferences. Seminars and conferences on computer applications to nursing are regular events at the local, regional, and national level. Some nursing programs have elective or required courses for computer literacy and computer appli-cations to nursing. Some nursing programs use computers for instruc-tion and/or management of the instructional process. In many nursing programs where computers are not yet being used for instruction, fac-ulty groups are discussing when and how to begin.

The aim of this chapter is to provide nursing educators who have had minimal or no prior computer experience with an overview of how the computer can be used to facilitate teaching and learning. The primary focus is on those educational functions involving direct interaction between a student and a computer. It is not concerned with such topics as computer programming or the intricacies of computer operations. The reader is directed to other references of choice for technical information and for discussions of the many instructional management functions of computers.

DEFINITIONS

A few basic definitions of computer terminology are given below. An effort has been made to state them in nontechnical language, while at the same time introducing a few common computer terms. The definitions are given in what seems to be a logical and sequential, rather than alphabetical, order. Key words within definitions are highlighted.

COMPUTER: The brains of an electronic system that has the ability to store and manipulate data by following a set of instructions; referred to as a *central processing unit* (CPU). Major types in terms of size, storage capacity, speed, and cost are *maxicomputer, minicomputer,* and *microcomputer.* The maxicomputer is the large, expensive mainframe computer found in large private, public, and governmental agencies for the purpose of collecting, storing, and processing extensive amounts of data for multiple users. The minicomputer is a smaller version of a mainframe and has medium size, cost, speed, and storage capacity. It serves a pool of several users and is found in smaller agencies and within departments of large agencies. The microcomputer is the small, relatively inexpensive, desktop or portable, one-user system that is also referred to as a "personal" computer. The trend is toward increasing miniaturization, increasing power, and declining costs.

TIME-SHARING: A situation in which one computer serves two or more users at the same time. Typically the users are at a site some distance from the computer and are communicating with the mainframe or minicomputer via telephone hookup using a device called a *modem.*

ON-LINE: A situation in which there is direct communication between the computer and a user when the user has immediate access to data generated by the computer.

COMPUTER NETWORK: Two or more computer systems linked together for the purpose of sharing information and programs.

INPUT: Data entered into a computer for storage or processing.

OUTPUT: Information that comes out of a computer.

TERMINAL: The devices used to interact with a computer, consisting of a televisionlike screen called a monitor, *cathode ray tube* (CRT), or *videodisplay ter-*

minal (VDT) and some mechanism, such as a keyboard, light pen, "mouse," or keypad for putting data into the computer. The user "talks to" the computer by using the input devices, and the computer responds by printing out messages or displaying them on the CRT.

HARDWARE: The physical and electronic equipment of a computer system, used to load, process, store, and report information. Basic hardware includes the CPU, terminal, disk drives, and printer. All hardware items, with the exception of the CPU, are referred to as *peripheral devices.*

INTERFACE: A connection between two kinds of hardware, such as a videocassette recorder/player with a microcomputer or a distant computer with a terminal.

PROGRAM: The set of instructions, usually on magnetic tape or disks/diskettes, that tells the computer what to do to accomplish specific functions or tasks. A program is also referred to as *software.*

PROGRAMMING LANGUAGE: The alphabetical and numerical symbols used to communicate instructions to a computer and develop a program. Examples are BASIC, FORTRAN, PILOT, COBOL, PASCAL, and TUTOR, each with unique applications, capabilities, and restrictions.

COMPUTER-BASED EDUCATION or COMPUTER-BASED INSTRUCTION (CBE or CBI): A general term that encompasses the full range of uses of the computer in any part of the educational process. Synonyms are computer-assisted learning (CAL) or computer-assisted education (CAE). Major subcategories are *computer-assisted instruction* and *computer-managed instruction.*

COMPUTER-ASSISTED (or -AIDED) INSTRUCTION (CAI): Instructional activities that use a computer as the primary vehicle for teaching content or processes in a one-to-one interaction with a student. Common categories are: *drill-and-practice, tutorial, simulation, games,* and *utility/problem solving.* Instructional software is called *courseware.*

COMPUTER-MANAGED INSTRUCTION (CMI): The use of the computer for overall management of instructional activities, such as outlining learning objectives, diagnosis of learning needs, prescription of learning resources, class scheduling, monitoring progress, generating and scoring tests, record keeping, and summarizing progress.

ERGONOMICS: The science of the relationships between humans and machines, particularly in the work or educational setting.

COMPUTER-ASSISTED INSTRUCTION

Computer-assisted instruction (CAI) involves the direct interaction between a student and a computer for the achievement of learning some specific task. Although some comments will be made about the management functions of computers (CMI), this chapter will focus primarily on CAI. The areas of discussion are the general interactive process, types of CAI, research about effectiveness, values, extent of use and barriers to adoption, examples of application in nursing education, and future possibilities.

The General Interactive Process of CAI

Imagine a computer that contains a program designed to teach a student about a particular topic. Then imagine a student seated at a station or carrel containing a computer terminal or microcomputer. The computer and terminal may be in close proximity to one another or they may be located some distance apart with the communication link provided by telephone lines or a communication satellite. With a computer in which numerous programs are stored, different students can be using different programs at the same time. However, since the computer can process data and respond to the student so quickly, each student has the impression that the computer is interacting solely with that student.

The basic pattern of interaction is that the student signs on by typing specific information, such as name or code word, which the computer has been programmed to recognize. If visual display is available at the terminal, the messages typed by the student appear on the screen as they are typed. Once the student signs on and the computer welcomes the student, selection of the desired program is made and the lesson begins. In some cases the student can send messages to the computer by touching an appropriate area on the display screen with a finger or special sensor pen. In the future, computers may be able to respond to voice commands. Regardless of the method of input, the computer responds to each student message according to the directions in the stored instructional program. The specific pattern of interaction varies depending on the type of instructional program being used. For example, drill-and-practice programs use a question and answer format, while simulation programs use a more conversational form of interaction that is typical of the usual teacher-student relationship. Messages from the computer to the student can be printed but they are more often displayed on the screen. Kinds of materials displayed include numbers (problems, numerical data); text (instructions, descriptions of clinical situations, information requested by the student, questions, feedback and messages of encouragement); and graphics (diagrams, charts, cardiograms). Auxiliary media—slides, videotape, audiocassette, microfiche—can be incorporated into the instructional program to provide variety of stimuli or allow student options. If the necessary hardware is available, these media are coordinated and controlled by the computer and presented at the terminal. If not, the student is directed by the computer to use the media located in the same station or carrel or to go to another location that has been designated for presentation of the media. Other supportive materials that provide a low-cost way of enhancing CAI without the need for expensive auxiliary equipment include visual materials (photographs, diagrams, charts); print materials (texts, articles, study guides); and anatomical models.

Throughout the process, the computer may keep track of student performance and provide that information to the teacher or student on demand. Depending on student performance, the computer may branch to previous or new material, generate a personally-designed assignment, or tell the student to consult with the instructor.

Types of CAI

Five types of CAI will be discussed. They are drill-and-practice, tutorial, simulation, games, and utility/problem solving. All are interactive in the sense that the student communicates with the instructional program stored in the computer; however, the "human" quality of that interaction varies from a very simple question and answer format to a more complex form of open, free "conversation" as would occur in an actual teacher-student encounter. All require active participation by the student since the student is being continually asked to respond to questions, solve a problem, or make a decision. The instructional sequence of some are primarily program or author controlled while others are learner controlled; all, however, allow the student to control the pace at which study occurs.

Descriptions of the types of CAI are often confusing and overlapping. Although the term "tutorial" could be applied to any situation in which a computer is used in a teaching mode, it is generally given as one of the categories of CAI. Furthermore, it is possible for a single program to incorporate more than one type, leading to some of the confusion regarding specific characteristics of "pure" types. The aim here is to present each type in its "pure" form as interpreted from the use of a variety of references (Alessi & Trollip, 1985, pp. 65–238; Chambers & Sprecher, 1983, pp. 3–6; Coburn, Kelman, Roberts, Snyder, Watt, & Weiner, 1982, pp. 21–36; Kuramoto, 1978; Mirin, 1981; Zemper, 1978, pp. 374–377).

Tutorial. In the tutorial mode of CAI, it is the function of the computer to present new information to the student. In its simplest form, the content is presented in a linear series of factual statements interspersed with predetermined questions and responses from the computer. Typically the computer will present a content statement or question to which the student will respond, and, then, the computer will analyze and evaluate that response before deciding what material to present next. Although usually straight presentation of content, the computer can also be programmed to provide coaching to students in discovering new information and concepts for themselves.

In a more complex form, parallel sequences at different levels of difficulty can be available or the program can branch to bypass familiar material or to provide supplementary and remedial work before returning to the main instructional sequence. Most tutorial programs follow a basic programmed instruction technique; however, much more sophisticated branching is possible with the use of the computer. In addition, the computer program can provide corrective feedback, recommend activities for remediation of important background knowledge, or refer a student to the teacher for personal assistance in problematic areas. At any rate, the sequence of instruction is predetermined and controlled by the program with the student having no direct impact on the sequence of the presentation. However, the tutorial program can be designed to present content at various levels. Thus, the student would be able to select the level of material to be presented based on individual learning needs. Other advantages of tutorial programs are that students receive one-to-one tutoring and regular feedback to indicate how well they are learning the material being presented. In addition, the student has a high degree of control over pacing and time of study. Examples of topics that can be taught by the tutorial mode include anatomy and physiology, calculation of intravenous rates, and physical assessment. Table 15-1 shows the text of part of a tutorial program on the calculation of intravenous fluid rates. The large type reflects computer statements and responses; student responses are in lower case type.

Drill-and-Practice. In drill-and-practice the computer presents a series of questions or problems about material that has been previously learned and provides the student with an opportunity to master the topic through repetitious practice. Such practice is thought to help embed the concepts being taught into the student's knowledge base. Drill-and-practice is the least complex form of CAI and is the most common type presently in use. Typically, the student is required to make simple responses, such as filling in blanks, choosing from a list of alter-

Table 15-1

Excerpt from a Computer-Assisted Instruction Program Using the Tutorial Mode

```
HELLO!  I HAVE SOME INFORMATION TO GIVE YOU ABOUT
CALCULATION OF INTRAVENOUS (IV) FLUID RATES.
PLEASE TYPE IN YOUR FIRST NAME AND THEN HIT THE
"RETURN" KEY WHEN YOU ARE READY TO CONTINUE.

mary

FINE, MARY.  LET ME BEGIN BY TELLING YOU THAT YOU
NEED TO HAVE BASIC MATH SKILLS AND THE ABILITY TO
SOLVE A MATHEMATICAL PROBLEM ONCE NUMERICAL VALUES
HAVE BEEN PLACED INTO A FORMULA IN ORDER TO BE
SUCCESSFUL WITH THIS PROGRAM.  NEXT, YOU NEED TO
KNOW THAT VARIOUS IV SETS HAVE VARIOUS DROP
FACTORS--THAT IS, HOW MANY DROPS THAT SET DELIVERS
FOR EACH ML. OF SOLUTION.  THE INFORMATION ABOUT
DROP FACTOR IS OBTAINED BY READING THE PACKAGE
THAT THE IV SET COMES IN.  FOR EXAMPLE, VARIOUS
ADULT IV SETS DELIVER 10, 15, OR 20 GTTS. PER ML.
DEPENDING ON THE MANUFACTURER OF THE SET WHILE
PEDIATRIC IV SETS USUALLY DELIVER 60 GTTS. PER ML.

YOU MAY WANT TO STUDY THE ABOVE EXPLANATION BEFORE
PROCEEDING.  HIT THE "RETURN" KEY WHEN YOU ARE
READY TO GO ON.

ALL RIGHT, MARY, LET'S LOOK AT THE FIRST FORMULA
FOR SOLVING IV RATE PROBLEMS.  FLOW RATE IS
EXPRESSED AS VOLUME OF FLUID TO BE DELIVERED PER
UNIT OF TIME, USUALLY ML. PER HR. OR GTTS. PER
MIN.  FIRST, YOU NEED TO DETERMINE HOW MUCH FLUID
IS TO BE GIVEN IN 1 HR.  SOMETIMES, THE DOCTOR'S
ORDER IS WRITTEN THAT WAY--GIVE 125 ML. PER HR. OF
5% DEXTROSE IN WATER.  HOWEVER, GENERALLY WITH THE
ADULT PATIENT, THE ORDER WILL READ: GIVE 1000 ML.
5% DEXTROSE IN WATER IN 8 HRS. AND THE NURSE WILL
NEED TO DETERMINE THE HOURLY RATE.  THIS IS DONE
BY DIVIDING THE TOTAL VOLUME OF FLUID TO BE
INFUSED (IN ML.) BY THE INFUSION TIME (IN HRS.).
WITH THE LATTER EXAMPLE, THEN, ONE CAN DETERMINE
THAT 1000 ML. DIVIDED BY 8 HRS. EQUALS 125 ML. PER
HR.

YOU MAY WANT TO STUDY THE ABOVE EXPLANATION BEFORE
PROCEEDING.  HIT THE "RETURN" KEY WHEN YOU ARE
READY TO CONTINUE.

LET'S SEE IF YOU HAVE LEARNED THE MATERIAL JUST
PRESENTED BY HAVING YOU DO A PROBLEM SIMILAR TO
THAT IN THE EXAMPLE.  IF THE DOCTOR'S ORDER READS:
```

```
GIVE 1000 ML. 5% DEXTROSE IN WATER IN 6 HRS., WHAT
WILL BE THE AMOUNT TO BE ADMINISTERED EACH HR.?
TYPE YOUR ANSWER WHEN YOU ARE READY.

167 ml.

VERY GOOD, MARY.  1000 ML. DIVIDED BY 6 HRS.
EQUALS 166.6, ROUNDED TO 167 ML.  LET'S GO TO THE
NEXT STEP BY CALCULATING GTTS. PER MIN.  TO DO
THIS, YOU MUST DIVIDE THE VOLUME OF FLUID ORDERED
(IN ML.) BY THE LENGTH OF TIME IT IS TO INFUSE
(IN MIN.) AND MULTIPLY BY THE DROP FACTOR OF THE
IV SET.  THUS, THE FORMULA IS


TOTAL VOLUME OF FLUID ORDERED (IN ML.)
──────────────────────────────────────
LENGTH OF TIME IT IS TO INFUSE (IN MIN.)

                    X DROP FACTOR OF IV SET


THUS, WITH THE PROBLEM YOU JUST CALCULATED (OF 167
ML. PER HR.) THE FORMULA WOULD BE FILLED IN AS
FOLLOWS WITH AN IV SET THAT DELIVERS 15 GTTS. PER
ML.

    167
    ─── X 15 = 41.7 or 42 GTTS. PER MIN.
     60
```

natives, supplying a missing phrase, or providing the answer to a problem. This format is most often used for simple, factual information requiring rote learning and repeated practice, such as medical terminology, abbreviations, definitions, and the calculation of drug dosages, body fluid needs, or caloric needs.

The rate of progress through a drill-and-practice program depends on individual student performance. Some students may progress rapidly; others may require extra practice; and others may need to be directed to remedial work if it is apparent that they do not know the material. Further, the level of complexity can be adjusted depending on individual student performance. These factors, along with the fact that the student has control over pacing and time of study, makes a drill-and-practice program at least somewhat individualized. However, control of sequencing and level lies with the program rather than with the student. Some educators think that CAI drill-and-practice programs are no better than what can be provided through traditional means. A computer program offers the additional benefits, however, of immediate feedback

Table 15-2

Excerpt from a Computer-Assisted Program Using Drill-and-Practice

```
PROBLEM 1.

    HOW MANY GRAMS OF GLUCOSE ARE THERE IN 1000
    ML. OF A 5% GLUCOSE SOLUTION?

    PLEASE TYPE YOUR ANSWER.

    5

    THE ANSWER GIVEN IS INCORRECT.  (HINT) DID YOU
    GIVE YOUR ANSWER IN RELATION TO 1000 ML.?
    LOOK AT THE PROBLEM AND TRY AGAIN.  PLEASE
    TYPE YOUR ANSWER.

    50

    THAT IS CORRECT.  1000 ML. X 0.05 (5% = 0.05)
    = 50 GRAMS.


PROBLEM 2.

    SINCE YOU HAD SOME TROUBLE WITH PROBLEM 1,
    LET'S HAVE YOU TRY ANOTHER ONE OF THE SAME
    TYPE.

    HOW MANY GRAMS OF GLUCOSE ARE THERE IN 250 ML.
    OF A 10% GLUCOSE SOLUTION?

    PLEASE TYPE YOUR ANSWER.

    25

    GOOD.  THE ANSWER IS CORRECT.  250 ML. X 0.10
    (10% = 0.10) = 25 GRAMS.
```

about performance and the opportunity to practice in a nonthreatening environment, both of which are known to enhance learning. Table 15-2 shows the text of part of a program using the drill-and-practice mode.

Simulation. The reader is referred to Chapter 3 for a general discussion of purposes, process, and types of simulation.

In a computer simulation, the computer is used as the vehicle to present a model of a real-life situation, provide data requested by the student, incorporate the student's decisions into the system, and provide the student with feedback about effects of decisions made. Computer simulations usually emphasize the importance of sufficient and accurate data collection before making critical clinical decisions. They help provide a total, more realistic picture of a clinical situation (from admission to discharge or from the beginning of a shift to the end of a shift) and help close the gap between abstract learning and application. Their real advantage is often in the development of critical thinking and problem solving rather than on learning the specific content being presented. The program is fully controlled by the student's questions and decisions, which are fed into the system. Once a decision is made, the computer responds with a new set of facts based on the consequences (both good and bad) of the decision. Thus, a computer simulation is a dynamic process reflecting many successive decisions over a period of time. As with any simulation, computer simulation helps to deal with the constraints posed by clinical education—time, patient safety, and limited availability of desired experiences. The student is able to gain a sense of the total picture by participating in patient care from beginning to end. All students can be provided with the desired experiences without dependence on clinical availability. The student can experiment with various alternatives without fear of doing something wrong or causing harm to a patient.

The interaction between the student and the computer program in a computer simulation is usually illustrative of either the inquiry or dialogue pattern of communication. Each can be incorporated depending on the specific purposes of the program. Inquiry involves a situation in which a student asks questions or requests data from a computer program. Only the specific information requested is provided. Inquiry is appropriate when the focus of the learning activity is on development of skills in precise data collection. Usually numerical or clinical data are provided so that the student can analyze data, determine relationships, and draw conclusions. After a patient situation is presented, the student is able to obtain various types of information—the patient's appearance, results of diagnostic tests, and physiological processes, signs, and symptoms. See Table 15-3 for an excerpt from a CAI program using inquiry.

In comparison with the inquiry form of interaction, dialogue takes on a more natural conversational quality. With dialogue the teacher (program) not only provides information requested but also guides the student in deciding what information is needed and focuses on desired learning by asking pertinent questions to help the student develop thinking and problem-solving skills. A student's input initiates several possible responses from the computer—a new question, coaching to try another approach, guidance in reviewing necessary material, or feedback about input. Thus, the "conversation" can move in different directions depending on student responses.

Table 15-3

Excerpt from a Computer-Assisted Program Using Inquiry

```
MRS. S., A 32-YEAR-OLD BLACK WOMAN WHO IS
SEPARATED FROM HER HUSBAND, HAS BEEN REFERRED FOR
PSYCHIATRIC CONSULTATION FROM THE DERMATOLOGY
CLINIC.  YOU MAY MAKE FIVE SELECTIONS FROM THE
DATA MENU GIVEN TO GATHER DATA ABOUT THE PATIENT.
ONCE YOU HAVE RECEIVED THE DATA IN THE FIVE AREAS,
YOU WILL BE ASKED TO GIVE YOUR DIAGNOSTIC
IMPRESSION.

     1.   REASON FOR M.D. OR N.P. REFERRAL FROM THE
          CLINIC.
     2.   PATIENT'S VERSION OF REASON FOR REFERRAL.
     3.   FINDINGS AT THE REFERRING CLINIC.
     4.   HISTORY OF SIMILAR PROBLEMS.
     5.   PATIENT'S DESCRIPTION OF THE PROBLEM.

     10.  APPEARANCE AND BEHAVIOR DURING INTERVIEW.
     11.  MENTAL STATUS.

     21.  CRYING SPELLS.
     22.  SUICIDAL THOUGHTS OR ATTEMPTS.

TYPE IN THE NUMBER OF YOUR FIRST SELECTION AND
THEN HIT THE "RETURN" KEY.

1

THE PATIENT COMES TO THE CLINIC COMPLAINING OF
"BODY ODOR" BUT THERE ARE NO UNUSUAL ODORS
APPARENT TO THE EXAMINING NURSE PRACTITIONER.
NEXT SELECTION?

2

I HAVE HAD A STRANGE ODOR FOR A LONG TIME AND
MANY DOCTORS HAVE TOLD ME THAT IT'S "ALL IN MY
HEAD".  NEXT SELECTION?

5

I HAVE EXPERIMENTED WITH MYSELF TO SEE IF
DIFFERENCES IN WEIGHT OR HOW MUCH I SMOKE MAKES
ANY DIFFERENCE IN THE ODOR.  IT DOESN'T SEEM TO
MATTER, BUT I THINK THERE IS LESS ODOR WHEN I AM
AT EASE AND RELAXED.  NEXT SELECTION?

11

MRS. S. IS ALERT, ORIENTED, INTELLIGENT, AND HER
MEMORY APPEARS INTACT.  HER EMOTIONAL EXPRESSION
IS APPROPRIATE BUT VERY LIMITED AND FLAT.  THERE
IS NO EVIDENCE OF PERSECUTORY DELUSIONS OR
HALLUCINATIONS.  NEXT SELECTION?

21

MRS. S. REPORTS THAT SHE CRIES A LOT--SOMETIMES IN
PUBLIC.  SHE IS UNABLE TO SAY WHAT PRECIPITATES
THE TEARS.  YOU HAVE COMPLETED GATHERING DATA ON
THIS PATIENT.  IN YOUR OPINION, DOES MRS. S. HAVE
A PSYCHIATRIC PROBLEM?  TYPE YES OR NO.

yes

RIGHT.  WHICH DIAGNOSTIC CATEGORY DO YOU THINK
WOULD BE MOST LIKELY?  TYPE THE NUMBER OF THE
CATEGORY FROM THE LIST BELOW TO INDICATE YOUR
CHOICE.
```

Whenever the dialogue method of interaction is used in a CAI program, the teaching-learning situation takes on greater flexibility. Therefore, it is necessary for the developer of the program to do extensive analysis of the subject so that the multiple possibilities in student questions and responses will be incorporated into the program. As program flexibility and branching increase, complexity and time for program development also increase. See Table 15-4 for an excerpt from a computer program using dialogue in a clinical problem-solving situation.

Educational computer simulations have been used for a number of years in such areas as business administration, economics, and medicine; however, they are relatively new to nursing education. At present, most computer simulations are done in a textual format, although some authors are beginning to incorporate various media in order to increase realism. Computer simulations have great potential usefulness in nursing education for both teaching and evaluation. Computer simulations can be used to teach problem-solving clinical skills for basic nursing education and training of nurse practitioners and for in-service and continuing nursing education. They provide an opportunity for the development of sound clinical judgment before actual clinical experience and for learning without fear of making a mistake and harming someone. In addition, they allow the same clinical situation to be presented to all learners without having to depend on availability of that situation in the clinical setting. In the area of evaluation, they can be used for end-of-course clinical evaluation, for evaluation of those with prior experience for credit and advanced placement, and for relicensure or certification/recertification. As technological capabilities increase, the cost of hardware declines, and quality of software improves, expanded use of computer simulations in nursing education will be possible.

The incorporation of various types of media is now occurring with the ability to interface the computer with videotape and videodisc players for the development of a new type of CAI—computer-assisted video instruction (CAVI) (see Saba & McCormick, 1986, pp. 397–398; Schwartz, 1984). Such advanced techniques are capable of incorporating all types of media, both still and motion, and add an efficiency and effectiveness to training and education that has not existed before. Graphics, slides, films, filmstrips, videotapes, and other media can become part of an integrated computer program. The computer drives the media and plays selected segments at designated points in the instructional program. Existing media may be used, or media can be developed to meet specific needs. Graphic displays of equipment readings, sounds and waveforms from various types of monitors, heart sounds and lung

Table 15-4
Excerpt from a Computer-Assisted Program Using Simulation of a Clinical Problem-Solving Situation Plus Dialogue

```
YOU ARE ON DUTY IN THE EMERGENCY ROOM WHEN A
6-YEAR-OLD CHILD IS BROUGHT IN BY HIS PARENTS.
THE CHILD APPEARS ALERT BUT WEAK, DOES NOT ATTEMPT
TO STAND OR WALK, AND HIS SKIN IS PALE AND COOL.
THE FATHER TELLS YOU THAT HE THINKS THE CHILD
SWALLOWED SOME PILLS FROM THE MEDICINE CABINET.
HE FURTHER TELLS YOU THAT THE CHILD'S MOTHER HAS
'HEART TROUBLE' AND SUFFERS FROM 'FUNNY BEATS' AND
THAT THE CHILD'S OLDER SISTER IS EPILEPTIC AND
TAKES MEDICATION FOR SEIZURES.  WHEN THE CHILD WAS
FOUND, ALL THE DRUGS WERE MISSING.  THE FATHER
ASSUMES THAT THE CHILD EITHER SWALLOWED THEM OR
POURED THEM DOWN THE DRAIN.  NEITHER PARENT CAN
GIVE YOU ANY MORE INFORMATION ABOUT THE TYPE OR
QUANTITY OF DRUGS THAT HAD BEEN STORED IN THE
MEDICINE CABINET.  PLEASE HIT 'RETURN' WHEN YOU
ARE READY TO CONTINUE.

AT THIS POINT, THE CHILD BECOMES RESTLESS AND
VOMITS.  LOOKING AT THE VOMITUS CONFIRMS THAT
THERE IS NO RECOGNIZABLE DRUG TO BE SEEN.  WHAT
TEST OR PHYSICAL FINDING DO YOU WANT TO CHECK
FIRST?  TYPE YOUR ANSWER.

respiration

GOOD, MAKE SURE THE PATIENT IS BREATHING WELL.
SINCE THE CHILD HAS JUST VOMITED, YOU SHOULD CHECK
HIS RESPIRATION TO MAKE SURE HE HAS NOT ASPIRATED
ANY VOMITUS.  INITIAL DATA ABOUT THE PATIENT . . .
RESPIRATION IS 20 PER MINUTE AND AIRWAY IS CLEAR.
RADIAL PULSE IS INITIALLY IRREGULAR IN STRENGTH
AND RHYTHM, THEN REGULAR AT 80 PER MINUTE.
REMEMBER, YOU HAVE NO OTHER PHYSICAL DATA SO FAR.
WHAT TEST OR PHYSICAL FINDING DO YOU WANT NOW?
TYPE YOUR ANSWER.

electrocardiogram

YES, THE CARDIOGRAM IS A VERY GOOD CHOICE, BUT
DON'T FORGET TO CHECK THE BLOOD PRESSURE, WHICH IS
IMPORTANT AND CAN BE DONE VERY EASILY.  THE BP IS
110/70.  THE ECG (LEAD II) SHOWS A SERIES OF SINUS
BEATS, SEVERAL PVC'S, DEPRESSED S-T SEGMENTS, AND
SLIGHTLY PROLONGED P-R INTERVALS.  PLEASE HIT
'RETURN' WHEN YOU ARE READY TO CONTINUE.

THE CHILD HAS NO PRIOR HISTORY OF CARDIAC PROBLEM
AND WE MAY ASSUME THAT HIS ARRHYTHMIA RESULTED
FROM INGESTION OF TOXIC AMOUNTS OF A DRUG.  THE
DRUG INGESTION TOOK PLACE 3 HOURS AGO.  THE
PARENTS DID NOT NOTICE ANY SYMPTOMS AFTER THE
INGESTION OR UP UNTIL THE TIME THEY BROUGHT THE
CHILD TO THE HOSPITAL.  WHAT DRUG GROUP DO YOU
SUSPECT AS THE MOST LIKELY CAUSE OF THIS DRUG
TOXICITY?  TYPE THE DRUG NAME.

digitalis

VERY GOOD.  YOU CORRECTLY INTERPRETED THE
ARRHYTHMIA, THE ECG SIGNS, AND THE VOMITING AS
CLASSICAL SIGNS OF DIGITALIS POISONING.  DON'T
FORGET, HOWEVER, THAT OTHER DRUGS CAN CAUSE
ARRHYTHMIAS AND VOMITING, INCLUDING THE
ANTIARRHYTHMIC AGENTS.  PLEASE HIT 'RETURN' WHEN
YOU ARE READY TO CONTINUE.
```

SOURCE: University of California, San Francisco. Used by permission of Martin Kamp, M.D., Computer Center.

sounds, and other data can be used to add the realism needed to narrow the gap between theory and practice and thereby provide learning that is more reflective of actual clinical experiences. For example, when the student needs to assess the patient's pupils, an image of pupils will appear on the monitor. When the student needs to assess the breath sounds, a sound recording of breath sounds will play while there is a visual image of a nurse placing the stethoscope on different areas of the chest while listening. The technique forces students to observe, listen, read, ask questions, and draw conclusions based on the specific data presented. The actual visual and auditory sequences presented depend on the learner's responses at critical decision points. The learner may be returned to a prior segment for review, go back to the data base for more information, or proceed to the next segment.

A few people around the country are developing CAVI. Most are using computer/videotape interface, such as that described by Fishman (1984), but more and more interest is being shown in the powerful potential of CAVI using computer/videodisc interface, such as that described by Parker (1984). The capacity and speed of access of the videodisc is astounding. A videodisc is similar in appearance and size to a 33 rpm record and is capable of holding 54,000 frames on each side. This means that one videodisc can hold the contents of 1,700 average books on each side, not to mention its capacity for nonprint media such as slides and videotape segments. It has been estimated that the entire *Encyclopedia Britannica* could be stored on part of one videodisc and that all material in a baccalaureate program, including lectures, reading assignments, and audiovisual media, could be stored on just eight videodiscs (Sweeney, 1985, pp. 80–81). The entire 54,000 frames can be searched in only 2 to 3 seconds. In most instances, the access time for a specific frame is less than 1 second. In addition, two sound tracks on the videodisc allow for the use of two languages or the ability to develop programs for entirely different audiences using the same videodisc.

Games. Both simulation games and nonsimulation games can be adapted for use with the computer. (The reader is referred to Chapter 3 for examples of simulation and nonsimulation games.) The gaming concept implies competition between two or more players (one of whom may be the computer program) to achieve a specific goal. In a computer game, the program is designed to assess strategies, give results or effects of decisions made, and introduce variables that alter the course of events. Computer games can involve either content (e.g., drugs and medical terminology) or process (e.g., developing strategies for decision making or changing attitudes). They are often incorporated with one of the other types of CAI and provide variety and increase motivation if they are used appropriately and not overused.

The most common applications of computer games in higher education have been in business, economics, and management areas. No computer game applications to nursing have been found; however, many games that have been developed for noncomputer use could be readily adapted for use with a computer. In addition, games developed for other fields can be adapted for use in nursing education or used, as designed, for purposes that are common with those of other disciplines. As an example of the latter, Metro-Apex,* a computerized simulation game, is designed to give participants an understanding of health care systems (Washburn & McGinty, 1977). Participants receive feedback about effects of decisions on the community and health care system. Each round lasting 3 to 8 hours is equivalent to 1 year. Roles include elected officials, public health department officials, environmental personnel, hospital administrators, representatives of special interest groups, and others. Although no nurses are included, Metro-Apex offers potential advantages for use with any group, such as graduate students in community health nursing, who need to develop insight about interrelationships among elements of the health care system, interaction between the health care system and the larger community, and long term health care planning.

Utility/Problem Solving.   Although not originally developed specifically for teaching, many computer programs designed for both general use and specific applications are of educational value. These programs do not present content directly to the student; however, the student learns related content and processes by involvement with the program. Applications software that allow the user to accomplish specific tasks include the general purpose software for spread sheets, database management, and word processing (Bellinger & Laden, 1985); database retrieval; authoring systems; and statistical packages. Each type of program helps the learner to accomplish specific tasks and, in so doing, also to achieve knowledge and understanding of the content and processes reflected in the program.

Spreadsheet programs are used to manipulate numerical or financial data and make automatic adjustments when any variable has been changed. They are helpful to those who need to do various types of planning, budgeting, personnel staffing and scheduling, and financial

*Available from the Center for Multidisciplinary Educational Exercises (COMEX), University of Southern California, Los Angeles, California 90007.

analysis and reports. Spreadsheet programs save time and decrease the possibility of errors in numerical calculations. "What if" situations can be devised by changing numbers and determining the consequences of that change. Use of such programs allows the learner to experience more fully the various situations involved in nursing service, education, and administration.

Database management programs allow the filing, storage, sorting, analysis, and retrieval of information of various types. Possible data sources are varied; examples include supplies, drugs, books, people, financial resources, and grades. Data in specific attribute areas, such as age, specialty area, and length of employment, can be recalled and used to generate reports as needed. A database management program may be used to generate tests by calling up test items by subject or key words, reviewing them, and printing those items selected. Database management also allows computerized maintenance of records of performance, course schedules, and student placement.

Word processing programs are probably the most used of all available general purpose software. They are useful for such tasks as writing, editing, and printing reports, papers, manuscripts, care plans, procedure manuals, and mailing lists. Significant time savings are realized with the capability of composing and editing on the screen. Changes can be made without having to redo the entire document. Many companion programs enhance the usefulness and timesaving ability of word processing programs by providing spelling and grammar checks, automatic formatting, hyphenation, footnotes, and other accessory functions.

On-line information services provide access to several databases relevant to nursing practice and nursing research. They are sometimes referred to as encyclopedic databases, since they provide in-depth information on a wide range of topics (Maher, 1984). Access is accomplished by the use of a computer, a modem, and standard telephone lines. Such services are available to subscribing agencies, such as libraries, research organizations, and hospitals, and now directly to individuals using a home computer. A fee is charged for each service depending on time of day and the specific database searched. Results of the search may be viewed on the screen, printed out, or sent in the mail. Examples of common computer databases (Clark & Clark, 1985; Grobe, 1984, pp. 126–129; Saba & McCormick, 1986, pp. 331–339; Stoia, 1983; Sweeney, 1985, pp. 265–267) include:

1. MEDLINE or MEDLARS Online (Medical Literature Analysis and Retrieval System Online), the National Library of Medicine's index to references from more than 3,000 international biomedi-

cal journals. Contains several databases, including *Index Medicus, Index to Dental Literature,* and *International Nursing Index.*

2. AVLINE, a catalog of nonprint instructional materials provided by the National Library of Medicine.

3. ERIC, the database of educational periodicals and reports provided by the Educational Resources Information Center of the National Institute of Education.

4. CINAHL (Cumulative Index to Nursing and Allied Health Literature) contains references to approximately 300 health-related journals printed in English, plus the publications of NLN, ANA, and state nursing associations. On-line access is available to subscribers.

5. DIALOGUE of Palo Alto, California, is an on-line commercial information service that provides access to specialized databases, including MEDLINE, ERIC, and CINAHL.

6. BRS (Bibliographic Retrieval Services) of Latham, New York, is an on-line commercial information service that provides access to bibliographic sources, including CINAHL, and an electronic card catalog for books in print. BRS After Dark offers the same services to individuals during noncommercial hours.

7. CompuServe of Columbus, Ohio, provides business-related and investor information and, now, educational materials from Ohio State University.

Particularly useful to nursing educators is the availability of authoring systems that allow those without programming skills to develop tests and CAI software (Beebe, 1983). Authoring systems ask the author a series of questions and, based on answers received, construct computer programs that teach or test content. Some authoring systems also allow the author to identify particular segments of a videotape or videodisc to be utilized at specific times in a program. Branching of presentation of content depending on student responses to questions permits increased flexibility and individualization of the program. Examples of authoring systems useful for the development of instructional materials for nursing education include:

1. NEMAS (Nursing Education Module Authoring System), available from J. B. Lippincott, allows the creation of patient simulations that incorporate both the nursing process and components of instructional design (Grobe, 1984, pp. 121–122; Saba & McCormick, 1986, pp. 366, 387).

Table 15-5
Summary of CAI Types, Purposes, Goals, and Point of Control of Lesson

CAI Type	Purpose	Goal	Control of Lesson
Tutorial	Presentation of new content	Acquisition of basic facts and concepts	Computer/author of program
Drill-and-Practice	Reinforcement and practice with previously learned content	Practice with material for fixing of concepts	Computer/author of program
Simulation	Presentation and manipulation of a model of real phenomena about which students can make decisions	Provide insight about actual situations; develop problem-solving skills; integration of knowledge and skills	Usually student/learner but can be combined
Game	Provide competitive situation in which outcome is defined	Development of insight into various strategies for reaching defined goal	Usually student/learner but can be combined
Utility/problem solving	Achievement of specific tasks	Acquisition of knowledge and insight about content and processes	Student/learner

2. Ghostwriter, available from CAVRI of New Haven, Connecticut, for development of interactive video programs.

3. Microinstructor, available from Mosbysystems, St. Louis, Missouri, for creation of branched CAI programs. The authoring system will interface with videotape or videodisc for development of CAVI.

4. Whitney System, available from Whitney Educational Services, San Mateo, California, can be used for developing CAVI.

Two test authoring programs are TESTAR from Mosbysystems and TAP (Test Authoring Package) from Addison-Wesley Publishers.

Computers also offer opportunities for teaching about the research process and completing statistical analysis of research data. Although many statistical packages have been available via use of a terminal and a mainframe or minicomputer system, statistical analysis software programs for microcomputers are now available. One example is CRISP, available from Crunch Software in San Francisco, for use on the IBM-PC.

See Table 15-5 for a summary of the purposes, goals, and amount of student control with each type of CAI.

Research Related to Effectiveness of CAI

Research about the effectiveness of using CAI in higher education settings is limited. However, several authors have provided summaries of research findings on the use of CAI in various fields and levels of education. They are presented here as a basis for comparison of studies done in nursing education.

1. Mahr and Kadner (1984) summarized research in basic education in which (a) computer use in a remedial basic mathematics course resulted in decreased attrition rates and an increased attendance rate, and (b) augmentation of classroom instruction with CAI brought about superior performance on standardized aptitude tests.

2. Braun (1980) presented a summary of results of 32 studies, in which the majority of students showed a savings in learning time, greater achievement in relation to time spent, and improved skills.

3. Kulik, Kulik, and Cohen (1980) presented an analysis of 59 studies at the college level in various fields comparing computer-based instruction with conventional methods. In 54 studies investigating student achievement on examinations, 37 showed superior performance by the CBI group while 17 favored conventional methods. In the 14 studies in which there was a significant difference, 13 favored CBI. In 11 of the 59 studies, student attitudes toward the instructional method and the subject matter were considered. Attitudes toward instructional method were more positive with CBI than with conventional methods in eight of the 11, with four being at a significant level. Attitudes toward subject matter were more positive with CBI than with conventional methods in five of the 11, with two being at a significant level. In eight studies in which time was considered, the CAI groups showed a substantial savings in learning time.

4. Edwards, Norton, Taylor, Weiss, and Dusseldorp (1975) summarized research results on the use of CAI at various educational levels. In those using CAI as a supplement to traditional methods (nine studies), all found that CAI supplementation was more effective, sometimes remarkably so, than normal instruction alone. In 20 studies in which CAI was used as a substitute for traditional instruction, CAI students achieved more than non-CAI students in nine. Of those studies investigating learning time (nine), all showed a significant time savings with CAI, even though it did not result in greater learning achievement. In the three studies inves-

tigating retention, one showed equal retention and two showed less retention with CAI learning than with non-CAI learning.

Relatively few studies are available that investigate the effectiveness of CAI in nursing education at the undergraduate or graduate level. Of those that are available, most compare CAI with traditional methods in relation to learning achievement while a few compare CAI with another autotutorial method or investigate retention and time for learning. Major findings of these studies are summarized below:

1. Bitzer (1966) compared the posttest scores of experimental and control groups in a diploma program during their study of the care of a patient with angina pectoris and myocardial infarction. The groups were matched in level of preinstruction knowledge. The experimental group received their instruction using tutorial CAI accompanied by a short film of a typical patient case history. Traditional methods, including lectures, readings, case histories, and nursing care plans, were used with the control group. The results showed that the computer taught group scored significantly better than the control group on the posttest.

2. A later study in the same setting (Bitzer & Boudreaux, 1969) investigated the effectiveness of CAI for teaching maternity nursing. The students in one course were divided into two groups that, according to pretest results, were matched in their preinstruction level of knowledge about the topic. The control group was taught in the conventional classroom manner while the experimental group received instruction using the computer system. While posttest scores showed that students in both groups made a significant gain in learning, final examination results showed no significant difference between the two groups. However, they found a major savings in time with those students using CAI.

3. Kirchhoff and Holzemer (1979), using a posttest design without a control group, examined the effectiveness of using a CAI program for teaching students in a baccalaureate program about postoperative nursing care. It was their conclusion that the students learned the material since posttest scores were significantly better than those on the pretest. Kirchhoff and Holzemer also determined that those students with an active experimentation learning style (using Kolb's learning style inventory) benefited most from the use of CAI.

4. Thiele (1984) found that baccalaureate nursing students using

CAI had a much lower failure rate than those using traditional methods (9 percent versus 38 percent and 33 percent).

5. Day and Payne (1984) compared CAI with lecture for teaching the theoretical components of health assessment to baccalaureate nursing students. They found no significant difference in learning.

6. In a study comparing CAI with traditional methods for teaching surgical nursing, Conklin (1983) provided evidence that CAI achieves equal learning in less time than traditional methods.

7. Boettcher, Alderson, and Saccucci (1981) found that CAI was as effective as printed programmed instruction for cognitive learning.

8. Neil (1985) compared two groups of baccalaureate nursing students in relation to cognitive learning and attitude toward instructional method. One group used a CAI module while the other used written text materials only. She found that the mean scores for the CAI group were slightly higher, although not at a level of significance. She also found a nonsignificant difference in relation to attitudes toward instructional method; however, a preference for CAI over reading was indicated by a majority of both groups.

9. Yoder and Heilman (1985) studied CAI for teaching nursing diagnosis to undergraduate and graduate students using a pretest-posttest research design. They determined that the CAI tutorial was effective since there was a significant difference between pretest and posttest scores.

10. Timpke and Janney (1981) found that CAI was highly successful for teaching drug dosage calculations. They also found that student anxiety and embarrassment was decreased and degree of confidence was increased with CAI.

11. Huckabay, Anderson, Holm, and Lee (1979) compared the use of CAI with lecture-discussion in relation to cognitive learning, transfer of learning, and affective behaviors with nurse practitioner students at the graduate level. Results showed no significant differences between the groups in cognitive learning, transfer of learning, or affective behaviors. However, the CAI group scored significantly higher on three posttests on cognitive learning and transfer of learning.

12. Schleutermann, Holzemer, & Farrand (1983) compared two formats (paper/pencil and CAI) for delivery of clinical simulations

to students in a graduate nurse practitioner program. They reported that students' reactions to both tools were very positive but that no preference for either was shown and that there was no difference in student performance. Students perceived CAI as providing more immediate feedback and being more time efficient; however, they viewed the paper/pencil format as more convenient since it could be studied at a personally selected time and place. Both methods were reported to be expensive to develop, produce, and use.

13. Van Dongen and Van Dongen (1984) reported that 85 percent of students preferred CAI to traditional lecture/reading and an even higher percentage stated that they would like more CAI experience.

A few studies using CAI with R.N.s are also available. They include:

1. Hoffer, Barnett, Mathewson, and Loughrey (1975), studied the application of CAI to instruction of hospital nurses in cardiopulmonary resuscitation. The results indicated that those nurses who used the computer increased their test scores in the cardiopulmonary resuscitation program while nurses in the control group using traditional in-service methods did not. They further demonstrated the importance of designing programs to meet the needs of a specific group since the nurses in this study objected to the use of criteria that clearly were developed for physicians.

2. Pogue (1982), using a pretest-posttest design with a CAI and a lecture group, found that the CAI group achieved significantly higher total posttest scores on cardiovascular drug content.

3. Fishman (1984) used three groups to compare learning about cancer chemotherapy. Groups included interactive video with computer, linear video with videotape, and traditional classroom lecture. She found that the interactive video group attained a significantly higher level of mastery on the posttest and retention test but that there was no reduction in learning time.

Although there are some variations among research results in nursing and, so far, rather limited evidence in some areas, the following tentative conclusions can be drawn about the use of CAI in nursing education:

1. CAI is an effective learning technique. Students using CAI learn at least as well, and often significantly better, than those using traditional classroom methods or other autotutorial methods.

2. Learning through the use of CAI requires less time than traditional methods.

3. The use of CAI results in improved retention and transfer of what has been learned.

These conclusions are comparable to those presented earlier in the summaries of research findings for general education. The consistency of findings among various disciplines lends support to the general conclusions presented.

Further research is needed in all of these areas, particularly student attitudes, learning retention, transfer of learning, and learning time required. In addition, other areas warranting investigation include cost effectiveness, impact on student attrition, relationships to learning styles and student preferences, extent of individualization of instruction achieved, and impact on the teacher-student relationship and their roles. CAI techniques also need to be compared with other autotutorial methods (Neil, 1985), as well as with those methods thought to develop skills in critical thinking and judgment.

Values of Using Computers for Instruction

The values of CAI regarding effectiveness, time-savings, and learning retention and transfer have been outlined in the research and conclusions presented above. It is also possible to identify other values, based on known learning theories and the principles of individualization presented in Chapter 12. In fact, some authors are of the opinion that the greatest potential strength of CAI is in its capacity to individualize instruction (Cross, 1976, p. 61; Magidson, 1977; Neher, 1975; Norman, 1982; Porter, 1978; Valish & Boyd, 1975). The following list is an outline of potential ways in which CAI can help to facilitate learning and increase individualization of the instructional process. The use of CAI can:

1. increase interactivity between the student and the learning situation and active participation of the student in learning.
2. provide enhanced use of all types of media with an increased richness of the sensory experience.
3. provide continuity to the learning experience.
4. help students develop new and creative ways of problem solving.
5. give immediate feedback about performance.
6. make adjustments in type and depth of content.
7. increase student control over time of study and pacing of lesson.
8. provide consistent, patient attention on a one-to-one basis.

9. provide the student with opportunities to experiment and be wrong without feeling embarrassed or fearful of harming someone.

10. permit students to repeat a learning activity as often as desired.

Another value that is indirectly related to individualization is that of freeing the teacher from routine, repetitive tasks so that greater attention can be given to more individualized aspects of the learning situation. When the teacher does not have to (1) give lectures on material that is widely accepted and noncontroversial, (2) participate in clerical tasks associated with record keeping about student performance and progress, (3) produce alternate test forms, and (4) administer and grade tests, more time can be given to personal attention to students, answering questions, leading discussions, providing guidance, and increasing the depth of learning experiences. Thus, there is more effective (and challenging) use of both teacher and student time; the teacher's attention can be focused on those activities that are uniquely human; and students can be provided the help needed to make the learning experience more productive in relation to achievement of curricular goals.

A value that is unrelated to individualization, except in the sense of curriculum improvements, is the ability to obtain feedback about courses and lessons for serious evaluation of instruction. Precise data about both individual and group performances can be generated in minutes. Data thus obtained can help the teacher to become aware of both the strengths and problems associated with CAI material. Programs can be revised to deal with any problems and improve the overall effectiveness of the material. When the emphasis is on mastery of objectives by all students, this type of activity is vital in providing instruction that, in fact, allows all students to achieve mastery.

COMPUTER APPLICATIONS TO EDUCATION

Early projects applying computers to instruction were mainly group efforts using mainframe systems with later expansion to the use of minicomputers and microcomputers. Some of the early developments have been outlined by several authors (Alessi & Trollip, 1985, pp. 47–50; Bork, 1978, pp. 199–203; Chambers & Sprecher, 1983, pp. 6–17; Sweeney, 1985, pp. 145–146). Several examples that seem particularly pertinent to nursing are included here in an effort to provide a historical perspective to current CAI applications.

PLATO

PLATO (Programmed Logic for Automatic Teaching Operations) was initiated at the University of Illinois in 1960 with the goal of designing a large, mainframe computer-based system for instruction. In the 1970s, funding by the National Science Foundation (NSF) and the Control Data Corporation (CDC) of Minneapolis resulted in the creation of interactive, self-paced CAI materials that were accessible from various regions of the United States using leased equipment and hookup with a mainframe time-sharing system. Entire courses and individual lessons were authored using TUTOR, the CAI authoring language of PLATO.

PLATO is now a commercial project of CDC. In addition to the educational software available through the use of time-sharing systems, some individual programs are available for use on certain microcomputers, and others are available to subscribers via CDC's Homelink telecomputing service. Many topics appropriate for nursing education are available (Index of nursing lessons, 1980), and the literature holds several examples of the use of PLATO in nursing (Bitzer, 1966; Bitzer & Bitzer, 1973; Bitzer & Boudreaux, 1969; Nabor, 1975; Schleutermann, Holzemer, & Farrand, 1983).

TICCIT

The TICCIT project (Time-shared Interactive Computer Controlled Information Television) was also funded by the NSF in the 1970s as a joint effort between the MITRE Corporation and Brigham Young University. The project focused on the use of minicomputers and television with an emphasis placed on team production of learner-controlled lessons for entire courses in math and English for undergraduate students. The system was implemented at two community colleges with varying degrees of success. It is presently marketed by Hazeltine Corporation. Two public domain TICCIT software programs for basic nursing skills are available (Hales, 1985, p. 34).

CONDUIT

CONDUIT, also begun in the 1970s, was a consortium effort among five universities in different states with its headquarters at the University of Iowa. CONDUIT's aim was to improve both quality and availability of software for instruction at the university level. The project was initially

funded by the NSF and later by the NSF and the Fund for the Improvement of Post-Secondary Education. Modestly priced CAI programs for
various microcomputer systems are available. An important role that
CONDUIT has played has been the dissemination of information about
computer programs that have been evaluated for educational soundness
(Mirin, 1981).

Ohio State University Projects

Another main participant in the development of CAI materials was Ohio
State University (OSU). Several OSU accomplishments will be highlighted. The OSU College of Medicine has been a leader in computer
applications to health sciences education (Pengov, 1978). The system
offers CAI to support teaching programs in medicine, nursing, and the
allied medical professions as well as for continuing professional education. All CAI types are represented. A variety of topics are available with
many indexed specifically to nursing education. Examples of programs
specific to nursing are (1) *Bottle,* on closed chest drainage systems, (2)
Veins, on venipuncture and IV therapy, (3) *CCNUR,* on cardiac anatomy
and physiology and pathophysiology of heart disease, and (4) *Nursims,*
for use in the evaluation of nursing care performance in a variety of
clinical areas (CAI program library, 1983). Although, at present, most
of the programs are only available on a time-sharing basis via the
CompuServe Network, efforts are underway to evaluate various microcomputer systems for the possible conversion of programs to a microcomputer format (J. Dale Brubeck, personal communication, June 25,
1984). Some programs, specifically *Nursims,* have already been converted
for use on certain microcomputers and are being marketed by J. B. Lippincott Company.

In the past, dissemination of OSU's CAI programs was through
CAIREN (Computer-Assisted Instruction Regional Education Network)
and HEN (Health Education Network). CAIREN was a regional network
for sharing CAI learning resources with Ohio health care facilities and
educational institutions (Forman, Pengov, & Burson, 1978). Its primary
aim was to provide accessible continuing education to medical, nursing,
and allied health personnel. Several professional groups, including the
Ohio Nurses' Association, approved selected programs for continuing
education credit.

HEN was established in 1975 as an outgrowth of the Lister Hill National Center for Biomedical Communications Network, an experimental CAI network supported by the National Library of Medicine. The

purpose of HEN was to "facilitate, maintain, and preserve economical, nationwide access to computer-assisted instructional materials for health education" (Tidball, 1978, p. 195). It was the first fully operational national network for the health sciences and provided access in many cities throughout the United States to the CAI program at OSU. Computerized clinical case simulations were available on a 24-hour basis to member medical, nursing, and dental schools, as well as to hospitals and other health care institutions (Held & Kappelman, 1976), thus expanding the educational opportunities in basic and continuing education in various health care fields.

In the late 1970s, the availability of microcomputers provided a potential mechanism for a revolution in the use of CAI. Although the potential for the revolution has been carried even further with declining costs and continuing improvement and expansion of technology, the widespread use of computers for instruction has not yet occurred.

Extent of Use of CAI in Higher Education

Earlier in this chapter the ability of CAI to provide overall improvement in the quality of learning and to increase individualization of learning was discussed. What, then, is the extent of use of CAI in nursing education? This question is difficult to answer precisely. Although individual examples of use are available in the nursing and related literature, data that establish a clear picture about extent of use among nursing programs are limited. The extent of computer use in the last few years is reflected in the following data:

1. Levine and Wiener (1975) cited research in which 7 percent of nursing schools used CAI, and 47.1 percent stated that use of CAI was being considered.
2. In a 1976 survey of National League for Nursing (NLN) accredited associate and baccalaureate degree nursing programs with an enrollment of 250 or more, Thompson (1980) found that 14.6 percent of the respondents were using CAI.
3. Knippers (1981) found that CAI was the least-used self-instructional method in nursing programs.
4. Thomas (1985) reported on a 1983 survey of NLN accredited baccalaureate and higher degree nursing programs regarding the place of computing in nursing education. Thomas found that 38 percent of the respondents were using computers for CAI and CMI. The extent of use for CAI alone was not reported.

5. Felton and Brown (1985) cited a study of baccalaureate nursing programs completed by the C. V. Mosby Company in 1983 in which almost 50 percent of programs reported that they owned or had access to at least one microcomputer. Although 35 percent indicated that applications for teaching, research, and administration had been developed, the extent of use for CAI alone was not reported. It was clear, however, that the extent of use was not great since about one-half indicated that they were just learning to use the hardware.

6. Thompson (1985) reported on a survey of NLN accredited associate and baccalaureate degree nursing programs completed in 1984 in which 44.9 percent of the respondents claimed to be using computers for instruction.

From these reports, it seems apparent that CAI in nursing education is steadily increasing although not yet widely used. In contrast, two-thirds of the U.S. medical schools were reported to be using computers for instruction as early as 1975 (Votaw & Farquhar, 1978). However, the extent of use of CAI within the individual medical schools was not reported.

General impressions about the status of computing in nursing has been offered by Heller, Romano, Damrosch, and Parks (1985). They cited several nursing authors to support their belief that "major gaps exist between the information processing power of the computer as a tool and the current use by nursing in practice, administration, education, and research" (p. 14). Although they were addressing the state of general computer literacy among nurses, their contentions apply equally well to the use of CAI in nursing education. If CAI is effective and has the power to individualize learning, what is it that impedes the widespread and immediate adoption of CAI methods?

Barriers to Adoption of CAI.   The answer to the question of why CAI is not yet widely used is no doubt complex and multifaceted. Several nursing authors have discussed factors that hinder the adoption of computers for instructional use in nursing education (Ackerman, 1982; Ball & Hannah, 1984, pp. 79–80; Heller et al., 1985; Kuramoto, 1978; Mirin, 1981; Porter, 1978; Thomas, 1985; Thompson, 1985). Four factors that seem particularly pertinent are identified and discussed here:

1. Lack of compatibility of hardware and software
2. Lack of appropriate software

3. Resistance of faculty
4. High costs

Lack of Compatibility of Hardware and Software.   Several computer languages, each with its own characteristics, limitations, and applications, are used to develop CAI materials. The language used tends to bind the user to one machine type. Companies can even change the language used for programming from one computer model to another. The result is that a program developed for one system cannot be used on other systems unless it is translated into compatible language. In addition, programs are produced in different formats (cassette tapes and diskettes), which limits their use to specific hardware systems. This lack of standardization prevents the ready sharing of materials or even the purchase of a desired software package. One of the most important considerations before purchase of a particular hardware system is the availability of software for that system. Once a system has been purchased, the nursing educator must carefully consider both content and format of software in order to make selections that are compatible with the hardware system to be used.

Several things need to take place in order to achieve the compatibility that would allow broader dissemination and usefulness of software. They include (1) setting up a software format that would make programs usable with a variety of hardware systems, (2) increasing the standardization of computer systems; (3) adopting a common language; and (4) establishing natural language authoring systems. With continued progress in these areas, access to high quality materials developed by subject experts would be possible for a greater number of institutions at less cost. Some efforts are underway to develop a common language, which will increase the possibility of using software on different hardware systems. However, results will probably not be seen at the implementation level for several years. As noted earlier, several authoring systems are now available that allow those without programming skills to develop instructional materials.

Lack of Appropriate Software.   A major obstacle to widespread use of CAI in nursing education is the limited availability of suitable high quality software. The problem of incompatibility just discussed results in programs that can be run only on a particular hardware system. Increasing the compatibility of software with various hardware systems would increase the quality of courseware, since programs could then be developed by experts and be more readily available to more people. Further, placing the emphasis on developing materials around broad concepts useful in all of nursing education regardless of setting would result in programs that could be more readily adapted to an individual curriculum.

One of the most significant problems affecting the use of CAI in nursing education is lack of high quality software (Thompson, 1985). Mahr and Kadner (1984) discussed the need for regulation and standardization of educational computer programs. They emphasized the importance of nursing educators, rather than manufacturers, setting the pace in the development of educational software. Ball and Hannah (1984, p. 77) also addressed the issue of quality by citing the lack of a formal mechanism for peer review, publication, and distribution of programs. As a result, most of the software that is currently available for nursing education, both commercial and in-house, is primarily drill-and-practice and tutorial, and much of it is of doubtful value. Some clinical simulation programs are available, but they most often display text only on the screen without the use of varied media or graphics. Some programs referred to by their authors as simulation are simulation only in the sense that they depict a real-life activity. When considering the learning process in which these programs involve the student, however, they are better classified as tutorial or drill-and-practice rather than simulation.

Nursing educators are exhibiting much interest in developing software on specific topics at the local curriculum level (Thompson, 1985). Although this is seen as a time-consuming, complex process, it is a route many have chosen in order to obtain software that is appropriate to their needs. In-house production is possible in some instances, but there are often problems since computers do not accept natural language programming, faculty do not have the required programming skills, or the incentives for faculty involvement with non-traditional strategies are lacking. Also, local development has resulted in software that is not readily available to others, is appropriate for local use only, and, possibly, is lacking in sound instructional design and programming (Grobe, 1984, p. 119).

Faculty who wish to become involved in the development of computer instructional programs need adequate support and assistance. Felton and Brown (1985) stressed the importance of the design team, including the faculty expert, instructional designer, graphics/media specialist, computer programmer, and systems analyst. Some faculty may wish to obtain basic programming skills or use available authoring systems to develop CAI materials. More faculty members are likely to be motivated in this direction when such activity receives consideration equal to that of research and publishing as evidence of scholarly and creative achievement in tenure and promotion decisions.

A few mechanisms are available by which faculty members can determine the quality of educational software. One of the most important is word-of-mouth recommendations from others who have used a program (Sweeney, 1985, p. 219). Other, more formal, methods are also becoming common. They include commercial advertisements of software publishers; publication of software catalogs (Bolwell, 1985); publication of software guides in professional journals (Hales, 1985; Worrell & Hodson, 1984a & 1984b); sections in textbooks on computers in nursing (Sweeney, 1985, pp. 307–322; Saba & McCormick, 1985, pp. 366–386); and the work of organizations like CONDUIT, which distribute information about computer programs that have been evaluated for educational soundness (Mirin, 1981).

Faculty Resistance.   The true potential for CAI cannot be realized without the support and involvement of faculty members. Faculty attitudes are thought to constitute one of the major barriers to the adoption of CAI. Resistance may be based on a variety of factors. One is that many faculty have had limited or no direct experience with computers and are intimidated by the technology they do not understand and the language they cannot use. Some do not know how to use CAI materials because the use of the computer as an instructional tool developed primarily in recent years. Even now most graduate programs do not include training in the use of CAI. Some faculty members feel threatened by technology that they fear could replace them. New methods that are thought to reduce one's own role in teaching may be resisted, especially by those who wish to keep the student in a dependent role and who wish to remain in a role as the primary transmitter of knowledge.

Many, particularly young faculty members, hesitate to become involved in activities that do not carry the same incentives in the tenure/promotion process as those available through traditional research and publication. When materials are used only at the local level, they are viewed as having less value than those that are published and widely distributed. Further, heavy teaching loads and related responsibilities, such as student advisement or committee work, may leave limited energy for the development of new materials and methods, especially when there is a lack of professional incentive.

Another element of faculty resistance may be based in the claim that CAI is impersonal and dehumanizing. Such an attitude may have developed as the result of administrative uses of the computer, personal experiences with computers in business settings, or the belief that any machine-based instruction is bad. Cross (1976, p. 63) cited studies that reject the claim that CAI is impersonal and dehumanizing—at least from a student's perspective. These studies show not only that student attitudes toward subject matter improve with CAI but also that some students, especially low achievers or those who do not respond well to conventional instruction, are especially enthusiastic about CAI. Others even view the computer as being "fairer" and more "likable" than the teacher.

Surveys by Ronald (1983) and Heller and associates (1985) indicated that both faculty members and students in nursing programs desire a high level of knowledge about computers. The issue of faculty development needs in relation to the use of CAI has been discussed by several authors (Armstrong, 1983; Felton & Brown, 1985; Kadner, 1984; Thompson, 1985; Ziemer, 1984). Faculty members especially need information that stresses the usefulness of the computer as a tool to help them in improving instruction. Structured, positive experiences with computers are required. Common methods recommended for facilitating faculty awareness and acceptance of implementation of CAI in the curriculum include workshops and short courses, agency support for enrollment in computer science courses, computer discount programs, and faculty committees focusing on various aspects of integration of computer concepts. In addition, Kadner (1984) commented on the relationship between the positive attitude of the program administrator toward CAI and the willingness of the faculty to participate, and Thomas (1985) stressed the importance of reassessing faculty work loads and current reward systems for increasing faculty involvement in the development of CAI materials. Faculty members who undertake the development of CAI materials will find references specifically helpful to the design process (Alessi & Trollip, 1985, pp. 271–312; Billings, 1985; Van Dongen & Van Dongen, 1984). Basically, the process involves adherence to the basic principles of instructional design with an integration of objectives, strategies, and evaluation, but with the added dimensions of flowcharting, programming, and branching called for with a CAI program.

High Costs. The costs associated with purchase or leasing of hardware systems, membership in computer networks, and purchase or production of software makes it impossible for many institutions to participate in CAI without outside funding. The availability of microcomputer systems has greatly reduced the costs; however, many educators and administrators are hesitant to invest in systems that may soon be modified or become obsolete, given recent technological advances, or that are incompatible with other systems. However, cost of hardware is expected to continue to decrease while computing capabilities increase.

Related to cost is the expenditure in relation to instructional hours. True figures are difficult to obtain since they are dependent on a number of factors—type of system, number of users, useful life of material, frequency of use, and cost of software purchase or production. Costs are expected to continue to decline with newer technology. Cost-effectiveness in fields that are considered to be more expensive, such as nursing and medicine, may be easier to achieve than in other disciplines that do not require a clinical component.

So far, the decreasing hardware costs have not been accompanied by comparable reductions in cost of software. Some of this is due to inflation and the increasing complexity and sophistication of programs. Software costs are likely to be a critical factor in the future. Nursing programs on limited budgets will not be able to purchase the more expensive programs. Unless costs decline, less wealthy schools will be unable to realize the advantages of computer technology. It is possible that, in the future, the demand for computer-based materials for instruction could be similar to that which now exists for textbooks if the expected advances in microcomputer technology occur, if the quality of software increases and the cost of software decreases, and if technology becomes more readily available to all. These factors may also allow an individual with a home computer to purchase or rent courseware or to access courseware via communication networks in order to achieve desired instructional goals. The resulting expansion of educational opportunity is obvious.

INDIVIDUAL APPLICATIONS OF CAI TO NURSING EDUCATION

Although use of CAI is not yet widespread, there are a number of examples of CAI being applied successfully to nursing education. Those applications that seem specifically directed at instruction (CAI rather than CMI) are listed in Table 15-6. The reader is also referred to the review of research earlier in this chapter for more examples of applications of CAI to nursing education. Those included in the earlier review of research have not been repeated here.

Many examples of CAI applications to in-service education and continuing education in nursing and to patient education are also available. In in-service education CAI programs have been used to teach staff nurses to document the nursing process by use of a computerized Medical Information System (Butters, Feeg, Harmon, & Settle, 1982), teach

Table 15-6

Examples of Individual Applications of CAI in Nursing Education

Author, Year	Title	Focus or Content Area
Ahijevych, Boyle, & Burger (1985)	Microcomputers enhance student health fairs	Health education, teaching plans
Barron (1985)	Using computer-based instruction to teach nursing ethics	Nursing ethics
Bitzer (1966)	Clinical nursing instruction via the PLATO simulated laboratory	Medical-surgical nursing
Bitzer & Bitzer (1973)	Teaching nursing by computer	Maternity and pharmacology
Bitzer & Boudreaux (1969)	Using a computer to teach nursing	Maternity nursing
Brennan (1981; cited in Grobe, 1984, p. 121)	Establishment of a CAI program to teach managerial decision making	Graduate nursing administration
Collart (1973)	Computer assisted instruction and the teaching-learning process	Medical-surgical nursing
Donabedian (1976)	Computer-taught epidemiology	Epidemiology in public health nursing
Estes (1976); Hall (1976)	The use of computer based instruction in an extended degree program for nurses leading to the Bachelor of Science degree; The development and utilization of mobile CAI for the education of nurses in remote areas	Self-assessment in seven basic nursing courses
Hannah (1983; cited in Grobe, 1984, p. 121)	CAI in nursing education: A macroscopic analysis	Immobility
Kamp & Burnside (1974)	Computer-assisted learning in graduate psychiatric nursing	Psychiatric nursing
Lambrecht (1985)	Computer-assisted learning: A vehicle for affective learning	Attitudes, beliefs, and feelings about death
Levine & Wiener (1975)	Let the computer teach it	Measurement systems
Nabor (1975)	Creative approaches to nurse-midwifery education	Nurse midwifery
Newman & O'Brien (1978)	Experiencing the research process via computer simulation	Research process
Reed, Collart, & Ertel (1972)	Computer assisted instruction for continued learning	Medical-surgical nursing
Sweeney, O'Malley, & Freeman (1982)	Development of a computer simulation to evaluate the clinical performance of nursing students	Myocardial infarction
Thiele (1984)	Use of computer-based instruction for dosage calculations	Drug dosage calculations

Table 15-6 (cont.)
Examples of Individual Applications of CAI in Nursing Education

Author, Year	Title	Focus or Content Area
Thiele & Baldwin (1985)	A simulated practice environment: Computerville Regional Hospital	Orientation of students to hospital
Timmer-Hawck (1985)	Computer-assisted interactive video use in nursing education	Maternal/child care
Timpke & Janney (1981)	Teaching drug dosage by computer	Drug dosage calculation
Tymchyshyn (1985)	Nursing and computers grow together in California adult education program	Computer terminology Hormonal, stress response Pathophysiology of starvation Test authoring
Van Dongen & Van Dongen (1984)	Using microcomputers to teach psychopharmacology	Psychopharmacology
Watson & Cabunoc (1985)	Computer-assisted instruction as a strategy for teaching psychomotor skills to nursing students	Psychomotor skills

physical assessment skills to community health nurses (Hagopian, Wemett, Ames, Gelein, Osborne, & Humphrey, 1982), teach pharmacology to staff nurses (Pogue, 1982), and teach case management skills to nurses providing care to children with chronic handicapping conditions (Parker, 1984). The last presents an interesting discussion on the use of computer-assisted interactive videodisc in an ongoing statewide educational undertaking.

Others discuss the use of CAI for continuing education (Meadows, 1977; Porter, 1978; Winter, 1978) and for patient education (Ellis & Raines, 1981; Ellis, Raines, & Hakanson, 1982; Lyons, Krasnowski, Greenstein, Maloney, & Tatarezuk, 1982; Sinclair, 1985).

FUTURE POSSIBILITIES

A wide range of predictions have been made about the future of technology and its impact on education (Ackerman, 1982; Butler, 1983; Chambers & Sprecher, 1983; Hassett, 1984; Podemski, 1984). The following prognostications are presented as a conservative estimate of what is possible by the year 2000. Whether or not they actually occur will depend to a great extent on whether the barriers to computer use in education discussed earlier are faced and dealt with. Areas of discussion include hardware, software, and the educational environment.

Hardware

Without a doubt, microcomputers will continue to play a major role in our society. The trend toward increased power and storage capabilities in smaller size microcomputers at lower prices is expected to continue. Virtually every home can be expected to have a microcomputer. Lap and handheld computers will be common in health care settings and the classroom. Expanding communication capabilities and ease of use will be enhanced by the use of natural language programming, voice input/output, and other output methods, such as Braille type. Increased standardization or the development of hardware simulators will permit a computer to run programs developed for other systems. Advances in related technology, particularly laser, holographic, and fiberoptic techniques, will further expand the capabilities and values of computer use. With declining costs and simplified techniques of production, it is possible that the videodisc could become a major force in education within the next 15 years. Holographic techniques will permit the transmission of three-dimensional images. Fiberoptic developments will result in the use of lightwave communication systems. Expansion of communication network capabilities will make it possible for every home to have an electronic link with schools, work settings, libraries, hospitals, and other agencies.

Software

The potential availability of software for educational use is closely tied to advances in hardware technology. However, it is clear that changes in software development, quality, and cost have not matched those of hardware technology. Software is expected to continue to be a major expense. Voice-activated computers and easy-to-use authoring systems will be commonplace. Software authoring will be seen as a legitimate example of creative achievement for tenure and promotion decisions. Professional associations and other groups will become involved in endorsing software as an element of higher quality education. Programs utilizing simulation will have replaced those using drill-and-practice and tutorial methods as the most common type of software available for nursing education. Computer-assisted interactive video instruction (CAIVI) using videodiscs will also be common if the above changes in ease and cost of production are realized. As a result, nursing education software will be of significantly higher quality and will be much more comprehensive than that available today. Extensive data banks will be available to every user of a microcomputer. It will be possible to transfer data from central databases to storage devices of the home computer.

Educational Environment

With the various changes in hardware and software outlined above, the environment in which learning will occur will also be drastically changed. Initially, the use of CAI will result in greater learning effectiveness and in increased individualization of learning for the general student population. Eventually, students with special learning needs and disabilities will have equal access to learning opportunities. The emphasis will be on development of mastery rather than on normative grading. The teacher will be a facilitator of learning and will see the student as an active partner in identifying learning goals and processes. Students will be required to have a computer just as they are now required to purchase texts. Computers will become as commonplace in faculty offices and homes as typewriters are now. Some learning will continue to take place in traditional ways, but new settings and opportunities for learning will be highly evident. There will be a great expansion of learning activity in the home, involving access to local, regional, national, and even international learning programs and networks. Programs will be available anytime the student wishes to use them. Individual programs and even complete courses from major universities will be available for rental or purchase as well as on-line via communication hookups with "electronic universities." Attendance at distant seminars and conferences will decline in favor of teleconferencing and on-line continuing education courses.

The definition of the word "literate" will include the ability to use computers as part of personal problem-solving and communication skills. Computer or electronic literacy will be a requirement for graduation from college, perhaps even for graduation from high school. Courses specific to computer applications in nursing will continue to proliferate. Content will include ethical and legal ramifications and ergonomic considerations, as well as basic applications to nursing service, administration, education, and research.

SUMMARY

The computer is a powerful tool for enhancing and individualizing the educational process. In spite of this, CAI has not yet been widely adopted in higher education. The extent of its use in nursing education is gradually increasing, although there are several recognized barriers to widespread adoption. At present the most common forms of CAI for nursing education are drill-and-practice and tutorial, although there has been much interest expressed in the increased use of the simulation form of CAI using videotape and videodisc. It is anticipated that significant changes will occur in the educational scene if the various barriers are overcome and the promise of advancing technology is realized.

References

Aavedal, M., Coombe, E., Fisher, C., Jones, M., & Standeven, M. (1975). Developing student-professor contracts in the clinical area. *International Nursing Review, 22*(4), 105–108.

Ackerman, W. (1982). Technology and nursing education: A scenario for 1990. *Journal of Advanced Nursing, 7,* 59–68.

Adams, D. E. (1980). Agency staff facilitate student learning. *Nursing Outlook, 28,* 382–385.

Ahijevych, K., Boyle, K. K., & Burger, K. (1985). Microcomputers enhance student health fairs. *Journal of Nursing Education, 24,* 16–20.

Alessi, S. M., & Trollip, S. R. (1985). *Computer-based instruction: Methods and development.* Englewood Cliffs, NJ: Prentice-Hall.

Allen, D., & Ryan, K. (1969). *Microteaching.* Menlo Park, CA: Addison-Wesley.

Anderson, H. E., White, W., & Wash, J. A. (1966). Generalized effects of praise and reproof. *Journal of Educational Psycholgoy, 57*(3), 169–173.

Archer, S. E., & Fleshman, R. P. (1981). Faculty role modeling. *Nursing Outlook, 29,* 586–589.

Armstrong, M. L. (1983). Paving the way for more effective computer usage. *Nursing and Health Care, 4,* 557–559.

Armstrong, M. L., Toebe, D. M., & Watson, M. R. (1985). Strengthening the instructional role in self-directed learning activities. *Journal of Continuing Education in Nursing, 16*(3), 75–79.

Atwood, A. (1979). The mentor in clinical practice. *Nursing Outlook, 27,* 714–717.

Backenstose, A. G. (1983). The use of clinical preceptors. In S. S. Stuart-Siddall & J. M. Haberlin (Eds.), *Preceptorships in nursing education* (pp. 9–23). Rockville, MD: Aspen Systems Corporation.

313

Bales, R. F., & Slater, P. E. (1955). Role differentiation in small decision-making groups. In T. Parsons & R. F. Bales (Eds.), *Family: Sociological and interactive process* (pp. 259–306). New York: The Free Press.

Ball, M., & Hannah, K. (1984). *Using computers in nursing.* Reston, VA: Reston.

Barnes, C. P. (1983). Questioning in college classrooms. In C. L. Ellner & C. P. Barnes (Eds.), *Studies of college teaching* (pp. 61–81). Lexington, MA: Lexington Books.

Barron, L. S. (1985). Using computer-based instruction to teach nursing ethics. In B. Thomas (Ed.), *Proceedings: Instructional computing in nursing education* (pp. 57–63). Iowa City: University of Iowa.

Barrows, H. S. (1968). Simulated patients in medical teaching. *Canadian Medical Association Journal, 98,* 676.

Bartol, G. (1984). Independent study in nursing education. *Journal of Nursing Education, 23,* 304–306.

Beare, P. (1985). The clinical contract—An approach to competency-based clinical learning and evaluation. *Journal of Nursing Education, 24,* 75–77.

Beebe, T. H. (1983). How to write your own instruction: Using a computer authoring system. *Instructional Innovator, 28*(6), 34–35, 48.

Bell, J., & Miller, M. (1977). A new concept of teaching-learning experience in trauma nursing. *Journal of Continuing Education in Nursing, 8,* 26.

Bell, S. K. & Marcinek, M. B. (1985). Nursing care analysis: A tool to develop problem solving. *Journal of Nursing Education, 24,* 118–121.

Bellinger, K., & Laden, J. (1985). Nurse use of general-purpose microcomputer software. *Nursing Outlook, 33,* 22–25.

Benner, P. (1984). *From novice to expert.* Menlo Park, CA: Addison-Wesley.

Benner, P., & Benner, R. V. (1979). *The new nurse's work entry: A troubled sponsorship.* New York: Tiresias Press.

Bevis, E. O. (1982). *Curriculum building in nursing* (3rd ed.). St. Louis: Mosby.

Billings, D. M. (1985). An instructional design approach to developing CAI coursework. *Computers in Nursing, 3,* 217–223.

Bitzer, M. (1966). Clinical nursing instruction via the PLATO simulated laboratory. *Nursing Research, 15*(2), 144–150.

Bitzer, M., & Bitzer, D. (1973). Teaching nursing by computer. *Computers in Biology and Medicine, 3*(3), 187–204.

Bitzer, M. D., & Boudreaux, M. C. (1969). Using a computer to teach nursing. *Nursing Forum, 8*(3), 234–254.

Blair, M. G. (1948). How learning theory is related to curriculum organization. *Journal of Educational Psychology, 29,* 161–166.

Blatchley, M. E., Herzog, P. M., & Russell, J. D. (1978). Effects of self-study on achievement in a medical-surgical nursing course. *Nursing Outlook, 26,* 444–447.

Bloom, B. S. (1956). *Taxonomy of educational objectives, Handbook I: Cognitive domaine.* New York: David McKay.

Bloom, B. S. (1968). Learning for mastery. *Instruction and curriculum* (Topical papers and reprints No. 1), Durham, NC: Regional Educational Laboratory for the Carolinas and Virginia, Mimeographed.

Bloom, B. S. (1980). The new direction in educational research: Alterable variables. *Phi Delta Kappan, 61,* 382–383.

Bloom, B. S., Hastings, J. T., & Madaus, G. F. (1971). *Handbook on formative and summative evaluation of student learning.* New York: McGraw-Hill.

Boettcher, E. G., Alderson, S. F., & Saccucci, M. S. (1981, August). A comparison of the effects of computer-assisted instruction versus printed instruction on student learning in the cognitive categories of knowledge and application. *Journal of Computer-Based Instruction, 8*(1), 13–17.

Boguslawski, M., & Judkins, B. (1971). Contemporary guidelines in teaching. *Journal of Nursing Education, 10*(1), 3–11.

Bolwell, C. (1985). *Software directory.* Saratoga, CA: Diskovery.

Bork, A. (1978). Computers in the classroom. In O. Milton (Ed.), *On college teaching* (pp. 184–211). San Francisco: Jossey-Bass.

Bouchard, J. & Steels, M. (1980). Contract learning: The experience of two nursing schools. *Canadian Nurse, 76*(1), 44–48.

Boyd, E. M. (1979). Contract learning. *Physical Therapy, 59*(3), 278–281.

Bradshaw, C. E. (1978). Concentrated experiential learning laboratories. *Journal of Nursing Education, 17*(2), 32–35.

Braun, L. (1980). Computers in learning environments: An imperative for the 1980's. *Byte, 5*(7), 7–10, 101–114.

Bredemeier, M. E., & Greenblat, C. S. (1981). The educational effectiveness of simulation games: A synthesis. In C. S. Greenblat & R. D. Duke (Eds.), *Principles and practices of gaming-simulation* (pp. 155–169). Beverly Hills, CA: Sage.

Brock, A. M. (1978). A study to determine the effectiveness of a learning activity package for the adult with diabetes mellitus. *Journal of Advanced Nursing, 3,* 265–275.

Brodie, G. (1969). Reexamination of reinforcement in the learning process. *Journal of Nursing Education, 8*(2), 27–30.

Bruner, J. (1966). *Toward a theory of instruction.* Cambridge, MA: Harvard University Press.

Brykczynski, K. (1982). Health contracting. *Nurse Practitioner, 7*(5), 27–31.

Bugelski, B. R. (1971). *The psychology of learning applied to teaching* (2nd ed.). Indianapolis: Bobbs-Merrill.

Burnside, I. M. (1971). Peer supervision: A method of teaching. *Journal of Nursing Education, 10*(3), 15–22.

Butler, D. W. (1983). Technological horizons. *Instructional Innovator, 28*(3), 14–17.

Butters, S., Feeg, V., Harmon, K., & Settle, A. (1982). Computerized patient care data: An educational program for nurses. *Nurse Educator, 7*(2), 11–16.

CAI program library. (1983). Columbus, OH: Ohio State University College of Medicine.

California Board of Registered Nursing. (1985). *Laws relating to nursing education-licensure-practice with rules and regulations manual.* Sacramento, CA: Department of Consumer Affairs, Board of Registered Nursing.

Cardarelli, S. M. (1972). The LAP—a feasible vehicle of individualization. *Educational Technology, 12*(3), 23–29.

Carnegie Commission on Higher Education. (1972). *The fourth revolution: Instructional technology in higher education—A report and recommendations.* New York: McGraw-Hill.

Chambers, J. A., & Sprecher, J. W. (1983). *Computer-assisted instruction: Its use in the classroom.* Englewood Cliffs, NJ: Prentice-Hall.

Chickerella, B. C., & Lutz, W. J. (1981). Professional nurturance: Preceptorships for undergraduate nursing students. *American Journal of Nursing, 81,* 107–109.

Chickering, A. W. (1975). Developing intellectual competence at Empire State. In N. R. Berte (Ed.), *Individualizing education through contract learning* (pp. 62–76). University, AL: The University of Alabama Press.

Chinn, P., & Hunt, V. O. (1975). Teaching child nursing by modules. *Nursing Outlook, 23,* 650–653.

Christman, L. (1979). The practitioner-teacher. *Nurse Educator, 18,* 8–11.

Clark, C. C. (1978). Teaching nurses group concepts: Some issues and suggestions. *Nurse Educator, 3*(1), 17–20.

Clark, M. D. (1981). Staff nurses as clinical teachers. *American Journal of Nursing, 81,* 314–318.

Clark, T. F. (1981). Individualizing education. In A. W. Chickering (Ed.), *The modern American college* (pp. 582–599). San Francisco: Jossey-Bass.

Clark, M. J., & Clark, P. E. (1985). Personal computers and database access. *Image, 17*(1), 21.

Coburn, P., Kelman, P., Roberts, N., Snyder, T., Watt, D., & Weiner, C. (1982). *Practical guide to computers in education.* Menlo Park, CA: Addison-Wesley.

Collart, M. E. (1973). Computer assisted instruction and the teaching-learning process. *Nursing Outlook, 21,* 527–532.

Collins, D. L., & Joel, L. A. (1971). The image of nursing is not changing. *Nursing Outlook, 19,* 456–459.

Conklin, D. (1983). A study of computer-assisted instruction in nursing education. *Journal of Computer-Based Instruction, 9*(3), 98–107.

The Consortium of the California State University (1984). *Undergraduate and graduate catalog, 1984–1985.* Long Beach, CA: The Consortium.

Cooley, C. H. (1909). *Social organization.* New York: Scribner's.

Cooper, S. S. (1979). Methods of teaching—revisited: Games and simulations,

Part 8. *Journal of Continuing Education in Nursing, 10*(5), 14; 47–48.

Cooper, S. S. (1980). Self-designed learning projects. In S. S. Cooper (Ed.), *Self-directed learning in nursing* (pp. 42–63). Wakefield, MA: Nursing Resources.

Cooper, S. S. (1982). Methods of teaching revisited: Experiential diaries and learning logs. *Journal of Continuing Education in Nursing, 13*(6), 32–34.

Cowart, M. E., & Burge, J. M. (1979). Evaluation by jury. *Nursing Outlook, 27,* 329–333.

Craeger, J. G., & Murray, D. L. (Eds.). (1971). *The use of modules in college biology teaching.* Washington, DC: The Commission on Undergraduate Education in the Biological Sciences.

Craig, A. S. (1975). Contracting in a university without walls program. In N. R. Berte (Ed.), *Individualizing education through contract learning* (pp. 77–96). University, AL: The University of Alabama Press.

Craig, J. L., & Page, G. (1981). The questioning skills of nursing instructors. *Journal of Nursing Education, 20,*(5), 18–23.

Crancer, J., Fournier, M., & Maury-Hess, B. (1975). Clinical practicum before graduation. *Nursing Outlook, 23,*(2), 99–102.

Crancer, J., & Maury-Hess, S. (1980). Games: An alternative to pedagogical instruction. *Journal of Nursing Education, 19*(3), 45–52.

Crancer, J., Maury-Hess, S., & Dunn, J. (1977). Contract systems and grading policies. *Journal of Nursing Education, 16*(1), 29–35.

Cranston, G. M., & McCort, B. (1985). A learner analysis experiment: Cognitive style versus learning style in undergraduate nursing education. *Journal of Nursing Education, 24,* 136–138.

Cross, K. P. (1976). *Accent on learning.* San Francisco: Jossey-Bass.

Crowley, D. M. (1965). Clinical diaries as part of the teaching-learning process. *Journal of Nursing Education, 4,*(4), 19–21.

Cudney, S. A. (1976). Mediated self-instruction of basic nursing skills. *Nurse Educator, 1*(2), 14–15.

Curtis, F. D., & Woods, G. G. (1929). A study of the relative teaching value of four common classroom practices in correcting examination papers. *School Review, 37,* 616–623.

Dale, E. (1969). *Audiovisual methods in teaching* (3rd ed.). New York: Holt, Rinehart & Winston.

Daniel, L., Eigsti, D., & McGuire, S. (1977). Teaching caseload management. *Nursing Outlook, 25,* 27–29.

Day, R., & Payne, L. (1984, January). *Comparison of lecture presentation versus computer-managed instruction.* Paper presented at the Conference on Research in Nursing Education, San Francisco.

Dearth, S., & McKenzie, L. (1975). Synoptics: A simulation game for health professional students. *Journal of Continuing Education in Nursing, 6.* (4), 28–31.

De Bella-Baldigo, S. (1984). Fostering nurses' participation in health care planning. *Journal of Nursing Education, 23,* 124–125.

De Cecco, J. P. (1968). *The psychology of learning and instruction.* Englewood Cliffs, NJ: Prentice-Hall.

De Cecco, J. P., & Crawford, W. R. (1974). *The psychology of learning and instruction* (2nd ed.). Englewood Cliffs, NJ: Prentice-Hall.

del Bueno, D. J. (1983). Doing the right thing: Nurses' ability to make clinical decisions. *Nurse Educator, 8*(3), 7–11.

Dell, M. S., & Griffith, E. (1977). Preceptor program for nurses' clinical orientation. *Journal of Nursing Administration, 7,*(1), 37–38.

Denson, J. S., & Abrahamson, S. (1969). Computer-controlled patient simulator. *Journal of the American Medical Association, 208,* 504–508.

de Tornyay, R. (1968). Measuring problem-solving skills by means of the simulated clinical nursing problem test. *Journal of Nursing Education, 7*(3), 3–8; 34.

Dewey, E. (1922). *Dalton laboratory plan.* New York: E. P. Dutton.

Diamond, R. M. (1977). Piecing together the media selection jigsaw. *Audiovisual Instruction, 22*(1), 50–52.

Dick, D. J. (1983). Teaching health assessment skills: A self-instructional approach. *Journal of Nursing Education, 22,* 355–356.

DiMinno, M., & Thompson, E. (1980). An interactional support group for graduate nursing students: A report. *Journal of Nursing Education, 19*(3), 16–22.

Dincher, J. R., & Stidger, S. L. (1976). Evaluation of a written simulation format for clinical nursing judgment: A pilot study. *Nursing Research, 25,* 280–285.

Dirr, P. J. (1976). Is our media program only skin deep? *Audiovisual Instruction, 21*(9), 24–26.

Dobbie, B. J., & Karlinsky, N. (1982). A self-directed clinical practicum. *Journal of Nursing Education, 21*(9), 39–41.

Donabedian, D. (1976). Computer-taught epidemiology. *Nursing Outlook, 24,* 749–751.

Dougan, M. A. (1980). Using "ICL" to meet the continuing learning needs of nurses . . . Individualized Contract Learning. *Journal of Continuing Education in Nursing, 11*(1), 3–7.

Dreher, R. E., & Beatty, W. H. (1958). *Instructional television project number 1: An experimental study of college instruction using broadcast television.* San Francisco: San Francisco State College.

Dreyfus, H. L., & Dreyfus, S. F. (1981). *The movement from novice to expert: What experience teaches.* Department of Health and Human Services, Public Health Services Grant # DIO NU 29024-03. San Francisco: University of California, San Francisco.

Duane, J. E. (1973). What's contained in an individualized instruction package. In J. E. Duane (Ed.), *Individualized instruction—programs and materials* (pp. 169–187). Englewood Cliffs, NJ: Educational Technology Publications.

Dunn, R., & Dunn, K. (1978). *Teaching students through their individual learning styles: A practical approach.* Reston, VA: Reston.

Eakes, G. G. & Finnen, R. (1985). Modification of a simulation game for use in a large group setting. *Journal of Nursing Education, 24,* 170–171.

Eaton, S. (1984). The influence of mental imagery on the performance of a complex psychomotor nursing skill using two learning approaches. (Doctoral dissertation, University of San Francisco, 1984). *University Microfilms International, 85,* 14988.

Eaton, S., Davis, G. L., & Benner, P. (1977). Discussion stoppers in teaching. *Nursing Outlook, 25,* 578–583.

Edwards, J., Norton, S., Taylor, S., Weiss, M., & Dusseldorp, R. (1975). How effective is CAI?: A review of the research. *Educational Leadership, 33,* 147–153.

Ellis, L., & Raines, J. (1981). Health education using microcomputers: Initial acceptability. *Preventive Medicine, 10,* 77–84.

Ellis, L., Raines, J., & Hakanson, N. (1982). Health education using microcomputers II: One year in the clinic. *Preventive Medicine, 11,* 212–224.

Ely, D., & Minars, E. (1973). The effects of a large scale mastery environment on students' self-concept. *Journal of Experimental Education, 41*(4), 20–22.

Engelke, M. K. (1983). Teaching the patient with a neurological deficit: A simulation experience. *Journal of Neurosurgical Nursing, 15,* 107–111.

Estes, C. A. (1976, April). *The use of computer based instruction in an extended degree program for nurses leading to the Bachelor of Science Degree.* Paper presented at the annual meeting of the American Educational Research Association, San Francisco.

Far Western Laboratory for Educational Research and Development. (1969). *Handbook for minicourse III: Effective questioning in a classroom discussion.* Berkeley, CA. (unpublished).

Farley, J. K., & Fay, P. (1983). Promoting positive attitudes among the caregivers of the elderly. *Nurse Educator, 8,* 43–45.

Feeney, J., & Riley, G. (1975). Learning contracts at New College, Sarasota. In N. R. Berte (Ed.), *Individualizing education through contract learning* (pp. 33–61). University, AL: University of Alabama Press.

Felton, G., & Brown, B. J. (1985). Application of computer technology in two colleges of nursing. *Journal of Nursing Education, 24,* 5–9.

Ferguson, M., & Hauf, B. (1973a). The preceptor role: Implementing student experiences in community nursing (Part 1). *Journal of Continuing Education in Nursing, 4*(1), 13–16.

Ferguson, M., & Hauf, B. (1973b). The preceptor role: Implementing student experiences in community nursing (Part 2). *Journal of Continuing Education in Nursing, 4*(5), 14–16.

Ferrell, B. (1978). Attitudes toward learning styles and self-direction of ADN students. *Journal of Nursing Education, 17*(2), 19–22.

Fishman, D. J. (1984). Development and evaluation of a computer assisted video module for teaching cancer chemotherapy to nurses. *Computers in Nursing,* 2, 16–23.

Foley, R. P. & Smilansky, J. (1980). *Teaching techniques: A handbook for health professionals.* New York: McGraw-Hill.

Forman, D. C., & Richardson, P. (1977). Open learning and guidelines for the design of instructional materials. *THE Journal—Technological Horizons in Education,* 4(1), 9–12; 18.

Forman, M. H., Pengov, R. E., & Burson, J. L. (1978). CAIREN: A Network for sharing health care learning resources with Ohio health care facilities and educational institutions. In E. C. DeLand (Ed.), *Information technology in health science education* (pp. 179–194). New York: Plenum Press.

Fuhrmann, B. S. & Grasha, A. F. (1983). *A practical handbook for college teachers.* Boston: Little, Brown and Company.

Gagné, R. M. (1965). *The conditions of learning.* New York: Holt, Rinehart & Winston.

Gagné, R. M., & Briggs, L. J. (1974). *Principles of instructional design.* New York: Holt, Rinehart & Winston.

Gall, M. D. (1970). The use of questions in teaching. *Review of Educational Research, 40,* 707–721.

Garity, J. (1985). Learning styles: Basis for creative teaching and learning. *Nurse Educator, 10*(2), 12–16.

Gentine, M. (1980). Methods of teaching revisited: Self-learning packages. *Journal of Continuing Education in Nursing, 11,* 58.

Gibb, J. R. (1951). The effects of group size and of threat reduction upon creativity in a problem-solving situation. *American Psychologist, 6,* 324. (Abstract).

Glaser, W. (1969). *Schools without failure.* New York: Harper & Row.

Godejohn, C. J., Taylor, J., Muhlenkamp, A. F., & Blaesser, W. (1975). Effect of simulation gaming on attitudes toward mental illness. *Nursing Research, 24,* 367–370.

Greenblat, C. S. (1981). Teaching with simulation games: A review of claims and evidence. In C. S. Greenblatt & R. D. Duke (Eds.), *Principles and practices of gaming-simulation* (pp. 139–154). Beverly Hills, CA: Sage.

Greenblat, C. S., & Duke, R. D. (1981). *Principles and practices of gaming-simulation.* Beverly Hills, CA: Sage.

Grobe, S. J. (1984). *Computer primer and resource guide for nurses.* Philadelphia: Lippincott.

Gudmundsen, A. (1975). Teaching psychomotor skills. *Journal of Nursing Education, 14*(1), 23–27.

Haggard, A. (1984). A disaster game that prepares you for the real thing. *RN, 47*(10), 22–25.

Hagopian, G., Wemett, M., Ames, S., Gelein, J., Osborne, F., & Humphrey, E. (1982). Methods to teach physical assessment skills to community health nurses. *Journal of Continuing Education in Nursing, 13*(5), 9–13.

Hales, G. (1985). Software exchange. *Computers in Nursing, 3,* 33–51.

Hall, K. A. (1976, April). *The development and utilization of mobile CAI for the education of nurses in remote areas.* Paper presented at the annual meeting of the American Educational Research Association, San Francisco.

Hanson, K. H. (1974). Independent study: A student's view. *Nursing Outlook, 22,* 329–330.

Hassett, M. R. (1984). Computers and nursing education in the 1980s. *Nursing Outlook, 32*(1), 34–36.

Haukenes, E., & Halloran, M. C. (1984). A second look at psychomotor skills. *Nurse Educator, 9*(3), 9–13.

Hawkins, J. W. (1981). *Clinical experiences in collegiate nursing education: Selection of clinical agencies.* New York: Springer.

Heatwole, R. (1984). Turning orientation into a game. *RN, 47*(10), 25.

Held, T. H., & Kappelman, M. M. (1976). *Continuing education through computer technology.* Paper presented at the Health Education Medical Conference, Miami, FL.

Heller, B. R., Romano, C. A., Damrosch, S., & Parks, P. (1985). Computer applications in nursing: Implications for the curriculum. *Computers in Nursing, 3,* 14–21.

Herje, P. A. (1980). Hows and whys of patient contracting. *Nurse Educator, 5*(1), 30–34.

Hilgard, E. R. (1956). *Theories of learning* (2nd ed.). New York: Appleton-Century-Crofts.

Hinthorne, R. (1980). Methods of teaching revisited: Self-instructional modules. *Journal of Continuing Education in Nursing, 11,* 37–38.

Hoban, J. D. (1978). Successful simulations for health education. *Audiovisual Instruction, 23*(9), 20–22.

Hoban, J. D., & Casberque, J. P. (1978). Simulation: A technique for instruction and evaluation. In C. W. Ford (Ed.), *Clinical education for the allied health professions* (pp. 145–157). St. Louis: Mosby.

Hodson, K. E. (1985). Cognitive style and the behavioral differences of nursing students in the clinical setting. *Journal of Nursing Education, 24,* 58–62.

Hoffer, E. P., Barnett, G. O., Mathewson, H. O., & Loughrey, A. (1975). Use of computer-aided instruction in graduate nursing education: A controlled trial. *Journal of Emergency Nursing, 1*(2), 27–29.

Holzemer, W. L., Schleutermann, J. A., Farrand, L. L., & Miller, A. A. (1981). A validation study: Simulations as a measure of nurse practitioners' problem-solving skills. *Nursing Research, 30,* 139–144.

Honey, G. M. (1975). *Independent study project for seniors.* New York: National League for Nursing, 78–84. (NLN Publication No. 16-1538)

Horn, R. E., & Cleaves, A. (Eds.). (1980). *The guide to simulations/games for education and training* (4th ed.). Beverly Hills, CA: Sage.

Horwitz, M. (1963). Hostility and its management in classroom groups. In W. W. Charters & N. L. Gage (Eds.), *Readings in the social psychology of education* (pp. 196–212). Boston: Allyn & Bacon.

Hubbard, J. P., Levit, E. J., Schumacher, C. F., & Schnabel, T. G., Jr. (1965). An objective evaluation of clinical competence. *New England Journal of Medicine, 272,* 1321–1328.

Huckabay, L. M. D. (1981). The effects of modularized instruction and traditional teaching techniques on cognitive learning and affective behaviors of student nurses. *Advances in Nursing Science, 3*(3), 67–83.

Huckabay, L. M., Anderson, N., Holm, D. M., & Lee, J. (1979). Cognitive, affective and transfer of learning consequences of computer-assisted instruction. *Nursing Research, 28,* 228–233.

Huntsman, A., & Thompson, M. A. (1977). Self-paced learning requires careful planning. *Cross-reference, 7*(2), 1–3.

Hyman, R. (1964). Creativity and the prepared mind: The role of information and induced attitudes. In C. W. Taylor (Ed.), *Widening horizons in creativity* (pp. 209–248). New York: Wiley.

Index of nursing lessons, University of Delaware PLATO project. (1980). Newark, DE: University of Delaware.

Infante, M. S. (1981). Toward effective use of the clinical laboratory. *Nurse Educator, 6*(1), 16–19.

Ingalls, Z. (1981, June 15). Of cells, seeds, and students and the "Professor of the Year." *The Chronicle of Higher Education,* pp. 5–6.

Ingalls, Z. (1986, February 5). To award winning teacher, giving praise is "heart of the matter." *The Chronicle of Higher Education,* p. 3.

James, W. (1908). *Talks to teachers on psychology: And to students on some of life's problems.* New York: Holt, Rinehart & Winston.

Jeffers, J. M., & Christensen, M. G. (1979). Using simulation to facilitate the acquisition of clinical observational skills. *Journal of Nursing Education, 18*(6), 29–32.

Jenkins, H. M. (1985). Improving clinical decision making in nursing. *Journal of Nursing Education, 24,* 242–243.

Joachim, G., & Karampelas, A. (1982). Head nurse and clinical instructor. *Canadian Nurse, 78*(2), 26–29.

Johnson, W. D. (1965). The effects of cognitive closure on learner achievement. (Doctoral dissertation, Stanford University, 1965). *University Microfilms International, 65,* 2861.

Jones, A. L., & Kerwin, E. (1978). A guided independent study program for nurses. *Community College Frontiers, 6*(2), 24–28.

Joos, I. R. (1984). A teacher's guide for using games and simulation. *Nurse Educator, 9*(3), 25–29.

Kadner, K. (1984). Change: Introducing computer-assisted instruction (CAI) to a college nursing faculty. *Journal of Nursing Education, 23,* 349–350.

Kamp, M., & Burnside, I. M. (1974). Computer-assisted learning in graduate psychiatric nursing. *Journal of Nursing Education, 13*(4), 18–25.

Kaye, W., Linhares, K. C., Breault, R. V., Norris, P. A., Stamoulis, C. C., & Kahn, A. H. (1981). The Mega-Code for training the advanced cardiac life support team. *Heart and Lung, 10,* 860–865.

Keller, M. L., & MacCormick, K. N. (1980). From graduate students to faculty: A simulation. *Nursing Outlook, 28,* 305–307.

Kemp, J. E. (1985). *The instructional design process.* New York: Harper & Row.

Kieffer, J. S. (1984). Selecting technical skills to teach for competency. *Journal of Nursing Education, 23,* 198–203.

Kilcullen, P. B. (1985). A learning experience in independent study. *Journal of Nursing Education, 24,* 30–31.

Kilty, J. (1982). Learning from practical experience. *Nursing Times, 78*(29), 2–5.

Kirchhoff, K. T., & Holzemer, W. (1979). Student learning and a computer-assisted instructional program. *Journal of Nursing Education, 18*(3), 22–30.

Knight, E. W. (1949). An improved plan of education, 1775. *School and Society, 69*(1799), 409–411.

Knippers, A. (1981). The use of self-instructional material in nurse education. (Doctoral dissertation, Indiana University, 1981). *University Microfilms International, 81,* 14959.

Knowles, M. (1978). *The adult learner: A neglected species* (2nd ed.). Houston: Gulf Publishing.

Kolb, D. A. (1978). *Learning style inventory: Technical manual* (Rev. ed.). Boston: McBer and Company.

Kolb, D. A. (1981). Learning styles and disciplinary differences. In A. W. Chickering (Ed.), *The modern American college* (pp. 232–255). San Francisco: Jossey-Bass.

Kolb, S. E. (1983). 3-North: A game for teaching concepts of patient care. *Nurse Educator, 8*(3), 12–15.

Kolb, S. E., & Shugart, E. B. (1984). Evaluation: Is simulation the answer? *Journal of Nursing Education, 23,* 84–86.

Kramer, M., Tegan, E., & Knauber, J. (1970). The effects of presets on creative problem solving. *Nursing Research, 19,* 303–310.

Krawczyk, R. M. (1978). Peer participatory conferences: A dynamic method of nursing instruction. *Journal of Nursing Education, 17*(8), 5–8.

Kruse, L. C., & Barger, D. M. F. (1982). Development and implementation of a contract grading system. *Journal of Nursing Education, 21*(5), 31–37.

Kulik, J. A., Kulik, C. C., & Cohen, P. (1980). Effectiveness of computer-based college teaching: A meta analysis of findings. *Review of Educational Research, 50*(4), 525–544.

Kuramoto, A. (1978). Computer-assisted instruction: Will it be used? *Nursing Leadership, 1*(1), 10–13.

Lambrecht, M. E. (1985). Computer-assisted learning: A vehicle for affective learning. In B. Thomas (Ed.), *Proceedings: Instructional computing in nursing education* (pp. 133–139). Iowa City: University of Iowa.

Laszlo, S. S., & McKenzie, J. L. (1979). The use of a simulation game in training hospital staff about patient rights. *Journal of Continuing Education in Nursing, 10*(5), 30; 35–36.

Layton, J. (1972). Students select their own grades. *Nursing Outlook, 20,* 327–329.

Layton, J. (1975). Instructional packaging. *Journal of Nursing Education, 14*(4), 26–30.

Leavitt, H. J. (1951). Some effects of certain communication patterns on group performance. *Journal of Abnormal Social Psychology, 46,* 38–50.

Lenburg, C. B. (1984). An update on the Regents External Degrees Program. *Nursing Outlook, 32,* 250–254.

Leveck, P. (1975). An extended master's degree program. *Nursing Outlook, 23,* 646–649.

Levine, D., & Wiener, E. (1975). Let the computer teach it. *American Journal of Nursing, 75,* 1300–1302.

Lewis, E. P. (1971). Secure in her skills. *Nursing Outlook, 19,* 519.

Lewis, L. C. (1978). Independent-individualized learning: The process and the processors. *Nursing Forum, 17,* 84–94.

Limon, S. (1984, June). Out of the classroom, into the hospital. *California Nurse,* p. 10.

Lincoln, R., Layton, J., & Holdman, H. (1978). Using simulated patients to teach assessment. *Nursing Outlook, 26,* 316–320.

Little, D., & Carnevali, D. (1972). Complexities of teaching in the clinical laboratory. *Journal of Nursing Education, 11*(1), 15–22.

Lord, A. S., & Palmer, W. R. (1982). Teaching psychiatric/mental health nursing via the contract for learning activities. *Journal of Nursing Education, 21*(4), 23–28.

Lowman, J. (1984). *Mastering the techniques of teaching.* San Francisco: Jossey-Bass.

Luchins, A. S. (1942). Mechanization in problem solving: The effect of "Einstellung." *Psychological Monographs,* No. 248.

Lyons, C., Krasnowski, J., Greenstein, A., Maloney, D., & Tatarezuk, J. (1982). Interactive computerized patient education. *Heart and Lung, 11*(4), 340–341.

Maatsch, J. L., & Gordan, M. J. (1978). Assessment through simulations. In M. K. Morgan & D. M. Irby (Eds.), *Evaluating clinical competence in the health professions* (pp. 123–138). St. Louis: Mosby.

Mager, R. F. (1968). *Developing attitude toward learning.* Palo Alto, CA: Fearon.

Magidson, E. M. (1976). Is your module good? How do you know? *Audiovisual Instruction, 21*(8), 43–44.

Magidson, E. M. (1977). One more time: CAI is not dehumanizing. *Audiovisual Instruction, 22*(8), 20–21.

Maher, W. (1984). A computer communications primer. *Computers in Nursing, 2,* 175–178.

Mahr, D. R. (1979). RN preceptors: Do they help students in the OR? *AORN Journal, 30,* 724–730.

Mahr, D. R., & Kadner, K. (1984). Computer-aided instruction: Overview and relevance to nursing education. *Journal of Nursing Education, 23,* 366–368.

Maidment, R., & Bronstein, R. H. (1973). *Simulation games: Design and implementation.* Columbus, OH: Charles E. Merrill.

Maraldo, P. J. (1977). Better nursing care through preceptorships. *RN, 40*(3), 69–71.

Marcus, M. T. (1983). Instructional strategy game: Navigating the inner sea. *Nephrology Nurse, 5*(5), 13–14.

Markle, S. (1977). Teaching conceptual networks. *Journal of Instructional Development, 1*(1), 13–17.

Martens, K. H. (1981). Self-directed learning: An option for nursing education. *Nursing Outlook, 29,* 472–477.

May, L. (1980). Clinical preceptors for new nurses. *American Journal of Nursing, 80,* 1824–1826.

McBride, H. (1979). Flexible process—An alternative curriculum option: Clinical evaluation. *Journal of Nursing Education, 18*(9), 20–25.

McCabe, B. W. (1985). The improvement of instruction in the clinical areas: A challenge waiting to be met. *Journal of Nursing Education, 24,* 255–257.

McClean, K. (1983). Closing: A new game show in the O. R. *Today's OR Nurse, 5*(7), 60.

McDonald, R. L. & Dodge, R. A. (1971). Audio-tutorial packages at Columbia Junior College. In J. G. Craeger & D. L. Murray (Eds.), *The use of modules in college biology teaching* (pp. 45–52). Washington, DC: The Commission on Undergraduate Education in the Biological Sciences.

McDowell, B. J., Nardini, D. L., Negley, S. A., & White, J. E. (1984). Evaluating clinical performance using simulated patients. *Journal of Nursing Education, 23,* 37–39.

McFarland, M. B. (1983). Contract grading: An alternative for faculty and students. *Nurse Educator, 8*(4), 3–6.

McGill, C., & Molinaro, L. (1978). Setting up and operating outreach centers for continuing education in nursing. *Journal of Continuing Education in Nursing, 9*(1), 14–18.

McGrath, B. J., & Koewing, J. R. (1978). A clinical preceptorship for new graduate nurses. *Journal of Nursing Administration, 8*(3), 12–18.

McGuire, C., & Babbott, D. (1967). Simulation techniques in the measurement of problem-solving skills. *Journal of Educational Measurement, 4,* 1–10.

McKay, S. R. (1980). A peer group counseling model in nursing education. *Journal of Nursing Education, 19*(3), 4–10.

McKeachie, W. J. (1963). Research on teaching at the college and university level. In N. L. Gage (Ed.), *Handbook on research on teaching* (pp. 1118–1172). Chicago: Rand McNally.

McKeachie, W. J. (1966). Procedures and techniques of teaching: A survey of experimental studies. In S. Sanford (Ed.), *The American college* (pp. 312–364). New York: Wiley.

McKeachie, W. J. (1978). *Teaching tips: A guidebook for the beginning college teacher* (7th ed.). Lexington, MA: Heath.

McLaughlin, F. E., Carr, J., & Delucchi, K. (1981). Measurement properties of clinical simulation tests: Hypertension and chronic obstructive pulmonary disease. *Nursing Research, 30*(1), 5–9.

Meadows, L. S. (1977). Nursing education in crisis: A computer alternative. *Journal of Nursing Education, 16*(5), 13–21.

Memmer, M. K. (1979). Television replay: A tool for students to learn to evaluate their own proficiency in using sterile technique. *Journal of Nursing Education, 18*(8), 35–42.

Merritt, S. L. (1983). Learning style preferences of baccalaureate nursing students. *Nursing Research, 32,* 367–372.

Mirin, S. (1981). The computer's place in nursing education. *Nursing and Health Care, 2,* 500–506.

Montag, M. (1951). *The education of nursing technicians.* New York: Putnam.

Moran, V. (1980). Facilitating self-directed learning: The role of the staff development director. In S. S. Cooper (Ed.), *Self-directed learning in nursing* (pp. 64–85). Wakefield, MA: Nursing Resources.

Morrow, K. L. (1984). *Preceptorships in nursing staff development.* Rockville, MD: Aspen Systems Corporation.

Murdock, J. E. (1978). Regrouping for an integrated curriculum. *Nursing Outlook, 26,* 514–519.

Nabor, S. (1975). Creative approaches to nurse-midwifery education. *Journal of Nurse Midwifery, 20*(3), 26–28.

National League for Nursing, Council of Baccalaureate and Higher Degree Programs. (1973). *Arrangements between an institution of higher education and agencies which provide learning laboratories for nursing education.* New York: National League for Nursing.

Neher, W. R. (1975). A plea for productive dialogue in the design of computer based education. *THE Journal—Technological Horizons in Education, 2*(2), 10–13; 22–23.

Neil, R. M. (1985). Effects of computer-assisted instruction on nursing student learning and attitude. *Journal of Nursing Education, 24,* 72, 74–75.

Newman, M. A., & O'Brien, R. A. (1978). Experiencing the research process via computer simulation. *Image, 10,* 5–9.

Norman, S. E. (1982). Computer assisted learning—its potential in nurse education. *Nursing Times, 78,* 1467–1468.

Novak, J. (1973). *The future of modular instruction.* Ithaca, NY: Cornell University Center for Improvement of Undergraduate Education. (CIUE Notes No. 6).

O'Connor, M. E., & Jones, D. (1975). An innovative teaching strategy for nursing education. *Journal of Nursing Education, 14*(4), 9–15.

Osborn, W. P., & Thompson, M. A. (1977). Variables associated with student mastery of learning modules. In M. V. Batey (Ed.), *Communicating nursing research* Vol. 9 (pp. 167–179). Boulder, CO: Western Interstate Commission for Higher Education.

Ostmoe, P., Van Hoozen, H., Scheffel, A., & Crowell, C. (1984). Learning style preferences and selection of learning strategies: Considerations and implications for nurse educators. *Journal of Nursing Education, 23*, 27–30.

Paduano, M. A. (1979). Introducing independent study into the nursing curriculum. *Journal of Nursing Education, 18*(4), 34–37.

Page, G. G., & Saunders, P. (1978). Written simulation in nursing. *Journal of Nursing Education, 17*(4), 28–32.

Parker, J. E. (1984). A statewide computer interactive videodisc learning system for Florida's CMS nurses. *Computers in Nursing, 2*, 24–30.

Parlocha, P., & Hiraki, A. (1982). Strategies for faculty teaching the RN student in a BSN program. *Journal of Nursing Education, 21*(5), 22–25.

Partridge, R. (1983). Learning styles: A review of selected models. *Journal of Nursing Education, 22*, 243–248.

Paynich, M. L. (1971). Why do basic nursing students work in nursing? *Nursing Outlook, 19*, 242–245.

Payton, O. D., Hueter, A. E., & McDonald, M. E. (1979). Learning style preferences of physical therapy students in the United States. *Physical Therapy, 59*, 147–152.

Pearson, B. D. (1975). Simulation techniques for nursing education. *International Nursing Review, 22*, 144–146.

Pengov, R. E. (1978). The evolution and use of computer-assisted instruction (CAI) in health sciences education at the Ohio State University College of Medicine. In E. C. DeLand (Ed.), *Information technology in health science education* (pp. 243–279). New York: Plenum Press.

Phillips, G. M. (1973). *Communication and the small group* (2nd ed.). New York: Bobbs-Merrill.

Pipes, L. (1980). Getting started with microcomputers. *Instructional Innovator, 25*(6), 10–11.

Plasterer, H. H., & Mills, N. (1983). Teach management theory through fun and games. *Journal of Nursing Education, 22*, 80–83.

Podemski, R. S. (1984). Implications of electronic learning technology: The future is now! *THE Journal—Technological Horizons in Education, 8*(11), 118–121.

Pogue, L. M. (1982). Computer assisted instruction in the continuing education process. *Topics in Clinical Nursing, 4*(3), 41–50.

Policinski, H. & Davidhizar, R. (1985). Mentoring the novice. *Nurse Educator, 10*(3), 34–37.

Porter, S. F. (1978). Application of computer-assisted instruction to continuing education in nursing: A review of the literature. *Journal of Continuing Education in Nursing, 9*(6), 5–9.

Postlethwait, S. N., & Russell, J. D. (1971). Minicourses—the style of the future? In J. G. Craeger & D. L. Murray (Eds.), *The use of modules in college biology teaching* (pp. 19–28). Washington, DC: The Commission on Undergraduate Education in the Biological Sciences.

Predd, C. S. (1982). Setting priorities: How to stay efficient in hectic nursing stations. *Nursing Life, 2*(3), 50–51.

Price, A. W. (1971). The effective use of the multimedia approach in staff development. *Journal of Nursing Administration, 1*(4), 38–45.

Price, G. E., Dunn, R., & Dunn, K. (1979). Productivity environmental preference survey. Lawrence, KS: Price Systems. (PEPS Manual)

Price, M. H., Swartz, L. M., & Thurn, K. E. (1983). The guided study: Self-directed learning for nurses. *Nurse Educator, 8*(4), 27–30.

Pullan, B., & Plant, S. M. (1978). Spot on!—that's the name of the game. *Nursing Mirror, 147*(23), 26–29.

Rauen, K., & Waring, B. (1972). The teaching contract. *Nursing Outlook, 20,* 594–596.

Ray, G. J., & Clark, C. E. (1977). The creation and use of an autotutorial learning system in a baccalaureate program in nursing. *THE Journal—Technological Horizons in Education, 4*(6), 32–34; 47–48.

Reed, S. (1968). The overhead projector and transparencies. *Journal of Nursing Education, 7*(2), 9–14.

Reed, F. C., Collart, M. E., & Ertel, P. Y. (1972). Computer assisted instruction for continued learning. *American Journal of Nursing, 72,* 2035–2039.

Reichman, S. L., & Weaver-Meyers, P. (1984). Glaucoma and cataracts: A nurse-patient simulation for nursing students. *Journal of Nursing Education, 23,* 314–315.

Reilly, D. E., & Oermann, M. H. (1985). *The clinical field: Its use in nursing education.* Norwalk, CT: Appleton-Century-Crofts.

Reinhart, E. (1977). Independent study: An option in continuing education. *Journal of Continuing Education in Nursing, 8*(1), 38–42.

Rezler, A. G., & French, R. M. (1975). Personality types and learning preferences of students in six allied health professions. *Journal of Allied Health, 4,* 20–26.

Richards, A., Jones, A., Nichols, K., Richardson, F., Riley, B., & Swinson, R. (1981). Videotape as an evaluation tool. *Nursing Outlook, 29,* 35–38.

Richardson, A. (1969). *Mental imagery.* New York: Springer.

Rochin, M., & Thompson, M. A. (1975). Strategies for independent learning in nursing. *THE Journal—Technological Horizons in Education, 2*(4), 15; 18–21.

Rockler, M. J. (1978). Applying simulation/gaming. In O. Milton (Ed.), *On college teaching* (pp. 286–313). San Francisco: Jossey-Bass.

Rogers, C. (1969). *Freedom to learn.* Columbus, OH: Charles E. Merrill.

Rogers, S. (1976). Testing the R.N. student's skills. *Nursing Outlook, 24,* 446–449.

Ronald, J. S. (1983). Learning needs and attitudes of nursing educators with respect to computers. In R. Dayhoff (Ed.), *Proceedings of the seventh annual symposium on computer applications in medical care* (pp. 771–775). Los Angeles: Institute of Electrical and Electronic Engineers Society.

Rose, J., & Riegert, E. (1976, March). *Looking at the instructional developer from the client's point of view.* Paper presented at the annual meeting of the Association for Educational Communications and Technology, Anaheim, CA.

Rose, T. L., Koorland, E. I., & Reid, B. (1978). Improving practicum performance: The CASE contract. *Contemporary Education, 50,* 18–23.

Rufo, K. L. (1985). Effectiveness of self-instructional packages in staff development activities. *Journal of Continuing Education in Nursing, 16*(3), 80–84.

Russell, J. D. (1974). *Modular instruction.* Minneapolis: Burgess.

Rynerson, B. C. (1980). Using videotapes to teach therapeutic interaction. *Nurse Educator, 5*(5), 10–11.

Saba, V. K., & McCormick, K. A. (1986). *Essentials of computers for nurses.* Philadelphia: Lippincott.

Sasmor, J. L. (1984). Contracting for clinical. *Journal of Nursing Education, 23,* 171–173.

Satterfield, J. (1978). Lecturing. In O. Milton, (Ed.), *On college teaching* (pp. 34–61). San Francisco: Jossey-Bass.

Schleutermann, J., Holzemer, W. L., & Farrand, L. (1983). An evaluation of paper and pencil and computer-assisted simulations. *Journal of Nursing Education, 22,* 315–322.

Schmidt, M. C. (1977). A self-paced ICU core curriculum. *Cross-reference, 7*(2), 4–5.

Schoffstall, C., & Marriner, A. (1982). Assessing the need and feasibility for an outreach baccalaureate program for RNs. *Nurse Educator, 7*(2), 25–33.

Scholdra, J. & Quiring, J. (1973). The level of questions posed by nursing educators. *Journal of Nursing Education, 12*(1), 15–20.

Schoolcraft, V., & Delaney, C. (1982). Contract grading in clinical evaluation. *Journal of Nursing Education, 21*(1), 6–14.

Schwartz, M. D. (1984). An introduction to interactive video systems. *Computers in Nursing, 2,* 8–13.

Schweer, J. E. (1972). *Creative teaching in clinical nursing* (2nd ed.). St. Louis: Mosby.

Seidl, A. H., & Dresen, S. (1978). Gaming: A strategy to teach conflict resolution. *Journal of Nursing Education, 17*(5), 21–28.

Selby, M. L. & Tuttle, D. M. (1985). Teaching nursing research by guided design: A pilot study. *Journal of Nursing Education, 24,* 250–252.

Shaffer, M. K., & Pfeiffer, I. L. (1980). You too can prepare videotapes for instruction. *Journal of Nursing Education, 19*(3), 23–27.

Sherer, B. K., & Thompson, M. A. (1978). The process of developing a learning center in an acute care setting. *Journal of Continuing Education in Nursing, 9*(1), 36–44.

Sheridan, A., & Smith, R. A. (1975). Student-family contracts. *Nursing Outlook, 23,* 114–117.

Sherman, J. E., Miller, A. G., Farrand, L. L., & Holzemer, W. L. (1979). A simulated patient encounter for the family nurse practitioner. *Journal of Nursing Education, 18*(5), 5–15.

Shockley, J. (1981). A multi-faceted program for continuing education in nursing. *Journal of Nursing Education, 20*(3), 20–26.

Shute, J. (1976). *Mastery learning and modules.* New York: National League for Nursing. (NLN Publication No. 23-1618)

Sim-Ed. (1978). *Catalog of educational simulations.* Tucson, AZ: The University of Arizona College of Education.

Simpson, E. J. (1966). The classification of educational objectives. *Illinois Teacher of Home Economics, 10*(1), 135–140.

Sinclair, V. G. (1985). The computer as partner in health care instruction. *Computers in Nursing, 3,* 212–216.

Skinner, B. F. (1968). *The technology of teaching.* New York: Appleton-Century-Crofts.

Slavin, R. E. (1977). Classroom reward structure: An analytical and practical review. *Review of Educational Research, 72,* 633–650.

Slavin, R. E., & Tanner, A. M. (1979). Effects of cooperative reward structures and individual accountability on productivity and learning. *Journal of Educational Research, 72,* 284–298.

Smith, C. M. (1980). Learning on your own for credit. *American Journal of Nursing, 80,* 2013–2015.

Smullen, B. (1982). Second-step education for RNs: The quiet revolution. *Nursing and Health Care, 3,* 369–373.

Sommerfeld, D. P., & Hughes, J. R. (1980). How independent should independent learning be? *Nursing Outlook, 28,* 416–420.

Sorensen, G. (1968). An honors program in nursing. *Nursing Outlook, 16*(5), 59–61.

Southin, J. L. (1984). Inquiry and explanation in introductory science. In K. I. Spear (Ed.), *Rejuvenating Introductory Courses* (pp. 99–108). San Francisco: Jossey-Bass.

Stadsklev, R. (1979). *Handbook of simulation gaming in social education.* University, AL: Institute of Higher Education Research and Services.

Steiner, M. J., & Rothenberg, S. (1980). Teaching home health care with video-tapes. *Nurse Educator, 5*(4), 5–7.

Stoia, J. P. (1983). Nursing instruction: Can data base searching enhance the practice?—A guide to the novice user. *Journal of Nursing Education, 22,* 74–79.

Stonewater, J. K. (1978). A process model for simulation design. *Audiovisual Instruction, 23*(5), 21–23.

Stuart-Siddall, S., & Haberlin, J. M. (Eds.). (1983). *Preceptorships in nursing education.* Rockville, MD: Aspen Systems Corporation.

Sullivan, H. J., Schutz, R. E., & Baker, R. L. (1971). Effects of systematic variations in reinforcement contingencies on learner performance. *American Educational Research Journal, 8,* 135–142.

Sullivan, K., Gruis, M., & Poole, C. (1977). From learning modules to clinical practice. *Nursing Outlook, 25,* 319–321.

Sweeney, M. A. (1985). *The nurse's guide to computers.* New York: Macmillan.

Sweeney, M. A., O'Malley, M., & Freeman, E. (1982). Development of a computer simulation to evaluate the clinical performance of nursing students. *Journal of Nursing Education, 21,*(9), 28–38.

Swendsen, L. A. (1981). Self-instruction: Benefits and problems. *Nurse Educator, 6,* 38.

Swendsen, L., Meleis, A., & Hourigan, J. (1977). Processes and strategies for implementing learning modules in a nursing curriculum. *The Journal of Biocommunication, 4*(2), 10–14.

Tansey, P. J., & Unwin, D. (1969). *Simulation and gaming in education.* New York: Barnes & Noble.

Thiagarajan, S., & Stolovich, H. (1978). *Instructional simulation games.* Englewood Cliffs, NJ: Educational Technology Publications.

Thibaut, J. W., & Kelley, H. H. (1959). *The social psychology of groups.* New York: Wiley.

Thiele, J. E. (1984, January). *Use of computer-based instruction for dosage calculations.* Paper presented at the Conference on Research in Nursing Education, San Francisco.

Thiele, J. E., & Baldwin, J. H. (1985). A simulated practice environment: Computerville Regional Hospital. *Computers in Nursing, 3,* 113–116.

Thomas, B. (1985). A survey study of computers in nursing education. *Computers in Nursing, 3,* 173–179.

Thompson, M. A. (1978). A systematic approach to module development. *Journal of Nursing Education, 17*(8), 20–26.

Thompson, M. A. (1980). Status of innovative programs in nursing education—a survey. *Proceedings and Evaluation of the Learning Resources Center Conference.* Bethesda, U.S. Department of Health and Human Services, *1,* 86–91.

Thompson, M. A. (1985). Computer-assisted instruction in nursing education:

A survey study. In B. Thomas (Ed.), *Proceedings: Instructional computing in nursing education* (pp. 31–41). Iowa City: University of Iowa.

Thorman, J. H., & Knutson, P. (1977). The option of retaking exams. *THE Journal—Technological Horizons and Education, 4*(7), 43.

Thorndike, E. L. (1911). *Animal intelligence.* New York: Macmillan.

Tidball, C. S. (1978). Health education network. In E. C. DeLand (Ed.), *Information technology in health science education* (pp. 195–209). New York: Plenum Press.

Timmer-Hawck, L. (1985). Computer-assisted interactive video use in nursing education. In B. Thomas (Ed.), *Proceedings: Instructional computing in nursing education* (pp. 141–152). Iowa City: University of Iowa.

Timpke, J., & Janney, C. P. (1981). Teaching drug dosage by computer. *Nursing Outlook, 29,* 376–377.

Tosti, D. T., & Addison, R. (1979). A taxonomy of educational reinforcement. *Educational Technology, 14*(9), 24–25.

Tough, A. M. (1981). Interests of adult learners. In A. W. Chickering (Ed.), *The modern American college* (pp. 296–305). San Francisco: Jossey-Bass.

Tuckman, B., Henkelman, J., O'Shaughnessy, P., & Cole, M. (1967, February). *The induction and transfer of search sets.* Paper presented at the meeting of the American Educational Research Association, New York.

Tymchyshyn, P. (1985). Nursing and computers grow together in California adult education program. *Input/Output, 1*(3), 1, 2, 4.

Ubben, G. C. (1971). The role of the learning package in an individualized instruction program. *Journal of Secondary Education, 46,* 206–209.

Ulione, M. S. (1983). Simulation gaming in nursing education. *Journal of Nursing Education, 22,* 349–351.

Valadez, A. M., & Heusinkveld, K. B. (1977). Teaching nursing students to teach patients. *Journal of Nursing Education, 16*(4), 10–14.

Valish, A. U., & Boyd, N. J. (1975). The role of computer assisted instruction in continuing education of registered nurses: An experimental study. *Journal of Continuing Education in Nursing, 6*(1), 13–32.

Van Dongen, C. J., & Van Dongen, W. O. (1984). Using microcomputers to teach psychopharmacology. *Journal of Nursing Education, 23,* 259–260.

Verplanck, W. S. (1955). The control of the content of conversation: Reinforcement of statements of opinion. *Journal of Abnormal and Social Psychology, 51,* 668–676.

von Oech, R. (1983). *A whack on the side of the head.* New York: Warner Books.

Votaw, R. G., & Farquhar, B. B. (1978). Current trends in computer-based education in medicine. *Educational Technology, 18*(4), 54–56.

Wales, C. E. & Nardi, A. (1984). *Successful decision making.* Morgantown, WV: West Virginia University, Center for Guided Design.

Wales, C. E. & Stager, R. A. (1977). *Guided Design.* Morgantown, WV: West Virginia University, Center for Guided Design.

Wales, S. K. & Hageman, V. (1979). Guided design systems approach in nursing education. *Journal of Nursing Education, 18*(3), 38–45.

Walljasper, D. (1982). Games with goals. *Nurse Educator, 7*(1), 15–18.

Walters, C. R. (1981). Using staff preceptors in a senior experience. *Nursing Outlook, 29,* 245–247.

Ward, P. S., & Williams, E. C. (1976). *Learning packets: New approach to individualizing instruction.* West Nyack, NY: Parker.

Washburn, A. W., & McGinty, R. T. (1977). The use of Metro-Apex in health administration and planning education and training. *Health Education Monographs, 5* (suppl. 1), 36–41.

Watson, L., & Cabunoc, J. (1985). Computer-assisted instruction as a strategy for teaching psychomotor skills to nursing students. In B. Thomas (Ed.), *Proceedings: Instructional computing in nursing education* (pp. 19–29). Iowa City: University of Iowa.

Weisgerber, R. A. (1973). Individualized learning through technology. *Audiovisual Instruction, 18*(3), 54–55.

Wenk, V. A. & Menges, R. J. (1985). Using classroom questions appropriately. *Nurse Educator, 10*(2), 19–24.

White, D. T., & Lee, A. S. (1977). A baccalaureate nursing program satellite. *Nursing Outlook, 25,* 394–398.

Wilson, S. R., & Tosti, D. T. (1972). *Learning is getting easier: A guidebook to individualized education.* San Rafael, CA: Individual Learning Systems, Inc.

Winter, J. M. (1978). Computer-assisted instruction in the continuing education of health professionals. *Journal of Allied Health, 7,* 206–213.

Witkin, H. A. (1973). *The role of cognitive style in academic performance and in teacher-student relations.* Princeton, NJ: Educational Testing Service.

Witkin, H. A., Moore, C. A., Goodenough, D. R., & Cox, P. W. (1977). Field-dependent and field-independent cognitive styles and their educational implications. *Review of Educational Research, 47,* 1–64.

Wolf, M. S., & Coggins, C. C. (1981). A workshop for development of simulation games in nursing. *Journal of Continuing Education in Nursing, 12*(3), 31–34.

Wolf, M. S., & Duffy, M. E. (1979). *Simulation/games: A teaching strategy for nursing education.* New York: National League for Nursing. (NLN Publication No. 23-1756)

Woodbery, P. M., & Hamric, A. B. (1981). Mock-emergency exercise. *Nursing 81, 11*(12), 32–34.

Worby, D. (1979). Independent learning: The uses of the contract in an English program. *Lifelong Learning: The Adult Years, 2*(6), 32–34; 42.

Worrell, P. J., & Hodson, K. E. (1984a). Computer software directory for nurse educators. *Nurse Educator, 9*(2), 32–34.

Worrell, P. J., & Hodson, K. E. (1984b). Software directory update. *Nurse Educator, 9*(3), 47–48.

Yoder, M. E., & Heilman, T. (1985). The use of computer assisted instruction to teach nursing diagnosis. *Computers in Nursing, 3,* 262–265.

Zangari, M., & Duffy, P. (1980). Contracting with patients in day-to-day practice. *American Journal of Nursing, 80,* 451–455.

Zebelman, E., Davis, K. B., & Larson, E. (1983). Helping staff nurses use learning modules. *Nursing and Health Care, 4,* 198–199.

Zemper, E. D. (1978). CAI at the Michigan State University Medical Schools. In E. C. DeLand (Ed.), *Information technology in health science education* (pp. 373–396). New York: Plenum Press.

Ziemer, M. (1984). Issues of computer literacy in nursing education. *Nursing and Health Care, 5,* 537–542.

Index

Aavedal, M., 254, 313
Abrahamson, S., 37, 318
Accomplishment, evidence of, 259–260
Ackerman, W., 301, 308, 313
Active participation, 31
Activities:
  learning, 8
  learning contract, 258–259
  learning module, 215–216
Adams, D. E., 161, 313
Addison, R., 7–8, 332
Adult learners, learning contracts,
  255–256
Adult learning theory, 193
Advanced placement, 211–212, 226
Affective gains, 191–192
Affective learning, 28
Ahijevych, K., 307, 313
Alderson, S. F., 294, 315
Alessi, S. M., 278, 297, 305, 313
Allen, D., 88, 313
Ames, S., 308, 320
Analog model, 21
Anderson, H. E., 5, 313
Anderson, N., 294, 322
Answers, discussion stoppers, 122–123
Approximation to reality, 37
Archer, S. E., 161, 313

Armstrong, M. L., 208, 228, 305, 313
Arousal, 79–80
Asking questions, *see* Questions
Attitudes, 9, 29
Atwood, A., 59, 313
Audiovisual aids, 105–108
  learning modules, 235
  motion pictures and television,
    108–109
  overhead projector, 106–107
  slides and film strips, 107–108
Authoring systems:
  for instructional programs, 290–291
    Ghostwriter, 291
    Microinstructor, 291
    NEMAS, 290
    TUTOR, 298
    Whitney System, 291
  for test construction, 291
Autonomous Leader Index, 183
Autotutorial study, 195
AVLINE, 290

Babbott, D., 32, 325
Backenstose, A. G., 160, 162, 313
Bafá bafá, 40
Baker, R. L., 11, 38, 331

For the new and experienced
nursing educator

HERE ARE THE TEACHING STRATEGIES YOU NEED TO MEET THE CHALLENGE

USE THIS BOOK TO:

- Learn about your options for helping students meet educational objectives

- Select effective teaching strategies that will *stimulate* and *motivate* students

- Discover new ways to help students learn, making their educational experience exciting as well as stimulating

WILEY MEDICAL
JOHN WILEY & SONS, INC.
605 Third Avenue
New York, New York 10158
New York • Chichester • Brisbane • Toronto • Singapore

ISBN 0-471-01197-5